"A key text within Golf academia, showcasing first-
Industry expert which brilliantly encapsulates the s
the game over recent decades. A must read for studen
Stuart Priestley, *PGA Advanced Pro~~fessional~~ & Lecturer in Golf*

Strength and Conditioning for Golf

The game of golf has changed dramatically over the last 20 years, with powerful, big-hitting players dominating at the elite level. With limitation and regulation of equipment being mandated by the R&A, players are increasingly looking to alternative options to increase their physicality to improve likelihood of winning. This is an area in which adding strength and conditioning training to a golfer's training programme will help to benefit performance. However, many players and coaches lack confidence or knowledge to train with strength and conditioning techniques, which is where this book, focusing on strength and conditioning and its application in golf, will help.

Strength and Conditioning for Golf provides golfers and coaches with the evidence and practical suggestions to ensure that the choices they make about their training are informed and objective.

This new volume examines why strength and conditioning techniques and principles are important for modern golf, blending scientific principles with real-world, practical advice and tips. *Strength and Conditioning for Golf* is of interest to golfers and coaches of all levels, as well as being of interest to researchers, students and coaches in the fields of; strength and conditioning, fitness and training, performance analysis, skill acquisition and other related sport science disciplines.

Alex Bliss is Associate Professor and Subject Lead for Strength and Conditioning Science at St Mary's University, Twickenham, UK. He has been a strength coach in golf for over 10 years and has supported amateur and professional players from European Tour, Challenge Tour, and within England Golf, where he is a regional S&C Coach for the South East. Alex is UKSCA- and BASES-accredited and has published research on training for golf and the determinants of golf performance.

Strength and Conditioning for Golf

A Guide for Coaches and Players

Edited by
Alex Bliss

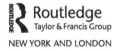
Routledge
Taylor & Francis Group

NEW YORK AND LONDON

Cover credit: Alex Bliss

First published 2023
by Routledge
605 Third Avenue, New York, NY 10158

and by Routledge
4 Park Square, Milton Park, Abingdon, Oxon, OX14 4RN

Routledge is an imprint of the Taylor & Francis Group, an informa business

Library of Congress Cataloging-in-Publication Data
A catalog record for this title has been requested

ISBN: 978-0-367-56785-9 (hbk)
ISBN: 978-0-367-56784-2 (pbk)
ISBN: 978-1-003-09932-1 (ebk)

DOI: 10.4324/9781003099321

Typeset in Bembo
by Newgen Publishing UK

"During the late typesetting stage of this book, the European Tour has changed to become the
DP World Tour. The case studies and references to the European Tour contained within this
book were accurately named at the time of writing. The Editor recognises the change to DP
World Tour, but felt for consistency at this late stage, and that reference to the European Tour
was accurate at the time of writing, that keeping the usage of European Tour throughout was
appropriate."

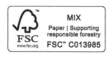

Printed in the United Kingdom
by Henry Ling Limited

For Freya, Eléna, and Zoë

Contents

Figures

Tables

Contributors

Alex Bliss is Associate Professor and Subject Lead for Strength and Conditioning Science at St Mary's University, Twickenham, UK. He has been a strength coach in golf for over 10 years and has supported amateur and professional players from European Tour, Challenge Tour, and within England Golf, where he is a regional S&C Coach for the South East. Alex is UKSCA- and BASES-accredited and has published research on training for golf and the determinants of golf performance.

Simon Brearley is a consultant S&C coach for the European Tour and an advisory board member for the European Tour Performance Institute. He is a co-founder of the Golf Performance Network. Simon is an accredited coach through the UKSCA and has been a regional S&C coach for England Golf since 2014.

David Brooks is a full-time professional golf coach with prominent roles for England Golf and the Professional Golfers' Association. He has a master's degree in Sport Coaching and became one of the first golf coaches in the UK to be awarded UKCC Level 4 status.

Orlaith Buckley holds a BSc. (Hons) in Physiotherapy and an MSc. in Sports Medicine and has been involved in golf for 20 years at both national and international levels. She has been a member of the ETPI Performance Team for 14 years and in this role she supports The Legends Tour. She owns and runs The Golf Physio Clinic in Dublin.

Dan Coughlan is Head of Strength and Conditioning for the European Tour and the National Lead for Sports Science and Medicine at England Golf. He was awarded his PhD in 2019 which focused on physical preparation and clubhead speed in junior golfers and is a co-founder of the Golf Performance Network.

Nigel Edwards is Performance Director for England Golf, a post he has held since 2012. Nigel oversees all aspects of performance within England Golf and was a key stakeholder in the development of a Strength and Conditioning service within the National Governing Body. A world-class amateur golfer and world number 2 in 2006, Nigel was capped 155 times by Wales and represented Great Britain and Ireland at four Walker Cups.

Alex Ehlert is an Assistant Professor of Exercise Science at North Carolina Wesleyan College. He has a PhD in Human Movement Sciences with a focus on strength and conditioning in golf. He has authored several peer-reviewed publications related to strength and conditioning practices for golfers, and has applied experience in golf as a competitor, coach, and sport science consultant.

Ben Evans is a professional golfer who currently plays on the European Tour. He has played in over 300 tournaments as a professional across the European Tour and Challenge Tour since 2005. He turned professional in 2007 with a +5 handicap having won a number of high-profile amateur events, including Faldo Series and the Sunningdale Foursomes.

Nicholas Jones is a strength and conditioning coach for the European Tour and formally England Golf. He has almost 20 years of experience coaching high performance athletes including British, European, World, Commonwealth and Olympic medallists in over 20 different sports. Nick was awarded a PhD in 2017 for his research into individual responses to training.

Ben Langdown PhD is Senior Lecturer in Sports Coaching at The Open University, UK. Ben's research focuses on athlete monitoring, warm-up protocols, and strength and conditioning interventions in golf. Over the past 15 years, Ben has provided golfers with sports science and strength and conditioning support and has delivered various invited international keynote workshops and presentations, with many organisations adopting his applied approaches.

Jamie North is Associate Dean for Research and Enterprise in the Faculty of Sport, Allied Health, and Performance Science at St Mary's University, UK. He has Psychology (undergraduate) and Sport Psychology (masters) degrees. His PhD investigated expert performance, the factors that differentiate skilled from less-skilled individuals, and how learning environments can expedite skill acquisition. He is Associate Editor for the *Journal of Sports Sciences* and the *International Journal of Sport Psychology*.

Emma Ross, PhD is a well-published sport and exercise physiologist, and former Head of Physiology at the English Institute of Sport. She developed the first Female Athlete Programme within the UK High Performance System, and has since founded The Well HQ to educate and empower women within sport. She was recently awarded the Change Maker award by the *Sunday Times* in the Sportswoman of the Year category.

Fiona Scott is Head of Physical Performance & Academic Liaison at Performance Herts. She is accredited through the UKSCA and NSCA and is a regional S&C coach for England Golf with over 15 years' experience in the sport and fitness industry.

Poora Singh is a Registered Osteopath and the Director of The Edgbaston Performance Clinic in Birmingham. He has worked on the European Tour as lead Therapist on Challenge Tour for 14 years and is active in facilitating research on Challenge Tour for the ETPI.

Jack Wells Jack is a Lecturer for Sport Science for the Professional Golfers' Association. He is a regional strength and conditioning coach for England Golf and a UKSCA accredited coach. He was awarded a PhD in 2020 which investigated the associations between clubhead velocity and kinetic variables during jumping and isometric mid-thigh pull in golfers.

Foreword

Nigel Edwards

As a golfer who is small of stature, I was always trying to find ways of hitting the ball further to help my ultimate aim of getting the ball in the hole as few shots as possible. Even as far back as the 1980's I could see the advantage of being "long" off the tee. As in many aspects of life including golf, the last 30 years have seen tremendous progress, an upskill of knowledge and a continual drive to get better.

Golf is a very demanding game, both physically and mentally. The sporting excellence and impressive physical presence of the likes of Tiger Woods, Adam Scott and Rory McIlroy in the male game and Anne van Damm, Nelly Korda and Lexi Thompson in the female game has reinvented how club golfers, aspiring elite golfers and professional golfers view the sport. It has also demonstrated what physical changes they are willing to explore in order to be the best they can be. As viewers, we are in awe of the prodigious distances and control the new style players display. All have shown the desire to become more explosive, stronger, flexible and stable in the search for even greater success. Professional golf is now so different, with increased media exposure, bigger sponsorships, bigger prize money, and the rise in golfer's profiles, it is no wonder the world of golf has changed. The days of hitting a few balls, a few forward and side bends and you're ready for the first tee are long gone.

Being fitter and stronger has become the norm in elite amateur and professional golf. However, it was once almost laughed at for a player to be seen "warming up" or even lifting weights. I can vividly remember in my first year as Performance Director with England Golf watching an amateur championship where the continental Europeans were definitely not shy of training and showing others that they were undertaking strength and conditioning programmes. Their warm up routines varied greatly but they were willing and focused on becoming the best they could be. Comparatively, I also noticed the lack of British players showing the same enthusiasm or athleticism. This was the pivotal moment for me, we had to change in order to keep contending. I'm glad to say that since that time, if you don't exercise or train physically for golf, at the elite level, you are now very much in the minority.

For England Golf the strength and conditioning programme was initially a bumpy ride, and we definitely had our detractors. I encountered common perceptions and concerns including: "focus being taken away from playing the game". "Players becoming too bulky...losing flexibility". "Players who lift weights get injured easily". These were the regular comments but the determination of the performance team to see the growth of the project has stayed strong and will reap long term benefits for those involved. Over the last ten years the programme has gained credibility by developing knowledge, practical experience and expertise, and the ultimate accolade of players buying in to strength and conditioning. More recently we have seen a growing number of golfers who have progressed through the regional programme arriving at national squad sessions and going to the gym of their own desire and motivation underpinned by good basics and understanding of gym use.

The benefits of a strength and conditioning programme are there for all to see. Golfers are now athletes rather than just golfers, they demonstrate increased clubhead speed, greater control, and reduced risk of injury. More widely however, there is also a feel-good factor for the players when undertaking strength and conditioning training, it promotes a healthy lifestyle, and the list goes on.

Alex Bliss has poured his heart and soul into this book and through his collaborations with other industry experts has compiled a resource that provides considerable detail and expert knowledge which aims to uncover and promote the benefits of physical training for golf for all. The book is an excellent example of both applied and academic expertise and will help support golfers both young and old, experienced and inexperienced to utilise physical training in their endeavours to play better golf.

Acknowledgements

A project of this nature does not come together without a large list of supporters. The entire list of acknowledgements, when I think deeply about the people who have made this possible, is vast. These people range from those with whom I share regular contact and a long-standing relationship, through to those that have had subtle, but important impacts on me both personally and professionally. I won't be able to name everyone here, but I can say with confidence that almost all of the connections I have made in the golf industry, whether fleeting or enduring, have helped to shape me as a practitioner and academic.

I would like to start by thanking all the contributors to this text. This textbook was compiled under extremely challenging conditions. Although originally work on this textbook began before the COVID-19 pandemic, much of the writing and editing of chapters took place at a time of great uncertainty for all involved. I commend my colleagues and friends for their dedication to this project and for persevering with it when it would have been easier not to have.

I would like to thank England Golf for taking such a proactive, visionary approach to embedding strength and conditioning support into their national programme, and for having me as part of that delivery structure for over five years. I have worked with and learnt from some incredible golf and strength coaches since 2015, but in particular Steven Orr with whom I share a long-standing relationship and who makes me a better coach every year.

I would also like to thank all of the players and coaches I have worked with throughout my career as a strength and conditioning coach in golf. While this will number well into the hundreds, each player and coach has helped challenge my practice and shape and hone my knowledge. I am grateful that they placed their trust in me to help support their golf careers.

I would like to thank all my friends and family who have been steadfast supporters of my academic and professional career. Particular mention should go to James Farrelly and Joel Tadman who ignited my love of golf when at university. Mark Packard for allowing me to try, fail, and improve as a strength coach supporting golfers in my early career. To Rob Harley and Dr. Neil Maxwell who took a chance on me in my first attempts to be a professional strength and conditioning coach and Dr. Dan Coughlan and Simon Brearley likewise from England Golf after what would have been a nervous interview performance!

And of course, to all my family, but particularly Mum, Dad, and Stacey who love and support me unconditionally, even if they are not always sure what I do in my academic and professional life! Lastly, I've dedicated this book to my children, Freya and Eléna, and my wife Zoë. I love you all immensely.

1 Strength Training for Golfers

Alex Bliss and David Brooks

The aim of this book is to provide golfers, coaches, and anyone with an interest in golf an insight into the role strength and conditioning (S&C) activities can play in supporting and enhancing golf performance. The contributing authors to this book (as outlined in the Contributors section) are either experienced S&C coaches who have applied their professional skills in golf for a number of years, or golf coaches, academics, players, medical staff, or a combination of these titles. The book, while grounded in scientific and coaching theory, is intended to be readable for a wide range of audiences. It will draw on objective, academic resources where possible, but will also encompass more experiential, subjective evidence from the various practitioners who regularly apply their knowledge and skills, and reflect on their support for golfers. This opening chapter, for example, is deliberately more subjective and philosophical, whereas subsequent chapters may be more grounded in academic theory, utilising subjective, experiential evidence where appropriate. Routledge recently published the *Routledge International Handbook of Golf Science*, which covers the application of scientific principles from the major sport science disciplines and how they inform and underpin golf performance. This textbook focuses exclusively on S&C.

S&C is the application of scientific principles to underpin the training processes of individuals, with the outcome of improving performance. The book will cover the "why, what, when, and how" questions that relate to S&C for golf in a scientific, but approachable manner. A novel aspect of this textbook is the inclusion of "practical application" sections within chapters. By drawing on the applied experiences of the authors, this text will help readers make informed decisions about whether to incorporate some of the strategies outlined into their own practices. S&C for golf has garnered considerable attention in recent years, particularly at the elite level, and as such, the development of this book is timely and will provide useful information on a range of topics.

A Rationale for Strength and Conditioning in Golf

Strength training and golf, until relatively recently, were widely considered to be incompatible. All sporting performance is a complex interplay between

DOI: 10.4324/9781003099321-1

psychological, tactical, physical, and skill components. Additionally, all sports exist somewhere along a continuum from high physical demand to high skill (fine motor skills) demand. Traditionally, golf was perceived as a game rather than a sport and emphasis was placed on golf "skill" rather than physical prowess. While this perception has changed in recent years, it is unlikely that coaches of physically precocious junior athletes will suggest that their physicality could make them a good golfer. For example, school-aged children undertaking physical assessment might be encouraged to try soccer, rugby, athletics, American football, and other physically demanding sports if they demonstrate impressive speed, power, and/or strength, or have physically impressive anthropometric characteristics, rather than take to the golf course. It will be interesting to see if this changes in the near future.

While some early pioneers of strength training for golf demonstrated that S&C routines could be used to support and enhance golf performance, the application of these principles to increase athleticism was not commonplace. As far back as the 1940s and 1950s, Frank Stranahan, who was described as the world's most prolific amateur champion of his era, followed a strength training regimen and had experience as a competitive weightlifter (Newton, 2007). However, it was not until the dominance of Tiger Woods in the men's game and Annika Sörenstam in the women's game in the late 1990s and early 2000s at the highest levels of the sport that S&C practices were thrust to the forefront of the golf mindset. In more recent times, the role S&C plays in golf continues to be seen at the elite level, with athletic, big-hitting players in the men's game such as Dustin Johnson, Brooks Koepka, and Bryson Dechambeau regularly performing well in major events. The success of players like Nelly Korda and others are demonstrating that athleticism in golf is important in the ladies' game too. Players such as Rory McIlroy and Lee Westwood have all had well-publicised strength training regimens. There are other players that have been able to maintain their longevity and competitive status across a range of tours by having robust physical training approaches. Notably, Bernhard Langer and Gary Player are excellent examples of successful ageing and have continued to be competitive and enjoy golf throughout their lives. S&C recommendations for the older athlete, and junior athlete, form bespoke sections of this text.

The ability to hit the ball further, particularly from the tee when driving and trying to achieve maximum distance, is a crucial component of the modern game. Drive distance has increased drastically in recent years, and is a critical determinant of performance (Bliss, 2021). Consequently, the golf swing itself has changed considerably to respond to these demands placed on the player. While technological improvements to golf balls and clubs have assisted the player in this regard, the ability for the player to use their body effectively to produce high forces over a short duration has become increasingly important to maximise the equipment advantage provided to all players. While golf's governing body (The R&A) set limits on the equipment produced, there is currently no limit on a player's physicality and therefore, those that are able to develop their golf fitness in such a way as to be able to generate higher clubhead and ball speeds are able to create an advantage for themselves over the field.

One approach to improve the player's potential to generate higher forces and transmit these to the clubhead has been to change the golf swing itself. While the traditional golf swing involved simultaneous rotation of the trunk and lower body towards the trail foot during the backswing, the modern swing involves resisting rotation of the pelvis in the backswing and affords for greater tension to be created in the trunk as it rotates towards the trail foot (Cole & Grimshaw, 2016). This increased rotation of the trunk relative to the pelvis is known as the "X-factor" or "x-factor stretch" (McLean, 1992; Cheetham et al., 2001). The combination of technological advances and alterations to the biomechanics of the swing have allowed players to generate greater distances. However, there is evidence to show that the golf swing places considerable strain on the player's physical structures: notably strain on the lumbar spine has increased. Indeed, studies have shown that compression forces up to 8 times bodyweight (Hosea & Gatt, 1996) and rotational forces of 10 times bodyweight (Sim, Choi, Lee, & Mun, 2017) are experienced in the lumbar spine when driving in healthy professional players. For context, these values are comparable to forces measured in the lumbar spine when blocking in American Football (Gatt, Hosea, Palumbo, & Zawadsky, 1997)

It is reasonable to contend therefore that utilising S&C techniques for golfers can not only develop physicality that can help improve performance, but can also help protect players against the high forces experienced during the swing. There are also physical and mental health benefits to regular participation in golf (Murray et al., 2017; Sorbie et al., 2021), and if following an S&C programme can allow players to have healthy bodies which are more resistant to injury, keeping them on the golf course, then this can only be a positive thing.

However, it is also important to outline the limitations of S&C in golf, some which are real, and some of which are misconceived. As a strength coach in golf for approximately 15 years at the time of writing, I now dedicate time in my initial player consultation around setting expectations and timeframes for changes to be observed. This is a critical aspect of the S&C support process for golfers, particularly those with limited physical training history.

A common frustration that the S&C coach experiences when working with golfers is managing players' expectations around the time-course of training adaptation. During the majority of my initial consultations with players when I ask "what are your goals for your S&C support?" the answers are invariably categorised into four responses or slight variations of these. They are:

- "I need to hit it 20 yards further" AND/OR
- "I want to put on more muscle mass to allow me to hit the ball further" AND/OR
- "I've been told I have limited mobility and need to improve this in my swing" AND/OR
- "I'm injured (or in pain) and I'd like to be able to play injury (or pain) free"

The inclusion of S&C support for a player can help, to varying degrees, all of these player aims. However, to improve the above usually requires a dedication of time (weeks or months at least) and consistency of training. When I respond to say "I can help with that, but to see lasting change will take time", it can come across as a sales pitch for more business! Conversely, highly skilled, knowledgeable, and experienced technical golf coaches can instigate incredible changes in just a few minutes of a single session. I have witnessed, both at the range and, crucially, in the heat of tournament preparation the dramatic effects a skilled coach can have on a player's performance. A drill, a cue, or a swing thought can help to "reset" a player back to better strike characteristics which will increase distance and/or accuracy, for example. Unfortunately, while certain training strategies can bring about acute changes in clubhead speed (CHS) (see Hebert-Loisier et al., 2021; Bliss et al., 2021, etc.) these changes are transient and short lasting. To experience more enduring physical change requires longer-term training. For example, an S&C training programme aimed at developing muscle size would typically last around six to twelve weeks and focus on a rough rule of 10 sets per week per muscle group targeted (Schoenfeld et al., 2021; 2017; Figuierdo et al., 2018). Again, this book contains bespoke chapters on training for speed, how to transfer gym training to the course, and will provide guidance on best-practice methods to achieve this.

Unless expectations are managed at the outset, this can be an unattractive proposition for players. Indeed, why should a player dedicate this amount of time to physical training to improve distance, mobility, or pain reduction, when there are faster "sticking plaster" alternatives? For example, a player hoping to increase CHS could try an equipment change (weight, length, shaft type of their clubs as examples). If mobility is an issue, skilled golfers can find "workarounds" that will allow them to still play to a high level (a player with limited torso rotation, for example, may manipulate the position of the club with their hands/wrists to increase the length of the swing if increased distance is the aim). If pain or injury is the reason for contemplating S&C, then paracetamol, ibuprofen, and other medications can achieve a level of pain reduction that is immediate and doesn't require any long-term dedication or consistency of training. The issue with all of these approaches is that they have a ceiling. There is only so much medication a person can take before it becomes dangerous to health. The design of a golf club is constrained by the Rules of Golf, as is the manufacturing process of all golf equipment. Once this is maximised no further gain can be made unless the rules are changed, or equipment manufacturers find subtle tweaks to design. Currently, there is no limit to a player's physicality on the golf course, and the only constraints to physical development are time, consistency of training, and the player's genetic potential. Therefore, the management and setting of expectations, both those of the player and of the S&C coach, form a crucial part of the initial consultation process. This is covered in greater detail in the Needs Analysis and Performance Profiling chapter.

With the above notwithstanding, there are players who defy current trends to improve athleticism as a mechanism to support their performance on the golf course. These players are able to exhibit "enough" physicality to perform and compete, and while they might not be long drivers of the ball, or possess a traditional athletic somatotype, they will likely possess considerable skills in other aspects of the game, whether these are technical/tactical skills, or personality/behavioural traits that offset and counter their lower levels of physicality in comparison to their peers. Additionally, players may be hesitant to engage with S&C. Despite the best efforts of the industry in recent years to combat some of the misconceptions of what S&C support is, there is still misinformation. I hope this book will address some of these concerns and enable golfers and golf coaches to achieve an enhanced understanding of how S&C can support golf performance.

There might be multifaceted and numerous reasons why a player may choose to avoid engaging with S&C, and these might not necessarily emanate from the player themselves. Perhaps more so than any other sport I have worked in during my career, my experience has been that golf is a referral sport and players will often seek S&C support, or be referred to a particular S&C coach because of a request from their technical coach, or other support staff. At the elite level, players may have management teams that will recommend particular S&C coaches, or the player might use a service provided by their respective tour. However, at a lower level, players and coaches might need to seek out an S&C coach. As the term "S&C Coach" is not yet a protected term (although this may change in time), the variety and quality of support staff who have this as their professional title can be vast. It is hoped that this book will again allow players and coaches to become more informed about evidence-based S&C support and allow for them to have high-quality conversations with their S&C coach about improving golf performance.

Lastly, and linked to the above, as S&C coaches will (particularly with high-performance golfers) work as part of a multidisciplinary team, it is useful to try to understand some of the concerns the coach may have about how S&C will impact their player. S&C coaches must recognise that they are there to support the coach to support the player and as such, managing that relationship through mutual understanding and agreed objectives is crucial. A golf coach places their reputation and relationship with their player under scrutiny with the recommendation of an S&C coach. As golf performance is transient and fleeting, with even the world's best players experiencing drops in playing level, players might attribute a downturn in scoring or ball striking to an S&C intervention, disrupting their belief in that intervention, and by extension, their coach's recommendation. Conversely, the opposite may also occur and an upturn in performance is observed after one or two S&C sessions, with the player attributing this to the new novel stimulus (physical training). The section below will provide a coach's perspective on S&C support for golfers, some of their observations throughout their career and discuss some of the benefits, but also risks for the player and coach.

A Golf Coach's Perspective on the Opportunities and Challenges of S&C

The global performance driver for any golfer will be control of their ball flight, with score, handicap, winnings, or simply an increasing sense of mastery, directly correlated to this. Ball flight can be distilled into four characteristics: direction, curvature, trajectory, and distance. These characteristics and their interpretation provide a framework under which the benefits of S&C for golf performance can be assimilated and discussed.

The most evident characteristic upon which S&C can have a direct and positive influence is distance, primarily via a meaningful effect on CHS (and by association, ball speed) from a gain in impulse, achieved through increasing force produced, predominantly through strength development (Wells et al., 2019). S&C may also assist by increasing the time the force can act over, but for this to hold true, it would have to be demonstrated that the S&C intervention had resulted in a positive technical adaption, most likely from improved kinematic sequencing.

Whether increasing impulse is best achieved by focusing on a golfer's force-producing capability, or from increasing the time over which that force can act, is a discussion which can inform the choice of coaching intervention, for example, technical adaptation, or S&C programmes with a focus on strength, and/or speed training. Which pathway to greater distance in ball flight is safer, faster, or more likely to be retained, is for other authors to argue later in this book, and for coaches and golfers reading this text to make an informed judgement from the information provided.

For competitors and coaches, the performance advantage from increasing distance is hard to ignore. Recent analysis from the governing bodies of the USGA and R&A (Distance Insights Report, 2020) demonstrated the spread (distribution of performance) of driving distance across the PGA Tour has grown by almost 25% between 1983 and 2018, while for all other performance statistics studied, the spread between competitors had reduced, including for driving accuracy (7%), greens in regulation (17%) and proximity to pin (12%). If aggregated with the known value of distance to a competitor's scoring (from an average stroke gain of 0.0049 per yard, per hole, for all drives, in the 15 years since the PGA Tour has collected Shot Link data), the potential for driving distance to create a clear performance differential over the competitive field is clear to see. However, findings from the European Tour also suggest an anomaly, drawn from the conclusion that while driving distance had increased from 2017 to 2019, and an average of almost 30 yards since the late 1990s/early 2000s (Ketzscher & Ringrose, 2002), overall stroke average remained stable (Bliss, 2021). This would suggest other mitigating factors are at play, potentially a negative weighting from course design and set up. Whatever the final statistical scoring benefits from this greater distance may be, S&C must be considered as a significant contributor (Ehlert, 2020).

A positive influence on the three other ball flight characteristics of direction, curvature, and trajectory are harder to attribute to S&C. This is simply because the intervention would need to be proven to adapt directly and positively, or at least facilitate the adoption of, an improved golf swing technique which feeds into a meaningful improvement of ball flight, through its influence on the impact relationships between the clubhead and the golf ball which relate to these characteristics. While further evidence for a direct correlation between S & C and other characteristics of ball flight may emerge, at this time, and except for a causative influence from CHS, there are still low levels of empirical substantiation.

As golfers embark on a personal journey of improving ball flight control, barriers in knowledge and skills will present themselves. This is when an individual coach, or a team of coaches, will be required by the golfer to guide and assist to find solutions to overcome these barriers. When distance is the primary performance concern, and for S&C training to be chosen as a recommended pathway to address it, much will depend on the personal experience and bias of the golf coach. Whereas the gains to be achieved from S&C are garnering increasingly compelling evidence for efficacy, and for which evidence will be presented throughout this book, it should be noted there are also challenges presented for both the golfer and the golf coach.

A golfer's technique may have adapted around a player's physical condition, and specifically their limitations, yet they may still demonstrate a relative level of success from a delicately balanced and dynamic system. A purely S&C-driven physical intervention can knock this system out of flux, by way of an unintended or poorly thought through consequence. For example, even if S&C training delivers a meaningful physical improvement, a golf swing is a complex motor pattern which will exhibit a level of automation, and these movement patterns may not simply and automatically adapt, just because the body can now move in a more efficient manner (Langdown, 2015).

Pursuing this line of associative or corollary links between physical limitations and golf swing faults and characteristics has been a philosophical cornerstone of several well-funded and high-profile providers of accredited career professional development (CPD) within the field of S&C. These have gained easy traction in coaching circles as they potentially provide convenient and ready-made solutions for coaches to diagnose and adapt swing faults, but in many cases the links between the physical and technical are at best tenuous, and at worst, completely unfounded.

As may be a danger for all experts working with athletes, for S&C coaches there will be a need to "justify" their position and effectiveness within the performance team, possibly for reasons of ego but primarily for economics. It will be in the interest of unscrupulous coaches to find a problem, because then they can provide a solution, at a financial cost to the consumer. This can result in S&C interventions being prescribed where one may not appropriate, or within that specific developmental period. It should be and is noted, that this not a dilemma only limited to S&C coaches, it can very much apply to golf coaches too.

For many golfers, there can be a challenge in identifying and accessing professionally qualified and experienced S&C coaches, rather than personal trainers or similar who have only undertaken a short "golf specific" accrediting course before starting to practice. It is difficult for adult golfers and their coaches, or perhaps even more pertinently, the parents of young golfers, to differentiate and evaluate the qualifications of providers all seemingly expert in this field.

Even when an appropriately qualified S&C provider has been appointed, integrating their support with existing technical and tactical support can present complications. Although it may be regarded as preferential for the golf coach and S&C coach to work together, the reality is often they will work independently, with an inevitable consequence of this polarity being a potential for conflict to arise. A motive for this may be that the golf coach feels they may lose their influence, or even authority, with the player, and are uncomfortable with delegating out, particularly if there is a longstanding coach–player relationship. Even if a professional working relationship, and accepted hierarchy, can be established, it will require a golf coach who can articulate what they really want a player to do and why, as well as then go further to give insight into how the S&C coach can help.

For even the most enlightened golf coach, there will also be concerns around whether their client will buy-in to an S&C approach. For some golfers, the time scale of meaningful improvement may be too great, the financial costs of the expertise and facilities required too high, or their athletic and physical development bias simply not aligned. It may even be a case of the golfer feeling that ship has already sailed, and they simply want to stay with a technical or tactical approach to their continuing golf development. This is an incredibly important consideration for the golf coach to make before recommending an S&C approach. If they get this judgement wrong, they risk losing a client, even if their intentions were sound.

Despite all the challenges highlighted above, this golf coach very much believes in the essential and intrinsic value of an integrated S&C involvement for any golfer's development. However, it is also a strong belief that it must be person centred, coach led, realistic and performance goal oriented. If the golf coach, S&C coach, and most critically the golfer, align in both their aims and delivery, the results can be both career, and life changing.

Concluding Remarks

Golf has changed drastically over the past 20 years. With the development of equipment, coaching and understanding of the golf swing, and changes to players' physicality at the elite level, performance metrics such as drive distance and the associated measures of CHS and ball speed have increased substantially. S&C in golf is becoming more commonplace and players may soon need to be able to demonstrate considerable physicality and athleticism in order to compete at the highest level. At a recreational level, the inclusion of an S&C

programme has also been demonstrated to aid improved performance and may also contribute to increased longevity, as will be discussed in other chapters in this book.

With that said, while our knowledge of how S&C can impact CHS has grown in the last 20 years, it is easy to overemphasise or become overly focused on this single measure, ignoring other potential benefits or impacts of the S&C intervention. Furthermore, not all performance measures in golf have changed to the same extent over that time period, and indeed some have remained very stable. While course design is a contextual factor that may account for this, the sport clearly retains a heavy "skill component", as is intended by the game's governing body (Distance Insights Report, 2020. www.randa.org). S&C interventions should be carefully considered before being implemented, even while having demonstrated efficacy in a range of empirical studies and as evidenced anecdotally or experientially by players or their coaches. Like any intervention, whether that is an S&C programme, or more golf-oriented approaches such as technical swing changes, equipment changes, or tactical changes, due consideration should be given to the desired outcome and a strong, well-reasoned rationale established. This rationale should consider the determinants of golf performance, but also, and most crucially, the desires and performance needs of the player. The following chapter in this book will detail how the player's needs, as well as the determinants of the sport, can be addressed with an effective needs analysis and profiling process.

References

Bliss, A. (2021). Modelling Elite Golf Performance: Predictors of Hole Score on the European Tour From 2017–2019. *International Journal of Golf Science.* 9(1).

Bliss, A., Livingstone, H., & Tallent, J. (2021). Field-based and overspeed potentiated warm-ups increase clubhead speed and drive carry distance in skilled collegiate golfers. *Journal of Sport and Exercise Science.* 5(2): 107–113.

Cheetham, P. J., Martin, P. E., Mottram, R. E., & St. Laurent, B. F. (2001). The importance of stretching the "X-Factor" in the downswing of golf: The "X-Factor Stretch". In P.R. Thomas (Ed.), Optimising performance in golf (pp. 192–199). Brisbane, Australia. Australian Academic Press. ISBN 1 875378 5.

Cole, M. H., & Grimshaw, P. N. (2016). The biomechanics of the modern golf swing: implications for lower back injuries. *Sports Medicine.* 46: 339–351. https://doi.org/10.1007/s40279-015-0429-1

Distance Insights Report (2020). R56 The Value of Distance. Available www.randa.org

Ehlert, A. (2020) The effects of strength and conditioning interventions on golf performance: A systematic review. *Journal of Sports Sciences.* 38(23): 2720–2731.

Figueiredo, V. C., de Salles, B, F., & Trajano, G, S. (2018). Volume for Muscle Hypertrophy and Health Outcomes: The Most Effective Variable in Resistance Training. *Sports Medicine.* 48(3): 499–505.

Gatt, C. J., Hosea, T. M., Palumbo, R. C., & Zawadsky, J. P. (1997). Impact loading of the lumbar spine during football blocking. *The American Journal of Sports Medicine.* 25(3): 317–321. https://doi.org/10.1177/036354659702500308

Hébert-Losier, K., & Wardell, G. L. (2021) Acute and persistence of the effects of the SuperSpeed Golf™ weighted-club warm-up on golf driving performance and kinematics. *Sports Biomechanics*, DOI: 10.1080/14763141.2021.1887344

Hosea, T. M., & Gatt, C. J. (1996). Back pain in golf. *Clinical Sports Medicine.* 15(1): 37–53.

Ketzscher, R., & Ringrose, T. J. (2002). Exploratory analysis of European Professional Golf Association statistics. *The Statistician.* 51(2): 215–228.

Langdown, B. (2015). *Movement Variability and Strength and Conditioning in Golf.* University of Birmingham. Ph.D/Doctoral thesis.

McLean, J. (1992). Widen the gap. *Golf Magazine.* 34(12): 49–53.

Murray, A. D., Daines, L., Archibald, D., Hawkes, R. A., Schiphorst, C., Kelly, P., Grant, L., & Mutrie, N. (2017). The relationships between golf and health: a scoping review. *British Journal of Sports Medicine.* 51: 12–19. doi:10.1136/bjsports-2016-09662

Newton, H. (2007). Effective Strength Training for Golf: What's the Right Approach? *International Journal of Sports Science & Coaching.* 2(1_suppl): 135–149. https://doi.org/10.1080/02640414.2016.1255345

Schoenfeld, B., Fisher, J. P., Grgic, J., Haun, C. T., Helms, R. R., Phillips, S. M., Steele, J., & Vigotsky, A. D. (2021). Resistance training recommendations to maximize muscle hypertrophy: position stand of the IUSCA. *International Journal of Strength and Conditioning.* https://doi.org/10.47206/ijsc.v1i1.81

Schoenfeld, B., Grgic, J., Ogborn, D., Krieger, J. W. (2017). Strength and hypertrophy adaptations between low- vs. high- load resistance training: a systematic review and meta-analysis. *Journal of Strength and Conditioning Research.* 31(12): 3508–3523.

Sim, T., Choi, A., Lee, S., & Mun, J. H. (2017). How to quantify the transition phase during golf swing performance: Torsional load affects low back complaints during the transition phase. *Journal of Sports Sciences.* 35(20): 2051–2059. https://doi.org/10.1080/02640414.2016.1255345

Sorbie, G., Richardson, A. K., Glen, J., Hardie, S., Taliep, S., Wade, M., Broughton, L., Mann, S., Steele, J., & Lavallee, D. (2021). The association of golf participation with health and wellbeing: A comparative study. *International Journal of Golf Science.* 9(1).

Wells, J. E. T., Charalambous, L. H., Mitchell, A. C. S., Coughlan, D., Brearley, S. L., Hawkes, R. A., Murray, A. D., Hillman, R. G., & Fletcher, I. M. (2019). Relationships between Challenge Tour golfers' clubhead velocity and force producing capabilities during a countermovement jump and isometric mid-thigh pull. *Journal of Sports Sciences.* 37(12): 1381–1386.

2   Meeting a Golfer's Needs

Needs Analysis, Profiling, and Coaching Considerations in Strength and Conditioning

Ben Langdown and Jack Wells

Introduction

There has been a considerable shift in recent years from the predominantly technical and tactical perspectives on performance gains in golf (Glazier & Lamb, 2018). While the technical and tactical aspects are undoubtedly important to success, the modern golfer, possibly alongside their coach and a support team, is pursuing methods of improvement that were rarely used in the past. Wells and Langdown (2020) highlighted that golfers perceive the engagement with strength and conditioning (S&C) as an opportunity to improve performance and reduce the risk of injury. In this regard, it is now common for elite amateur and professional golfers to employ fitness or S&C coaches as part of their support team. Sustained engagement in S&C may also place the golfer in a better position to adapt their behaviours to the various performance demands and constraints on the course.

The change in culture

Traditionally, golfers refrained from engaging in S&C based on the outdated misconceptions that these training modalities would decrease range of motion (ROM) / flexibility (Álvarez et al., 2012). However, recent research has highlighted that, of a sample of 430 highly skilled golfers, 79.3% (341 of 430) disagreed that S&C would reduce flexibility (Wells & Langdown, 2020). As such, S&C is now seen as a fundamental tool that can help golfers of all levels succeed within the sport. These changes in perspective are likely due to the growing body of research supporting S&C for golf and underpinning practitioners' knowledge. In addition, statements from high-profile golfers openly advocating the benefits training has had on their game increase the trust and the reputation of S&C for performance enhancement. For the S&C practitioner who is currently working with (or aspiring to work with) golfers, it is important to recognise the needs of the individual. For instance, research has highlighted that the top three qualities golfers looked for when working with an S&C coach were that they had 1) previously worked with golfers, 2) a developed understanding

DOI: 10.4324/9781003099321-2

of the swing and 3) suitable qualifications (Wells & Langdown, 2020). It is advisable for an S&C coach to work closely with Professional Golfers' Association (PGA) golf coaches to develop further understanding of swing biomechanics, the 'coaching language', and the ability to create an intervention matched to the golfer's goals. It is critical that well-coordinated, interventions be put in place to optimise the golfer's availability and readiness to train. Lack of communication among the team of coaches can easily result in overloading the golfer's schedule with inappropriate training and practice volumes, thus increasing the risk of injury, overtraining and fatigue.

Optimising the golfer's availability to train and compete

Through a systematic and robust needs analysis process, it is possible to gain insight into the moderators that impact upon the golfer's daily, weekly, and monthly training load, and specifically, their internal load (the body's ability to cope with, and its response to, the prescribed external load). These moderators (Figure 2.1) should be highlighted as part of the discussions around the establishment of training environments conducive to effective functional adaptations and should include general health, nutrition and hydration, sleep and recovery strategies. It is the S&C coach's role to use the needs analysis to establish a systematic programme that is both organised and provides a prescribed plan with quality exercises, completed in the required quantities, to elicit the desired internal load following a critical analysis and understanding of the moderators impacting on the individual golfer. While this chapter is not focusing on the measurement of internal or external loads, it is important for the needs analysis to consider the moderators of the internal load, i.e., the body's psychophysiological response. The European Tour Performance Institute (ETPI) developed a theoretical Probability of Performance Impact model indicating the different benefits S&C could have on golfers' performance (see Chapter 10) (Brearley et al., 2019). The model suggests that the greatest benefits from S&C provision would be through maximising the golfer's availability and readiness to play the game. This can be achieved by ensuring the moderators of load are optimised for each individual in order to reduce the risk of injury, susceptibility to illness and fatigue, and therefore maintain their S&C engagement. Consistent engagement allows the principles of training to be applied effectively through progressive overload and suitable rest, resulting in the efficient achievement of adaptations, and minimising the impact of reversibility. Suboptimal golfer behaviours will present opportunities for the S&C coach to educate and inform the subsequent training programme based on the golfer's current needs and development. S&C coaches should prioritise optimisation of the moderators of internal load as a goal of the S&C programme, alongside providing an organised, quality intervention with correct quantity to elicit functional adaptations.

From a needs analysis perspective, it is initially important to understand the demands of golf (Figure 2.1 'determinants'). These decisions are advocated through recognising the demands of the swing and the stress that this can

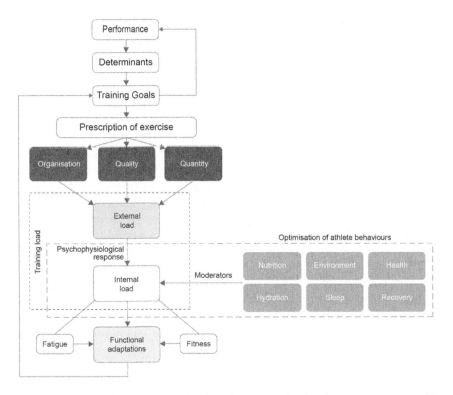

Figure 2.1 The theoretical framework of training load split into 2 measurable components: external (training load) and internal load (psychophysiological response)
Note: The figure visualises how this is relevant to the systematic programming of exercises in response to the needs analysis process, the fitness–fatigue model, and the other characteristics which can moderate the internal response.
Source: Adapted from Impellizzeri, Marcora & Coutts (2019).

place on the body. As such, recognising the most common injuries within golf are of upmost importance (see Chapter 9). Increases in the collection of performance stats on professional and amateur tours / events, statistical methods for analysing the sport (Broadie, 2014), development of new technology, such as launch monitors (Stefanyshyn & Wannop, 2015), and an increased financial incentive for success at the elite levels (Farrally et al., 2003) has driven an increased understanding and influenced the approach taken in profiling protocols and how to elicit performance enhancements. As an example, this includes generating greater drive distances through training interventions (e.g., Alvarez et al., 2012; Bliss, McCulloch & Maxwell, 2015; Cummings et al., 2018) and measurement of impulse and vertical force production (e.g., Wells et al., 2019).

Coach's perspective: The coach–golfer relationship

Before coaches begin to apply their professional S&C knowledge, it is essential to understand that professional knowledge (i.e., coaching knowledge), interpersonal knowledge (i.e., relationships with golfers and the educational community) and intrapersonal knowledge (i.e., a coach's own reflections, ethics and coaching dispositions) are not independent of each other (Côté & Gilbert, 2009). Coaches need to understand the individual(s) in front of them. Having extensive professional S&C knowledge and conducting a needs analysis with a golfer is potentially redundant if coaches cannot effectively communicate their knowledge to, and with, the golfers they are coaching, in order to meet their needs. Here is where effective coaching is required. Understanding the needs of an individual, whether in a golf or S&C context, is paramount to being able to work effectively with them. Szedlak et al. (2015) reported that coaches' actions, values and the relationship the coach built with the athletes were three fundamentally important behaviours of successful S&C coaches. Coaches will need to reflect and adapt their practice to facilitate the golfer's achievement of their optimum performances and reduction of injury risk through effective coaching experiences.

Needs analysis: A multi-disciplinary approach

A needs analysis forms the ideal starting point when working with golfers of any level (see Figure 2.2). It allows coaches to identify the demands of the sport and the specific requirements for each individual within their S&C sessions and golf practice/performance. It should also take on the form of a multi-disciplinary approach to consider all aspects of sport and exercise science. When considering individual disciplines, the S&C coach must seek to establish ways in which a golfer is less likely to incur an injury. Additionally, the S&C coach should enhance performance variables that are associated with decreased scoring and, in the professional game, increased prize money. The disciplines and considerations that an S&C coach could include, but are not limited to, are:

Anatomy and physiology: The demands that golf places on the golfer's body. An S&C coach can gain greater understanding of their resilience to these demands through the individual's current profiling test scores – e.g., force producing capabilities and joint ROM compared to normative data to allow a training programme to focus on the strengths and weaknesses as required. For instance, for a golfer to swing the club to the top of the backswing, it requires adequate mobility in the hips and thoracic spine. Indeed, research has suggested that the pelvis and torso rotate to approximately 49° and 98° in the backswing

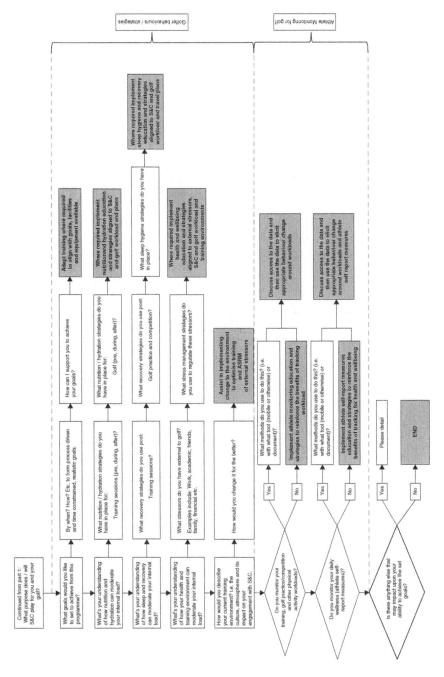

Figure 2.2 A needs analysis template for strength and conditioning coaches working with golfers

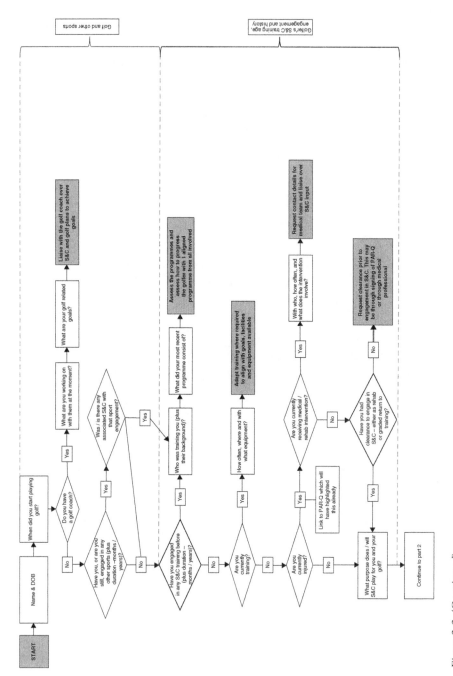

Figure 2.2 (Continued)

respectively (Chu, Sell & Lephart, 2010). It is important to recognise that the rotational values presented here are mean values with requirements varying among individuals. If this level of rotation is unattainable, the golfer may then produce a 'shorter' backswing or is forced to make adaptations in their swing (e.g., by lifting the arms, standing out of posture, extending the trail knee, increasing radial deviation (wrist cocking), or flexing the lead elbow). Having a 'short' backswing may negatively affect the carry distance a golfer can achieve. Increasing the length of the backswing by 12 cm (as represented by the path of the hands) has been suggested to increase clubhead speed (CHS) by 2.7 mph (Mackenzie, McCourt & Champoux, 2020). Therefore, alongside potential technical adjustments (where physical constraints have been overcome), an S&C intervention may support the golfer to meet their need for an increased length of backswing. Furthermore, golf coaches should consider the ball flight and liaise with the S&C coach on how the anatomy and physiology may be impacting this. The authors would not recommend the opposite approach whereby the S&C practitioner attempts to achieve arbitrary thresholds (e.g., 98° torso rotation) to produce a 'model swing'.

Aside from the golf swing itself, a round of golf can exceed four hours. However, it would be erroneous to assume that golf should be classified as an endurance-based sport. Blood lactate responses of 0.8–1.1 mmol/L, which are typically representative of resting levels, and peak heart rate responses below anaerobic thresholds have been recorded following the completion of 18 holes (Unverdorben et al., 2000). Indeed, Unverdorben et al. (2000) reported that golfers only reached 55.3 $\pm$ 9.1% of $VO_{2\,Max}$ during their round, which is obviously dependent on course topography. Given the requirements to protect the golfer from golf related injuries, while trying to enhance key performance measures such as CHS, the provision of S&C programmes should focus on these aspects rather than prioritising any endurance training.

Training demands: Current and future training demands should result from appropriate assessment of the individual's training age, history and status and linked to the results of profiling tests. The systematic training programme should then be implemented to help the athlete meet the demands of golf and their specific needs and goal(s). Anecdotally, we know that there can also be increased demands placed on the golfer by themselves, golf coaches and parents (especially if they are juniors). This can lead to an increase in the number of balls hit within practice sessions. Langdown et al. (2018) highlighted that golfers engaged in a regional and national performance programme had large fluctuations in practice volumes, particularly around school holidays, such as Easter and summer. There are numerous factors that could elicit significant increases ('spikes') in a golfer's practice volume. For instance, a dip in form for a professional golfer may lead to an increase in time spent on the driving range (e.g., number of long game shots played) in an attempt to improve their performance prior to subsequent competitive rounds. With large spikes in volume and intensity providing cause for concern over injury risk, it is critical that sustained engagement in S&C be encouraged and made viable for golfers to protect them from such risks.

With increased engagement in S&C comes an increased athlete training load. Measures of training load can be through the external load (e.g., volume load lifted in the gym), and internal load (e.g., the perceived exertion required to complete the session). With large fluctuations in volumes seen in Langdown et al.'s (2018) performance squad sample (n = 111), it is evident that practice strategies have large inter- and intra-individual fluctuations. Average monthly total volumes can be dictated by the time available to the golfer, pressures external to golf (e.g., work, family or academic) and motivation to practice. With better weather comes an increase in short game and putting practice durations. In contrast, with poor weather and reduced daylight hours, during the autumn and winter months there is an increase in long game practice (Langdown et al., 2018). With this in mind, Penner (2003) highlighted that the force created during the impact between the club and ball reaches 10 kN (1020 kg). With the hands and wrists being the first anatomical location to experience the result of this impact between club and ball it is unsurprising that injuries in this area are common (Murray et al., 2017). With many shots being played from range mats, increasing the forces experienced through the wrists in comparison to practice on softer turf, it is important that both S&C coaches and PGA Professional golf coaches collaborate in the facilitation of monitoring and management of training and practice volumes (e.g., through structuring effective practice schedules). Considerations should also include the impact of other external factors (e.g., other physical activity besides golf, non-golf stress and pressures etc.), monitored through athletes' self-report measures such as wellness surveys and training load logs (including volume/duration and intensity). As previously mentioned, to increase tolerance against the demands of high volumes of practice and tournament play, golfers should engage in a systematic and well-conceived S&C programme.

Biomechanical demands: While hierarchical or deterministic models can provide us with the biomechanical understanding of the golf swing and the influences on ball flight (e.g., see Hay, 1993), S&C coaches need to focus their attention on which aspects are within their control and remit within the gym environment. Glazier and Lamb (2018) stated that while these hierarchical models can provide information about performance (i.e., ball flight physics), they are limited in their ability to provide information on what the body is doing to achieve the shot outcome. They argue that much of the golf research that looks at, for example, peak values of a movement variable (e.g., peak angular velocity of the pelvis and torso) does little to inform coaches of what is really occurring at a coordination and motor control perspective.

Each golf swing places a significant stress on the body, and when considered over time, the cumulative load theory (see Kumar, 2001) suggests that repeated loading through the golf swing, with high forces, increases the overall stress experienced by the golfer's body, which can damage musculoskeletal tissues. For example, compression forces in the spine are in excess of 6.5 (Lim, Chow & Chae, 2012) and eight times body weight (Dale & Brumitt, 2016) immediately after impact, or 6.1 kN (621 kg) and 7.6 kN (773 kg) when an amateur and professional player, respectively, hits a 5-iron (Hosea & Gatt, 1996). Shear forces, although not as large as compressive forces, are also present within the swing with anterior-posterior and medio-lateral loads peaking during mid-follow through at ~1.6 and 0.44 times body weight, respectively, when using a driver (Lim, Chow & Chae, 2012). As such, the spine is another common site of injury within golfers (Murray et al., 2018) and although the lumbar spine in particular is able to cope with these forces, junior golfers are particularly susceptible to defects in the pars interarticularis (e.g., spondylolysis and spondylolisthesis) (Brearley et al., 2021). For older golfers, the spine will degenerate with age and lose its shock-absorbing capabilities (Hosea & Gatt, 1996), leaving older golfers more susceptible to injury. It would be advisable, for S&C interventions to prioritise exercises that develop strength and mobility in and around this region. The following exercises may be advantageous in this regard:

- Hip mobility (e.g., 90–90 rockovers)
- Trunk mobility (e.g., open book stretch and elbow reach backs)
- Anti-extension (e.g., roll out and anti-extension overhead press)
- Anti-rotation (e.g., Pallof press and plank rows or pull through variations)
- Anti-lateral flexion (e.g., overhead Pallof press or exercises with added perturbation, such as offset step ups).

With a growing interest for golfers to increase drive distance, the interaction between the golfer and the ground during the swing is an important consideration for S&C. Highly skilled golfers have been shown to generate >1.6 times their body weight in ground reaction forces (GRF) when hitting a driver, with these vertical GRF (vGRF) significantly related to CHS (Han et al., 2019). Therefore, S&C interventions and profiling procedures targeting vGRF are preferential (e.g., vertical jumps and isometric mid-thigh pull; Wells et al., 2018, 2019).

Nutrition and hydration demands of the activity: These demands can be based on the climate in which the golfer is training (usually an indoor environment), the typical conditions for competition, as well as current habits and behaviour modification through monitoring of the individual over time. Nutrition and hydration are two of the moderators of internal load (Figure 2.1), and, although beyond the scope of this chapter, assessing and optimising strategies here, to remain fuelled and hydrated, can allow more effective training adaptations and an optimised psychophysiological response to prescribed exercises in a given S&C programme.

Athlete monitoring: While there are protective benefits of training for golf, the individual needs to have an awareness and understanding of how to monitor fatigue, wellbeing and performance. It is critical that the golfing population embrace lessons learned from other sports in athlete monitoring. Maintaining training, practice, tournament and wellness logs allows coaches to assess acute training status (i.e., how they present to each session as an individual in comparison to their norm or optimal state [i.e., readiness]) and longer-term readiness. Measures can include, but not limited to, energy levels, perceived recovery from previous training, muscle soreness, impact of menstrual cycle (for female athletes), and, in line with the psychological demands of each session, their motivation to train, and non-golf related stress etc. Athlete self-report measures are a useful addition to any systematic training to allow both acute and chronic alterations to the frequency, intensity, and volume of interventions across the completion of a periodised plan. A lack of measurement here leaves uncertainty over the appropriateness of the application of training to that individual and their needs on each specific training (and rest) day.

Goal(s) of the individual golfer: Arguably the most important area for the golfer. Recognising the needs of the golfer is important in developing specific goals, however small or large these may be. It is the role of the coaches to ensure discussions take place to agree on suitably structured goals and to plan for all aspects of sport and exercise science to feed into this process (where appropriate). For instance, it may be that you are delivering S&C provision to a junior golfer to achieve longer-term goals of reducing the risk of overuse injury and to enhance specific process goals and ultimately, performance goals. However, to attain these longer-term goals, the player will need to engage in the training programme set for them. The player and S&C coach should discuss and agree a realistic number of sessions per week that, alongside other physical activity loads, should be completed to help achieve the long-term goal(s).

There are other areas of sport and exercise science that may be considered along with those highlighted above here and S&C coaches may also find themselves working alongside other professionals to create the needs analysis and a plan to reach a specific goal (e.g., sports medicine professionals where a golfer is injured and returning to training). When working with a golfer in an S&C environment it is critical that coaches understand them from a holistic perspective as an individual athlete. Agreement must be reached on the goals to be set and achieved and how this aligns to the demands of their golf.

Conducting a needs analysis

In scenarios where an S&C coach is working with any level of golfer, the programme goals must be to prescribe exercises that optimise the psychophysiological response (i.e., internal load) to elicit adaptation in the body in relation

to their training goals. With the golfer performing S&C sessions systematically, adaptations will occur through changes at a cellular level (through functional capacity, structure and metabolic processes), and in the tissues, organs
and the body's functional capacity, all of which lead to enhanced muscular
activity (Viru & Viru, 2000). To achieve targeted adaptations, the planning of
S&C interventions must reflect the needs analysis process coaches undertake
with the golfer. This process initiates the formation of a relationship between
the demands of the sport, the coach, the golfer and their goals. It acts to establish factors such as training age, access to facilities / equipment, availability to
train, injury, and health history (dealt with through a Pre-Activity Readiness
Questionnaire [PAR-Q]), goals, motivation etc. (see Figure 2.2). Testing of
adaptations through specific profiling tests (see 'Physical profiling' section)
will allow for alterations in the exercise intervention to be administered. In
this regard, the first session with an athlete can often provide a lot of information to guide the systematic planning of the S&C interventions. Gathering
this information can be done through discussion with the golfer and their
support team (including parents for junior golfers) as well as assessing their
profiling results and any monitoring data available to the coach to establish their current training status. Figure 2.2 provides a framework to ensure
coaches can gather the initial information they may need through a flow of
the key questions to prompt an extensive, but not exhaustive, needs analysis
in golf.

Physical profiling

Having established the underpinning demands on the golfer (e.g., training loads
from other sports, availability, impact of their current behaviours – moderators of
internal load), the S&C coach can then look to physically profile the golfer. This
allows the S&C coach to establish a baseline of physiological attributes within
the selected tests. This baseline helps to identify areas of weakness that can be
addressed through physical interventions. For example, if a golfer demonstrates
undesirable results on an isometric mid-thigh pull or a repetition maximum
test, a key focus for an intervention would be to target an increase in strength
in line with the training goals. Profiling also facilitates the monitoring of progression while encouraging increased engagement through accountability for
the golfer in the knowledge that post-intervention testing will take place to
monitor any changes in physical performance. It is important for an S&C coach
to match the demands of the sport to the tools they have available to profile
the golfer ensuring that there is a strong rationale for the collection and use
of each specific metric. At this point, it is worth noting that the monitoring of
maturation is critical when working with junior golfers to allow insights into
their growth, years from peak height velocity and to control for this when comparing profiling results over time (see Chapter 6).

Whichever profiling tools a coach chooses to use with a golfer, it is essential
that the S&C coach has a clear and defendable rationale for utilising these profiling procedures. Not only should this rationale be supported by research, but

it is also important to clearly explain the links between the profiling procedure and the demands of golf performance. Additionally, it is essential to ensure robust testing protocols are used to allow for accurate comparisons across pre- and post-interventions. Only when measurement reliability and validity are achieved does the data provide effective evidence to feed into the needs analysis and determine the new goals for training.

Range of motion and movement assessments

It is our belief that, where appropriate, tests to establish a golfer's ROM should be used, but coaches should not be fixated on measuring every joint used in the golf swing or try to predict specific swing characteristics based on a physical limitation. Instead, the PGA Professional and S&C coach should work together to establish the causes of undesirable ball flights, impact factors, swing faults and potential movement assessments to identify any ROM limitations.

Coach's perspective: The sequence of detection

When analysing the golfer, it is preferential to work from the ball flight backwards:

Ball flight → Impact factors → Swing mechanics

Here we show a hypothetical example of the ways in which a PGA Professional and S&C coach, working together, may seek to assess the ROM in a golfer.

Case study: Right-handed golfer

1. Ball flight: The golfer lacks distance with their driver and long irons.
2. Impact factors: CHS is likely to be the issue as it accounts of 75% of the variance in ball speed (Sweeney et al., 2013).
3. Swing mechanics: The golfer appears to have limited rotation in their thoracic spine and their club is short of horizontal at the top of the backswing.
4. Assessing ROM: Given the short backswing and limited thoracic rotation in the swing, an S&C coach may wish to assess the ROM using the seated thoracic rotation test. Golfers who perform better in this test have greater spine rotation at the top of the backswing (Gould et al., 2021).
5. Limitation found – the S&C coach can provide interventions to increase ROM. Where no limitation is found – the PGA Professional can provide technical interventions to increase the length of the backswing.

The sequence of detection offers great value when assessing ROM, especially compared to assessing the full body before observing the golf swing. Therefore, rather than predicting what movements may occur in the swing based on the results of a full screening battery, coaches could simply observe the ball flight and golf swing and target the movement assessments that may be of relevance to the golfer's and PGA Professional's technical goals. Additionally, the S&C coach should consider focusing more on observing and developing effective movement patterns within the gym environment, thus allowing safe and progressive S&C to take place, in line with the individual's goals.

As an example, it has been claimed by the Titleist Performance Institute that if a golfer is unable to perform an overhead squat (OHS), it is 'almost impossible' for them to maintain their posture in the swing (Rose, 2013). Despite these claims, evidence from Langdown et al. (2012) suggests otherwise given that the overhead squat was only a small significant predictor of loss of posture in the golf swing. Specifically, Langdown et al. (2012) reported that at the top of the backswing only 30% of the variance in upper body lift is attributable to the measure of OHS torso lean when profiling the golfer using this test. At impact even less of the variance could be accounted for. The highest variance was OHS torso lean accounting for just 11.9% of spine flexion/extension (i.e., loss of posture angles in the torso at impact). Furthermore, Langdown et al. (2022) used an intervention to significantly improve the OHS depth but reported no significant changes to subsequent in-swing posture. This emphasises that S&C is only one aspect of performance enhancement and that, where new strength/ ROM/speed etc. goals are achieved in the S&C environment, it is vital that golf coaching supports the application of these gains into the swing and performance where appropriate. Research tells us that a delay often exists between improvements in physical capacity and its translation to improved sport-specific performance (Suchomel, Nimphius & Stone, 2016). For example, Alvarez et al. (2012) reported significant gains in muscle strength and power after six weeks of training, but associated golf measures did not significantly improve until after 12 weeks.

Vertical jumps

The interaction between the ground and the golfer is fundamental in producing a golf swing and maximising this interaction can lead to increased CHS and distance gains. Although both medial-lateral (left-right) and anterior-posterior (forwards-backwards) GRF affect swing mechanics, the greatest magnitude of force is produced vertically (Lynn & Wu, 2018). Indeed, these vGRF are typically very large (>2.5 times body weight) for golfers who achieve long drive distances (e.g., >300 yards) (Lynn & Wu, 2018). Exercises such as the countermovement jump (CMJ) and squat jump (SJ) are commonly used to profile golfers given that these are focused on producing vGRF. Research has highlighted significant relationships between CHS and both CMJ height and SJ height (Hellström, 2008). This is advantageous in applied settings as jump height is easy to measure through contact mats or from mobile applications that have been validated against force platforms (Balsalobre-Fernández, Glaister & Lockey, 2015). Unfortunately, solely relying on jump height as a metric is problematic. Jump height is affected and thus confounded by the mass of the golfer. For instance, if two golfers (with masses of 70 kg and 85 kg) both jumped 0.3 m, it is evident that the 85 kg golfer needed to produce greater vGRF to attain the same jump height as the 70 kg golfer. Recent research assessed the relationships between 50 highly skilled golfers' CHS and CMJ height, peak force, average power, peak power, force at zero velocity, net impulse and positive impulse (Wells et al., 2022). Each variable presented strong significant relationships with CHS, apart from jump height which was not statistically significant. This is in contrast to Hellström (2008) and therefore raises questions as to the validity of using jump height as a metric when profiling golfers. Specifically, although research has found significant relationships between CHS and jump height, the authors recommend that S&C practitioners consider the use of other metrics to ensure validity.

In this regard, peak power in a CMJ and SJ are often utilised as an alternative profiling metric, especially given that Hellström (2008) reported strong significant relationships with CHS. There is a general belief that power is a cause-and-effect variable. For instance, if a golfer generated greater power in a vertical jump, it may be assumed that there would also be an increase in their jump height. However, a more powerful golfer in a jump test may not necessarily jump higher (Table 2.1).

As seen in Table 2.1, golfer A has a greater average power, a larger mass and greater relative power (average power / body mass) than Golfer B, but a lower jump height by 0.06 m (6 cm). It is essential that practitioners recognise that power does not directly cause a change in jump height. Consequently, it is recommended that impulse (which is the force generated over a given duration [force x time]) be utilised when profiling golfers (Knudson, 2009; Winter et al., 2016).

Research from Wells et al. (2018) reported a strong significant relationship between highly skilled golfers' (handicap ≤5) CHS and positive impulse generated during a CMJ and SJ. Indeed, 37.9% of the variance in Challenge Tour golfers' CHS can be accounted for by CMJ positive impulse (Wells et al., 2019). However, the investigations of Wells et al. (2018, 2019) utilised force

Table 2.1 The average power, mass, relative power and jump height in a countermovement jump for two golfers

	Golfer A	Golfer B
Average power (W)	2010.12	1344.87
Mass (kg)	90.02	70.93
Relative power (W.kg^{-1})	22.33	18.96
Jump height (m)	0.25	0.31

plates which are not always readily available to practitioners. Where an S&C coach only has a jump height mobile application and a set of scales available, inverse dynamics has been suggested as a valuable method to calculate net impulse (Wells et al., 2022). Here, a hypothetical example of a golfer who jumps 0.35 m and has a body mass of 73.3 kg is used to demonstrate how this could be applied in practice:

1. Calculate the take-off velocity of the centre of mass:

    Take-off velocity = $\sqrt{(\text{Jump height}*(2*\text{Gravity}))}$
    Take-off velocity = $\sqrt{(0.35*(2*9.81))}$
    Take-off velocity = 2.62 m.s^{-1}

Note: gravity is always 9.81 m.s^{-2} and jump height is always in metres not centimetres for this calculation.

2. Calculate net impulse:

    Net impulse = Mass * Take-off velocity
    Net impulse = 73.3 kg * 2.62 m.s^{-1}
    Net impulse = 192.08 N's

The calculation of net impulse is of great value to the practitioner since this is easily accessible and has a strong relationship with CHS. When considering the examples in Table 2.1, the net impulse is 199 N's for golfer A and 175 N's for golfer B.

As a benchmarking guide for S&C coaches using the above equations, the authors have observed mean values for net impulse of ~180 N's and ~190 N's for highly skilled male (handicap <5) and Challenge Tour golfers, respectively.

Coach's perspective: Assessing clubhead speed, ball speed and distance

While this section is focused upon the profiling within an S&C environment, it is important to note that CHS, ball speed and distance testing also needs rigorous assessment methods to allow accurate analysis of the impact of S&C on drive performance measures. In this regard, here we present a method for maintaining reliability in testing:

1. Use a launch monitor where possible and consider the inherent measurement error for the specific make and model of the system being used (Leach et al., 2017).
2. Set up ensuring the alignment and target selection are known to the golfer.

3. Ensure the golfer performs a standardised warm-up to maintain reliability of testing.
4. Ask the golfer to hit three drives as if playing a par five tee shot – i.e., aiming for maximal distance while maintaining accuracy to hit the fairway. Ensure 60 s rest is taken between each shot.
5. Ask the golfer to play three maximal drives with the only concern being maximum CHS. Ensure 60 s rest is taken between each shot.
6. Record the highest CHS, ball speed and distance from each condition to demonstrate results from maximum effort and controlled shots.

Run this protocol pre-intervention alongside any profiling where relationships are to be drawn to CHS, ball speed and distance. Then repeat post-intervention or before any major amendments to training programmes to understand S&C's impact.

Repetition maximum assessment

The most utilised method for assessing maximum strength is a repetition maximum (RM) test where the athlete (under qualified supervision) completes the chosen number of reps at an increasing load, with adequate rest between sets, until failure. Where >1 rep is used in the assessment, calculations are performed to estimate 1RM, the values of which can then inform programme design and setting of loads for specific exercises. Research that links RM testing to golf has reported significant relationships between CHS and the load lifted in a 1RM back squat (Hellström, 2008). Additionally, Parchmann and McBride (2011) reported that the relative load (load lifted/body mass) lifted in a back squat significantly related to golfers' CHS, supporting the notion that strength is an important component in this regard. This is of no great surprise given the aforementioned suggestion that the greatest magnitude of GRF are in the vertical direction (Lynn & Wu, 2018). However, conducting a RM test is only of value if the golfer can execute the lift proficiently and safely. As such, the limitations in a golfer's ability to perform a RM test in, for example a back squat, may be masking the true relationship between strength and CHS. From a practical standpoint, if the S&C coach is only able to assess strength through a RM test (due to limited access to force plates), it is essential to initially develop the golfer's lifting technique through an intervention. Once the golfer is proficient in their technique, this will provide a better representation as a profiling tool. Where golfers are unable to use a direct 1RM testing, a predicted 1RM can be calculated from the number of reps at an appropriate weight where >1 rep can be completed. Typical alternatives include a 3RM through to 10RM predictive test.

There are some notable considerations and disadvantages of using a RM test when assessing golfers. For instance, Stone et al. (2019) suggested that these are time consuming and fatiguing. This is especially true where the goal is to test maximal strength (1RM) as opposed to predictive tests (see Niewiadomski et al., 2008). A further consideration for the S&C coach is the standardisation of the squat depth as it is easier to lift a greater external load when reducing the depth of the squat. Ensuring a consistent squat depth (e.g., thighs parallel to floor) over each repeat testing session controls for this and increases the confidence that successful lifts of greater external load are due to physiological adaptation.

Isometric mid-thigh pull

Given the limitations with RM tests, alternative methods such as an isometric mid-thigh pull (IMTP) can be employed. The IMTP pull is utilised extensively by S&C researchers and coaches to measure peak force and rate of force development (RFD). Evidence has highlighted that peak force generated in an IMTP has a strong significant positive relationship with 1RM back squat strength (McGuigan et al., 2010; Wang et al., 2016). Furthermore, research has reported a significant positive relationship between highly skilled golfers CHS and IMTP peak force (Wells et al., 2018). As guidance, mean IMTP peak force values of ~1600 N and ~2100 N have been reported for category-1 and Challenge Tour players respectively (Wells et al., 2018, 2019). Please note that these values represent average values for different skill levels and depending on the training goals, a golfer and their S&C coach would likely want to exceed these. There have also been suggestions that developing a golfer's ability to enhance RFD would be advantageous for generating CHS (Read & Lloyd, 2014). While theoretically this appears plausible, research has highlighted that measuring RFD during an IMTP is unreliable (Wells et al., 2018), with the authors strongly cautioning against the use of this metric. It is appreciated that IMTP testing does require access to force plates and that this may prohibit widespread use. However, where they are available, S&C coaches should consider the following applied set-up: Setting up an isometric rig can be performed without a Smith Machine by using a squat rack instead. In this scenario the 'J-hooks' can be turned upside down and pulled against with an Olympic bar. This is further applicable if heavy resistance bands are used to attach the Olympic bar to a 'pull-up' bar at the top of the rack, meaning that the athlete does not have to support the weight (Figure 2.3).

There are advantages of using an IMTP set-up (when available), to establish deficits in vGRF production, over RM testing. With the IMTP, technique is less likely to confound the results. Additionally, golfers are more likely to engage in an IMTP assessment, as there is reduced muscle soreness, less fatigue affecting the rest of the session and they may perceive this as a safer alternative compared to maximally loaded lifts (Stone et al., 2019). These advantages have led to the IMTP being employed by organisations such as England Golf and the European Tour to objectively profile golfers.

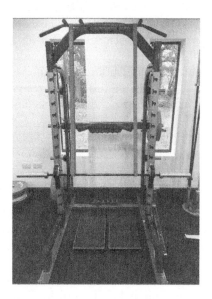

Figure 2.3 A gym-based set-up of an isometric mid-thigh pull

Medicine ball (MB) throws

It is very common for S&C coaches to use MB throws with golfers given that there is an element of visual similarity with the golf swing. While it would be erroneous to select assessments purely on this basis, research has highlighted significant relationships between various MB throws and CHS. Gordon et al. (2009) reported a significant relationship between a standing rotational MB throwing distance and CHS in adult golfers. Results from Read et al. (2013) supported this with significant relationships between both a standing rotational MB throw and seated MB chest throw with CHS. These findings were also observed by Lewis et al. (2016) for golfers >30 years of age, but for golfers <30 (mean = 25.6 ± 2.9) years of age, only the seated MB chest throw had a significant correlation with CHS. For junior golfers on a performance pathway (aged 15.1 ± 0.8 years of age) there were significant relationships reported between both the seated single arm and the standing rotational MB throws with CHS (Coughlan et al., 2020). A note of caution: an eight-week plyometric intervention noted significant improvements in a MB chest and rotational throw in both the intervention group and control. Therefore, it is likely that changes in throwing distance are partially due to learned effects (Bliss et al., 2015). MB throw testing provides S&C coaches with a useful field-based protocol to profile golfers of all ages, however, coaches must ensure a consistent technique is used with the same weight MB at pre- and post-testing sessions (3–4 kg is suggested). Additionally, familiarisation trials should be offered to the golfer before recording a measurement.

Conclusion

Establishing the needs and goals of each individual golfer is paramount to the effectiveness of any S&C intervention. In doing so, the S&C coach needs to understand the demands of the sport and the athlete to ensure an appropriate, systematic programme can be developed as part of a periodised plan. Adopting a holistic, multi-disciplinary approach to the needs analysis and subsequent interventions will allow the optimisation of training load to elicit functional adaptations to improve performance and reduce the risk of injury. In order to benchmark and assess the impact of prescribed S&C interventions it is important that time efficient and appropriate profiling protocols are utilised in the field. This chapter has recommended the use of various methods and encouraged the application of tests most appropriate to equipment accessibility and the golfer's needs. With the shift in culture towards S&C engagement within golf, research has demonstrated the importance of assessing vGRF (i.e., impulse) with a view to enhanced functional adaptations leading to greater drive performance measures. Where physical restrictions are impacting on the ball flight and swing characteristics, ROM testing may have a place, but it is important that these tests are used as part of an assessment and not relied on to predict why specific movements are occurring in the swing. Above all, the S&C coach implementing the tests should be aware of how to ensure reliability and validity and use the data to adapt S&C programmes effectively rather than collect the data for no reason. Optimal functional adaptation will only occur through the systematic S&C programme when an exhaustive needs analysis process, reliable profiling tests, effective coach–athlete relationships, and monitoring of each golfer's availability and readiness to train and compete are in place and adapted, as appropriate, to meet the needs and goals of each individual.

References

Álvarez, M., Sedano, S., Cuadrado, G., & Redondo, J. C. (2012). Effects of an 18-week strength training program on low-handicap golfers' performance. *Journal of Strength and Conditioning Research, 26*(4): 1110–1121.

Balsalobre-Fernández, C., Glaister, M., & Lockey, R. A. (2015). The validity and reliability of an iPhone app for measuring vertical jump performance. *Journal of Sports Sciences, 33*(15), 1574–1579. https://doi.org/10.1080/02640414.2014.996184

Bliss, A., McCulloch, H., & Maxwell, N. S. (2015). The Effects of an Eight-Week Plyometric Training Program on Golf Swing Performance Characteristics in Skilled Adolescent Golfers. *International Journal of Golf Science, 4*(2): 120–135. https://doi.org/10.1123/ijgs.2015-0009

Brearley, S., Coughlan, D., & Wells, J. (2019). Strength and Conditioning in Golf : Probability of Performance Impact. *Sport Performance & Science Reports, May* (June): 1–3.

Brearley, S. L., Buckley, O., Gillham, P., Clements, B., & Coughlan, D. (2021). Inter-Disciplinary Conservative Management of Bilateral Non-United Lumbar Pars Defects in a Junior Elite Golfer. *International Journal of Sports Physical Therapy, February*. https://doi.org/10.26603/001c.18873

Broadie, M. (2014). *Every Shot Counts.* Avery Publishing Group, New York, USA

Chu, Y., Sell, T. C., & Lephart, S. M. (2010). The relationship between biomechanical variables and driving performance during the golf swing. *Journal of Sports Sciences,* *28*(11): 1251–1259. https://doi.org/10.1080/02640414.2010.507249

Côté, J., & Gilbert, W. (2009). An Integrative Definition of Coaching Effectiveness and Expertise. *International Journal of Sports Science & Coaching,* *4*(3): 307–323. https://doi.org/10.1260/174795409789623892

Coughlan, D., Taylor, M. J. D., Jackson, J., Ward, N., & Beardsley, C. (2020). Physical Characteristics of Youth Elite Golfers and Their Relationship With Driver Clubhead Speed. *Journal of Strength and Conditioning Research,* *34*(1): 212–217. https://doi.org/10.1519/JSC.0000000000002300

Cummings, P. M., Waldman, H. S., Krings, B. M., Smith, J. W., & McAllister, M. J. (2018). Effects of Fat Grip Training on Muscular Strength and Driving Performance in Division I Male Golfers. *The Journal of Strength & Conditioning Research,* *32*(1): 205–210.

Dale, R. B., & Brumitt, J. (2016). Spine biomechanics associated with the shortened, modern one-plane golf swing. *Sports Biomechanics,* *15*(2): 198–206. https://doi.org/10.1080/14763141.2016.1159723

Farrally, M. R., Cochran, A. J., Crews, D. J., Hurdzan, M. J., Price, R. J., Snow, J. T., & Thomas, P. R. (2003). Golf science research at the beginning of the twenty-first century. *Journal of Sports Sciences,* *21*(9): 753–765. https://doi.org/10.1080/0264041031000102123

Glazier, P. S., & Lamb, P. F. (2018). Inter-and intra-individual movement variability in the golf swing. In M. Toms (Ed.), *Routledge International Handbook of Golf Science* (pp. 49–63). Routledge. https://doi.org/10.4324/9781315641782-6

Gordon, B. S., Moir, G. L., Davis, S. E., Witmer, C. A., & Cummings, D. (2009). An investigation into the relationship of flexibility, power, and strength to club head speed in male golfers. *Journal of Strength and Conditioning Research,* *23*(5): 1606–1610.

Gould, Z. I., Oliver, J. L., Lloyd, R. S., Neil, R., & Bull, M. (2021). The golf movement screen is related to spine control and x-factor of the golf swing in low handicap golfers. *Journal of Strength & Conditioning Research,* *35*(1): 240–246.

Han, K. H., Como, C., Kim, J., Lee, S., Kim, J., Kim, D. K., & Kwon, Y. H. (2019). Effects of the golfer–ground interaction on clubhead speed in skilled male golfers. *Sports Biomechanics,* *18*(2): 115–134. https://doi.org/10.1080/14763141.2019.1586983

Hay, J. G. (1993). *The biomechanics of sports techniques* (4th ed.). Prentice Hall, New Jersey, USA

Hellström, J. (2008). The Relation between Physical Tests, Measures, and Clubhead Speed in Elite Golfers. *International Journal of Sports Science & Coaching,* *3*(1_suppl): 85–92. https://doi.org/10.1260/174795408785024207

Hosea, T. M., & Gatt, C. J. (1996). Back Pain in Golf. *Clinics in Sports Medicine,* *15*(1): 37–53.

Impellizzeri, F. M., Marcora, S. M., & Coutts, A. J. (2019). Internal and external training load: 15 years on. *International Journal of Sports Physiology and Performance,* *14*(2): 270–273. https://doi.org/10.1123/ijspp.2018-0935

Knudson, D. V. (2009). Correcting the use of the term 'power' in the strength and conditioning literature. *Journal of Strength and Conditioning Research,* *6*(23): 1902–1908. https://doi.org/10.1227/01.NEU.0000297070.90551.DF

Kumar, S. (2001). Theories of musculoskeletal injury causation. *Ergonomics,* *44*(1): 17–47. https://doi.org/10.1080/00140130120716

Langdown, B. L., Bridge, M, W., & Li, F, X. (2022). The influence of an 8-week strength and corrective exercise intervnetion on the overhead deep squat and golf swing kinematics. *The Journal of Strength and Conditioning Research*. doi: 10.1519/JSC.0000000000004254

Langdown, B. L., Burnett, S., Jones, N., & Coughlan, D. (2018). Practice And Tournament Volumes Of Young Golfers In Regional And National Squads. *World Scientific Congress of Golf.* http://oro.open.ac.uk/id/eprint/55982

Leach, R. J., Forrester, S. E., Mears, A. C., & Roberts, J. R. (2017). How valid and accurate are measurements of golf impact parameters obtained using commercially available radar and stereoscopic optical launch monitors? *Measurement: Journal of the International Measurement Confederation, 112*(August): 125–136. https://doi.org/10.1016/j.measurement.2017.08.009

Lewis, A. L., Ward, N., Bishop, C., Maloney, S., & Turner, A. N. (2016). Determinants of Club Head Speed in PGA Professional Golfers. *Journal of Strength and Conditioning Research, 30*(8): 2266–2270. https://doi.org/10.1519/JSC.0000000000001362

Lim, Y. T., Chow, J. W., & Chae, W. S. (2012). Lumbar spinal loads and muscle activity during a golf swing. *Sports Biomechanics, 11*(2): 197–211. https://doi.org/10.1080/14763141.2012.670662

Lynn, S. K., & Wu, W. (2018). The use of the ground reaction forces and pressures in golf swing instruction. In M. Toms (Ed.), *Routledge international handbook of Golf Science* (pp. 15–25). London and New York: Routledge.

Mackenzie, S., Mccourt, M., & Champoux, L. (2020). *How Amateur Golfers Deliver Energy to the Driver, 8*: 1–21.

McGuigan, M. R., Newton, M. J., Winchester, J. B., & Nelson, A. G. (2010). Relationship between isometric and dynamic strength in recreationally trained men. *Journal of Strength and Conditioning Research, 24*(9): 2570–2573.

Murray, A. D., Daines, L., Archibald, D., Hawkes, R. A., Schiphorst, C., Kelly, P., Grant, L., & Mutrie, N. (2017). The relationships between golf and health: a scoping review. *British Journal of Sports Medicine, 51*(1): 12–19. https://doi.org/10.1136/bjsports-2016-096625

Murray, A. D., Robinson, P. G., Murray, I. R., Oliver, C. W., Tilley, N. R., Glover, D., Hawkes, R., Duckworth, A. D., & Hillman, R. (2018). Systematic review of musculo-skeletal injuries in professional golfers. *British Journal of Sports Medicine, 53*(1): 13–18. https://doi.org/10.1136/bjsports-2018-099572

Niewiadomski, W., Gąsiorowska, A., Cybulski, G., Laskowska, D., & Langfort, J. (2008). Determination and Prediction of One Repetition Maximum (1RM): Safety Considerations. *Journal of Human Kinetics, 19*(June): 109–120. https://doi.org/10.2478/v10078-008-0008-8

Parchmann, C. J., & McBride, J. M. (2011). Relationship between functional movement screen and athletic performance. *The Journal of Strength & Conditioning Research, 25*(12): 3378–3384.

Penner, A. R. (2003). The physics of golf. *Reports on Progress in Physics, 66*(2): 131–171. https://doi.org/10.1088/0034-4885/66/2/202

Read, P. J., & Lloyd, R. S. (2014). Strength and conditioning considerations for golf. *Strength and Conditioning Journal, 36*(5): 24–33. https://doi.org/10.1519/SSC.0000000000000062

Read, P. J., Lloyd, R. S., Croix, M. D. S., & Oliver, J. L. (2013). Relationships between field-based measures of strength and power and golf club head speed. *Journal of Strength and Conditioning Research, 27*(10): 2708–2713. https://doi.org/10.1519/JSC.0b013e318280ca00

Rose, G. (2013). *The Overhead Deep Squat Test*. Www.Mytpi.Com. www.mytpi.com/articles/screening/the_overhead_deep_squat_test

Stefanyshyn, D. J., & Wannop, J. W. (2015). Biomechanics research and sport equipment development. *Sports Engineering*, *18*(4): 191–202. https://doi.org/10.1007/s12283-015-0183-5

Stone, M. H., O'Bryant, H. S., Hornsby, G., Cunanan, A., Mizuguchi, S., Suarez, D. G., South, M., March, D. J., Haff, G. G., Ramsey, M. W., Beckham, G. K., Santana, H. A. P., Wagle, J. P., Stone, M. E., & Pierce, K. (2019). Using the isometric mid-thigh pull in monitoring of weightlifters: 25+ years of experience. *Profesional Strength and Conditioning*, *54*: 19–26.

Suchomel, T. J., Nimphius, S., & Stone, M. H. (2016). The Importance of Muscular Strength in Athletic Performance. *Sports Medicine*, *46*(10): 1419–1449. https://doi.org/10.1007/s40279-016-0486-0

Sweeney, M., Mills, P., Alderson, J., & Elliott, B. (2013). The influence of club-head kinematics on early ball flight characteristics in the golf drive. *Sports Biomechanics*, *12*(3): 247–258. https://doi.org/10.1080/14763141.2013.772225

Szedlak, C., Smith, M. J., Day, M. C., & Greenlees, I. A. (2015). Effective behaviours of strength and conditioning coaches as perceived by athletes. *International Journal of Sports Science and Coaching*, *10*(5): 967–984. https://doi.org/10.1260/1747-9541.10.5.967

Unverdorben, M., Kolb, M., Bauer, I., Bauer, U., Brune, M., Benes, K., Nowacki, P. E., & Vallbracht, C. (2000). Cardiovascular load of competitive golf in cardiac patients and healthy controls. *Medicine and Science in Sports and Exercise*, *32*(10): 1674–1678. https://doi.org/10.1097/00005768-200010000-00002

Viru, A., & Viru, M. (2000). Nature of training effects. In W. E. Garret & D. T. Kirkendall (Eds.), *Exercise and Sport Science* (pp. 67–95). Lippincott Williams & Wilkins. Philidelphia, USA

Wang, R., Hoffman, J. R., Tanigawa, S., Miramonti, A. A., La Monica, M. B., Beyer, K. S., Church, D. D., Fukuda, D. H., & Stout, J. R. (2016). Isometric mid-thigh pull correlates with strength, sprint, and agility performance in collegiate rugby union players. *Journal of Strength and Conditioning Research*, *30*(11): 3051–3056.

Wells, J.E.T., Charalambous, L. H., Mitchell, A. C. S., Coughlan, D., Brearley, S. L., Hawkes, R. A., Murray, A. D., Hillman, R. G., & Fletcher, I. M. (2019). Relationships between Challenge Tour golfers' clubhead velocity and force producing capabilities during a countermovement jump and isometric mid-thigh pull. *Journal of Sports Sciences*, *37*(12): 1381–1386. https://doi.org/10.1080/02640414.2018.1559972

Wells, J.E.T., Mitchell, A. C. S., Charalambous, L. H., & Fletcher, I. M. (2018). Relationships between highly skilled golfers' clubhead velocity and force producing capabilities during vertical jumps and an isometric mid-thigh pull. *Journal of Sports Sciences*, *36*(16): 1847–1851. https://doi.org/10.1080/02640414.2018.1423611

Wells, J.E.T., Mitchell, A. C. S., Charalambous, L. H., & Fletcher, I. M. (2022). Relationships between highly skilled golfers' clubhead velocity and kinetic variables during a countermovement jump. *Sports Biomechanics*. https://doi.org/10.1080/14763141.2022.2041709

Wells, Jack E T, & Langdown, B. L. (2020). Sports science for golf : A survey of high-skilled golfers' 'perceptions' and 'practices'. *Journal of Sports Sciences*, *38*(8): 918–927. https://doi.org/10.1080/02640414.2020.1737350

Winter, E. M., Abt, G., Brookes, F. B. C., Challis, J. H., Fowler, N. E., Knudson, D. V., Knuttgen, H. G., Kraemer, W. J., Lane, A. M., Van Mechelen, W., Morton, R. H., Newton, R. U., Williams, C., & Yeadon, M. R. (2016). Misuse of 'Power' and Other Mechanical Terms in Sport and Exercise Science Research. *Journal of Strength and Conditioning Research*, *30*(1): 292–300. https://doi.org/10.1519/JSC.000000000 0001101

3   Planning the Season

Alex Bliss and Ben Evans

Introduction

Golf is a sport that can be played year-round. At the recreational level, the only impediments outside of socioeconomic factors and injury on the ability to play all year are weather, course conditions, and physical fitness. At the elite level, where players are on tour and generally play golf in countries where weather conditions are good, this is less of a concern. Indeed, the continual nature of touring in elite golf can be observed by the tournament schedule. On the European Tour for example, tournaments are scheduled from November through to October, culminating in the Tour School. Subsequently, players will need to plan their season to ensure they have a viable schedule.

From a strength and conditioning (S&C) perspective, the planning process will involve an initial consultation with the player and coach to set training goals for the year. This is covered extensively in Chapter 2. Once this process has been completed, the S&C coach will traditionally employ a periodisation strategy and separate the competitive season into chunks or "cycles". These cycles can be categorised into three cycle types. A long-term cycle is referred to as a "macrocycle" and is usually a year or longer (for example a quadrennial cycle in the Olympics/Paralympic sports). A medium-term cycle will typically last a month or multiple months and is referred to as a "mesocycle". A short-term cycle might last from a single session to a few weeks and is referred to as a "microcycle". This compartmentalising of the year into cycles is referred to as periodisation and will be covered later in this chapter.

The rationale for compartmentalising the player's year in this way is that it allows for the pursuit of either the overall goals of the plan, or to focus on the attainment of more precise, shorter-term targets and prioritise particular areas of their physical development. This is important if there is a sequential emphasis on the development of the player's physical or technical skill or capacity. For example, a player might wish increase their clubhead speed to improve their proximity to the hole from tee shots. A strategy for this could be to initially train for increased muscle mass to promote greater muscle cross-sectional area and therefore improved force producing capacities in the athlete, and then subsequently focus on applying these forces quickly i.e. speed training.

DOI: 10.4324/9781003099321-3

An additional reason for segregating training into specific foci could be to manipulate some of the training variables (volume, intensity, density etc. described in detail below) to allow for the pursuit of particular adaptations and to limit interference with technical training. As an example, if a golfer wishes to train for increased muscle size (hypertrophy), they may be encouraged to do this in the off-season or outside of competition weeks as this type of training can (but does not have to, and arguably should not (Damas et al., 2018)) result in high fatigue levels that will influence how hard or how comfortably the player can perform their technical on-range or on-course training. Again, as mentioned in Chapter 1 and Chapter 2, if the player is made aware of some of the likely outcomes from particular training cycles then this should not cause any issues and a plan can be made to allow for increased recovery time or fluctuations in the volume and intensity of other training.

Determinants of Performance

Any training plan should have a sound rationale. It should have clear aims and objectives and these, where possible, should follow the SMART principle (Figure 3.1). A critically reasoned and well-rationalised training plan is desirable as it will ensure that adaptations from the training stimuli provided are understood and targeted, rather than random and intangible. Essentially, it should give insight into "cause and effect". But how do we know what aims and objectives we should set? How do we know that if we set a goal, it is going to have a beneficial impact on performance, and will the effort required to achieve it be worth it?

One method to adopt is a fundamental "first-principles" approach, which is to initially identify the key determinants of the sport are and crucially, in the case of S&C, what physical skills and capacities the athlete needs to provide the greatest potential for high performance. It is now well known that a crucial determinant of performance in golf is drive distance, across all levels of performance. At the elite level, Hellström and colleagues showed that on the PGA Tour, there was a relationship between drive distance (and remaining distance to the pin) and score. This relationship was evident across hole types, but particularly for par 5 holes (Hellström et al., 2014). For recreational golfers, there is a strong relationship between a player's clubhead speed, a crucial component of drive distance, and their handicap, with lower-handicap players possessing higher speeds (Fradkin et al., 2004). From a physical perspective, upper and lower body strength and power have the strongest correlations with clubhead speed, while anthropometrics and muscular endurance have weaker relationships (Ehlert, 2021). S&C interventions can support the development of clubhead speed (Ehlert, 2020) and through improving strength and power qualities in golfers. However, adding S&C interventions into the existing playing and practice schedules of golfers requires due consideration.

In skill-based sports like golf this cause-and-effect model is not always linear or as clear as it might be in other sports where physical precocity is a more

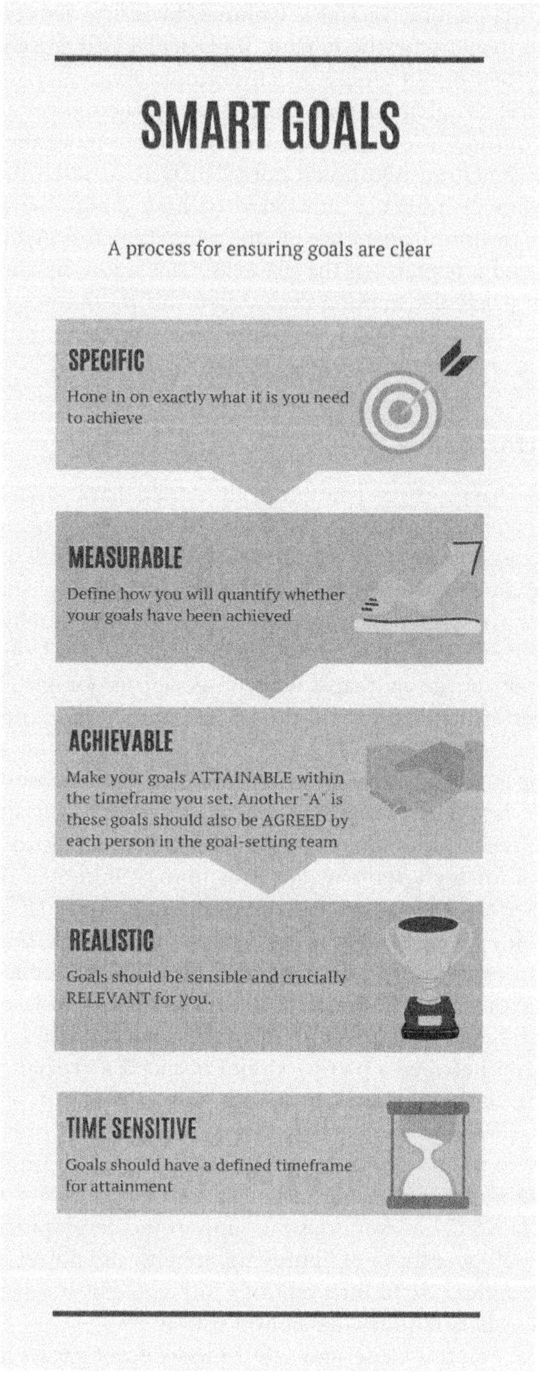

SMART GOALS

A process for ensuring goals are clear

SPECIFIC

Hone in on exactly what it is you need
to achieve

MEASURABLE

Define how you will quantify whether
your goals have been achieved

ACHIEVABLE

Make your goals ATTAINABLE within
the timeframe you set. Another "A" is
these goals should also be AGREED by
each person in the goal-setting team

REALISTIC

Goals should be sensible and crucially
RELEVANT for you.

TIME SENSITIVE

Goals should have a defined timeframe
for attainment

Figure 3.1 SMART goals guidance descriptors

dominant aspect of high performance. For example, in weightlifting, improving an athlete's maximal strength (force-producing capabilities) is clearly a desirable outcome as there is an obvious and well-demonstrated relationship between force-producing capabilities and success in the two lifts (Joffe et al., 2021). In golf, improving aspects of physical conditioning might not always immediately transfer into performance (see Chapter 10 for a thorough overview of this topic). For example, it has been shown that strength and conditioning strategies that improved drive distance acutely by increasing clubhead speed (the physical component), did not simultaneously improve ball-striking and the player's ability to apply their newly acquired speed to the ball (the skill component) (Bliss et al., 2021). Therefore, to ensure the season is well structured and training is organised to allow for the greatest chance of transfer to performance, a brief discussion of training theory is provided below. This will allow for readers to understand traditional S&C practices before they are discussed in relation to golf in the "practical applications" section of this chapter.

Training Theory and Periodisation

Before outlining some of the complexities and nuances involved in planning strength training specifically for the golf season, it is worth briefly detailing some of the theory behind periodisation and the organisation of training. Periodisation is a widely recognised concept that supports athletic training and is considered to be crucial when attempting to optimise and understand training and expected adaptations (Haff, 2021), although this viewpoint has been contested (Kiely, 2017). While periodisation can be confusing owing to the many and varied athletic training models proposed by numerous coaches and authors, fundamentally, all periodisation is concerned with is incorporating variation into training (Haff, 2021) and dividing the annual plan into smaller phases (Bompa & Buzzicheli, 2019). The type of periodisation approach chosen will depend on situational and contextual factors, but effective modern programming is a science and an art and requires a degree of flexibility and adaptability, particularly when unexpected situations (injuries, competition changes, personal issues etc.) arise (Verkhoshanksy & Siff, 2009). Typically, the various prominent periodisation models divide training into early/pre-season general preparation exercise, followed by mid-season specific preparation exercises, strength maintenance, and competition phases, and then off-season, transition or recovery phases, each with a pre-determined focus on developing targeted physical attributes. For golfers and coaches reading this chapter, a simple summation of periodisation approaches is that training will have different foci depending on a range of factors including, but not limited to: time of the season, proximity of competition, the training status of the athlete, and their physical development goals. There are entire textbooks dedicated to periodisation so this chapter gives a brief overview. For in-depth discussions of periodisation theory, readers are encouraged to explore some of the references provided herein.

Adaptation to Exercise

While there are a range of models utilised to explain the adaptive response to training (including the fitness-fatigue paradigm and the stimulus-fatigue-recover-adaptation theory), Selye's (1951) General Adaptation Syndrome (GAS) model is widely adopted to explain what happens when a living organism experiences stressors. The GAS provides a mechanistic model to understand stress, adaptation, and fatigue, and their interrelationships (Cunanan et al., 2018). Although the model was originally devised to explain the phase-response to the introduction of damaging substances in mice, it provides a basic model to understand responses to athletic training in humans (Jones & DiMenna, 2011). These are highlighted in Figure 3.2.

Selye's model describes that, after an initial training stimulus, there is an "alarm phase" where the body experiences fatigue and the subsequent performance level will decrease. The magnitude of the alarm phase will depend on myriad factors and it may last a few hours or days. Contributors to this phase will include whether the training is novel and the athlete is accustomed to it, and whether the stimulus applied is more intense (maybe through more eccentric loading or lifting heavier external loads for example). If the training stimulus is new to the athlete, and/or is at an intensity that is greater than they have previously experienced then the magnitude of the alarm phase will be greater (Haff, 2016).

Following the initial alarm phase, the body will begin to recover and adapt ("resistance phase") before returning to baseline, and if training is appropriately designed, there will be a "supercompensation" phase where a greater performance level (greater training intensity for example) is achieved. After the supercompensation phase, if no training stimulus is provided, the "reversibility" training principle (outlined later in the chapter) will determine that performance level will return to baseline.

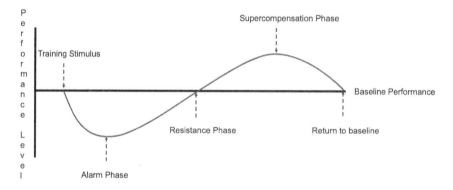

Figure 3.2 Selye's General Adaptation Syndrome
Source: Selye (1951).

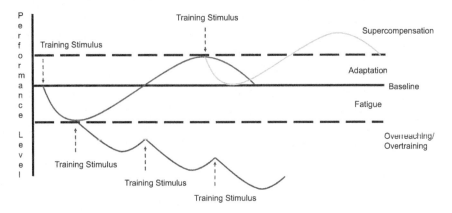

Figure 3.3 A theoretical model for well-timed (above baseline) and poorly timed (below baseline) provision of additional training stimuli in the development of supercompensation or overtraining

The GAS model helps to conceptualise what is possible with repeated exposures to training stimuli and how (with reference to physical development through S&C) new performance levels are achieved, or conversely, how athletes can become overtrained. Figure 3.3 shows a theoretical example of how repeated training stimuli, if well timed and provided once an athlete has fully recovered during the athlete's supercompensatory phase, can lead to sustained increases in the performance level above baseline. However, if training stimuli are repeatedly provided when the athlete is still in an alarm phase and has not recovered from the previous training exposure, this will initially lead to the athlete's being functionally overreached, before subsequently becoming overtrained and exhibiting reduced performance levels if training stimuli continue to be provided.

While there may be instances where repeated, frequent training stimuli might be provided (pre-season for example) to encourage specific adaptations (i.e. cardiovascular fitness or strength endurance), this process is complex and will require a skilled S&C coach to be able to manage the process to ensure the athlete does become overtrained. To do so, qualified S&C coaches as part of their training and experience will be aware of the "Principles of Training" and how to manipulate training variables to manage training and recovery processes. These training principles and variables are briefly outlined below.

Principles of Training

The fundamental reason why athletes strength train is to improve their physical qualities (strength, speed, robustness etc.) which will support and enhance their sporting performance. Deciding which physical qualities to train will depend on the determinants of performance in the sport and the needs analysis process (see Chapter 2 for more detail). In untrained individuals, the application of any physical training stimulus will likely create an improvement in physical performance. However, humans are adaptive organisms and over time, once they are exposed to training stimuli consistently and become more well trained, the same training stimulus will no longer provide sufficient challenge to elicit such a response. Therefore, it is crucial that, in order to make physical improvement, training is organised so that it provides the opportunity for variation in the training stimulus that challenges the athlete. To help organise the training process, S&C coaches will ensure that their training adheres to the principles that follow the SPORT acronym:

- **S**pecificity
- **P**rogression
- **O**verload
- **R**eversibility
- **T**edium Avoidance

Specificity is one of the more misunderstood aspects of training, but for the purposes of this section, a simple definition is that training needs to reflect, at least in part, the physical characteristics exhibited in the sport to allow for training to transfer (Fleck & Kraemer, 2014). Specificity does not mean that all S&C training for golf needs to involve gym movements that look like the golf swing, which is a common misconception. For a detailed insight into specificity and training transfer please see Chapter 10.

Progression and Overload are arguably the two most important training principles. As outlined above, if athletes become overly familiar with their training and it does not create sufficient challenge then their physical development will stall (and may even reverse – more on this shortly). Progression is self-explanatory. S&C coaches need to create opportunities for their athletes to progress in their training. This is achieved using the overload principle which can be combined with progression to refer to "Progressive Overload". Progressive overload is the process of continually increasing the training stress placed on the athlete as their physical qualities improve as a result of training (Fleck & Kraemer, 2014). Progressive overload will be achieved through the manipulation of training variables which are outlined later in this chapter.

Reversibility encapsulates the phenomena that, without sufficient and regular stimulus (not achieving progressive overload, for example) an athlete's physical condition will plateau and then begin to revert to their pre-training baseline. Training adaptations induced from S&C interventions are transient and can disappear when training stops or is performed without sufficient volume or intensity (French, 2016). The reversibility principle is therefore inexorably linked to the effects of "detraining" which is defined as the partial or complete loss of training-induced adaptations from insufficient training stimulus (Mujika & Padilla, 2000). Reversibility from detraining can be pronounced, can occur over relatively short duration, and can affect athletes of all fitness levels. Indeed, research has shown that after only eight weeks of inactivity, when exercising at peak oxygen uptake an Olympic champion rower lost 20% of their pre-training power output, and experienced an 8% decrease in the key marker of aerobic fitness (Godfrey et al., 2005). This reversibility principle, as will be demonstrated later on in the case study, is particularly important for elite golfers who have a high number of competitive tournaments scheduled, which may limit time for S&C training if not programmed appropriately around their golf.

Lastly, tedium is the state of being bored and can be attributed to monotony in a training programme (Farrow & Robertson, 2017). Programme monotony can be avoided by ensuring one or more training variables are altered to provide variety and new stimulus. This approach has been linked to greater adaptations in physical fitness than non-varied approaches (Fleck, 1999). Therefore, once an athlete feels that their programme is no longer challenging, they feel they have exhausted their development with a particular exercise or exercises, or have observed a performance plateau, the S&C coach should ensure that exercises within programmes are modified or changed, or that variation through manipulation of volume and/or intensity is achieved to avoid athletes becoming disinterested in their programmes through lack of challenge or improvement. However, it is important to recognise that meaningful physical change does not happen immediately and consistency of training is crucial to ensure adaptations have the best chance of becoming realised.

Training Variables

The three primary training variables are volume, intensity, and frequency. Frequency refers to how often training takes place (greater training frequency being more training sessions completed with subsequently shorter rest periods between sessions over a given time period. i.e. seven days). Volume refers to amount of the training completed, and intensity refers to the effort required in the session. Quantifying both of these variables can be complicated (particularly intensity) but at its essence volume refers to "how much" training has been undertaken, and intensity refers to "how hard" the training was (Cleather, 2018).

Volume of training in some sports can be quantified by the number of minutes or hours spent training, or the distance covered (e.g. endurance sports). For golf, overall "training volume" can be categorised into two main areas: 1) golf activities 2) S&C activities. Training volume of golf activities will relate to the number of golf balls hit, the duration of practice sessions, or the number of holes played. For S&C activities, volume will be quantified at the exercise and session levels, as well as micro, meso, and macrocycle levels. Volume will be identified by the number of repetitions performed in exercises within the session, multiplied by the load lifted per repetition.

Volume Load = Total repetitions x load per repetition

For example, a player performing three sets of five repetitions for a back squat, with a barbell loaded to 60 kg will have a volume load of 900 kg ((3 x

5) x 60 kg) for that exercise. This can then be conducted for all the exercises within a session and repeated for the number of sessions in a week to give session and weekly volume load, respectively, or for the number of sessions across a month for the monthly volume load and so on.

Intensity is more difficult to quantify. Again, if we separate intensity into golf activities and S&C activities, then the most "intense" or effortful golf activity is a maximal effort swing with a driver. If the player's maximum clubhead speed is known, then we could calculate how "intense" their golf practice is as a percentage of that. From an S&C perspective, intensity is typically characterised (although many variations exist, see Suchomel et al. (2021) for a review) by how much load is being lifted as a percentage of the athlete's single (one) repetition maximum (1RM) for that exercise. An athlete that has a 1RM for a deadlift of 100 kg, if lifting 90 kg for a single repetition is lifting at 90% of 1RM. However, as the number of repetitions increases, the maximum number of repetitions the athlete will be able to perform will go down. An athlete who has the same 1RM of 100 kg in the deadlift, might be able to perform five repetitions at 85 kg, which is 85% of their 1RM, but it is 100% of their 5RM.

Alternatively, there are more subjective approaches for estimating intensity. Athletes might be given the freedom to choose the weight they lift against a predetermined rating of perceived exertion (RPE) for the exercise or session within a given rep range. For example, the coach might programme five repetitions of an exercise, with a load that the athlete "feels" equates to an effort of 8 out of 10. A related concept for gauging intensity subjectively is the "repetitions in reserve" method that, rather than being based around RPE, is anchored by how many repetitions the athlete "felt" they would have left at a set load in a predetermined repetition range. For example, a coach might programme that the athlete chooses a load on the bar that, when performing three repetitions, they felt they would have two repetitions "in reserve": i.e. if they had to, they could perform five repetitions at that load. This method has been shown to be comparable and even more effective against traditionally RM-based programmes (Graham & Cleather, 2021). However, a caveat of the repetitions in reserve method and the RPE based method is that both require the athlete to have good experience of S&C and the exercises being performed. A novice lifter would likely not be able to accurately estimate their RPE or how many repetitions they might have left to perform.

Lastly, there is an inverse relationship between volume and intensity whereby when one is "high" or prominent within the phase of training, then the other must be reduced, as shown in Figure 3.4. The rationale for this approach is that it is not possible to train with both high volume and high intensity concurrently. If we consider running as an example, if an athlete performs a truly high-intensity effort, such as an all-out sprint, the corresponding volume (distance or time) of that exercise will be low (100 m or approximately 10 seconds in an elite sprinter). If the athlete increases their volume of exercise, they must decrease the intensity of the effort as they would not be able to maintain their 100 m intensity (maximal or mean running speed) for any longer. If the exercise volume increases to 400 m, the intensity, expressed via maximal or mean running speed would be

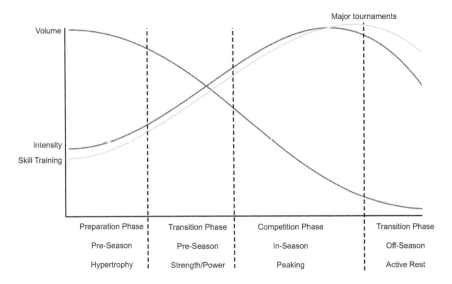

Figure 3.4 Linear periodisation of volume and intensity of training, and skill training, throughout a competitive season. This is adapted from Fleck & Kraemer's model (2014) but a key difference is that golfers will likely retain at least a moderate level of "skill training" year round, as opposed to the original model where skill training is very low in the preparation phase

Source: Adapted from Fleck & Kraemer (2014).

lower, and lower still over 5 km, and even lower over 42 km for the marathon for example. For golf, training intensity is highest when hitting full-effort driver swings. When intensity is high, volume will need to be low, and so the player might only be able to hit 20–50 or so driver swings before fatiguing and being unable to continue at the desired intensity. Conversely, when intensity is low, for example putting, a player might be able to hit hundreds of putts without experiencing physical fatigue (the mental/psychological "intensity" might be high, depending on the aim of the task, but this is a separate consideration). From an S&C perspective, when intensity is high (at or close to RM, high RPE etc.), training volume will need to decrease to accommodate, and vice versa.

When planning the year, a traditional periodisation model would dictate that volume of training is high in pre-season, reduces in mid-season, and is low during competition phases, with the reverse being true for intensity (Figure 3.4). However, as golf is played year-round, and there are competitions almost weekly, this presents a considerable challenge to the S&C coach and the player. Perhaps owing to the individual nature of the sport, or that the application of S&C in golf has not been commonplace until relatively recently, there is extremely limited empirical evidence to demonstrate how best to periodise the golf year, or even if it is necessary. In the practical applications section, we discuss an elite player's thoughts and approach to planning the year and the inclusion of S&C training within that plan.

Regardless of the approach taken, players and coaches reading this chapter should be aware that there is an inverse relationship between volume and intensity and that volume-dominant programmes will lead to different adaptations than those that are intensity-focused. The SAID principle (Specific Adaptations to Imposed Demands) describes that the physical adaptations that an athlete experiences will be as a result of the "imposed demands" or simply, the type of training they are exposed to. A high-volume programme will impose demands that are different to high-intensity training, and the athlete's body will adapt specifically to that demand. As an example, a recent meta-analysis demonstrated that high-load training (greater than 60% 1RM) promoted greater changes in maximal strength, as where both low load (less than 60% 1RM) and high-load training improved muscle size (Schoenfeld et al., 2017).

Practical Applications

Amateur vs professional

How the season is planned will invariably be dictated by the player's tournament schedule. "Reverse engineering" the year is one approach whereby the player's "intended" season plan is diarised first, and then S&C and other coaching sessions are inputted. For amateur players in the UK, there is a substantial off-season from around October to March when there is limited high-profile tournament golf. This allows for a consistent block of training to be undertaken, without concern for how the athlete will perform in immediate competition. For elite professional golfers, the tournament schedule can quickly become filled and there is a very limited off-season, meaning the approach to planning the year will need bespoke consideration. An example of an athlete's (Ben Evans, see below) intended annual plan is displayed in Figure 3.5. For the player, once the season started in February, the longest break the player had between competitions was four weeks, until October. This presents challenges around the prescription of training with regards volume and intensity. In competition weeks, total golf training volume will be high as the player will be practising and competing. Therefore, it is pertinent to limit the volume of S&C work at these times. Just practising and competing may not provide sufficient training stimulus to maintain adaptations that were driven by intensity. While volume is kept low, S&C training intensity can be elevated during competition weeks to ensure maintenance of physical qualities, and perhaps even drive new adaptation. Example sessions are provided in Table 3.1 with subjective exercise intensity descriptors in Table 3.2.

A Player's Perspective on Planning the Season

Background

This interview was conducted in December 2021. Ben Evans (BE) and Alex Bliss (AB) worked closely together from 2016 to 2018, and after a hiatus, began

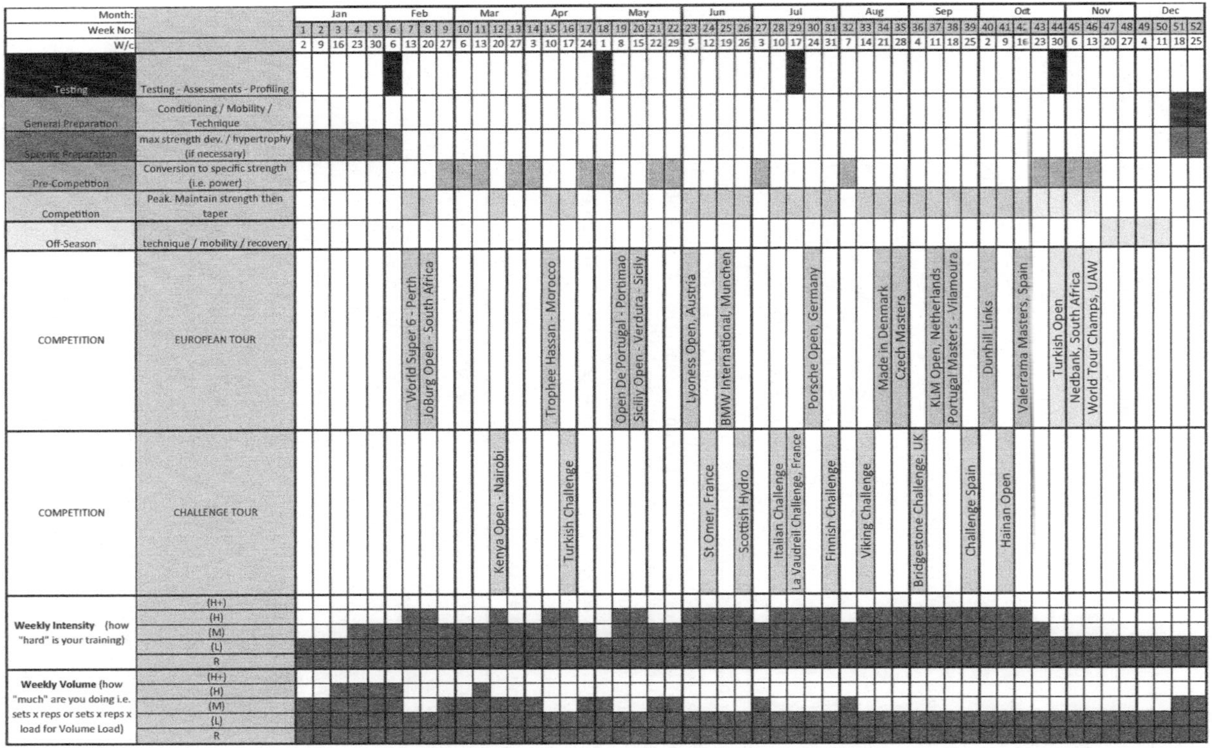

Figure 3.5 Example season plan for professional touring golfer

Note: November tournaments are subject to qualification based on performance. Volume of training is low during competition weeks, intensity high, and vice-versa. Testing weeks involve CHS measures, jumps, force profiling etc. Although the "intensity" for these is high, the overall intensity for the week is displayed as a testing session might only take 30 minutes or so.

Table 3.1 Example S&C Sessions with a volume (above) or intensity (below) focus

Example off-season, volume-focused training programme

Exercise	Sets	Reps	Rest	RPE	RIR	Estimated %1RM
Deadlift	4	6-8	60-90 s	5-6	6-4	~75%
Lateral lunge	4	3-4 es	60-90 s	5-6	6-4	~75%
Bench press	4	6-8	60-90 s	5-6	6-4	~75%
Bent over row	4	6-8	60-90 s	5-6	6-4	~75%
Landmine rotations	3	3-4 es	60-90 s	5-6	6-4	~75%
Farmer's Carry	3	20 m	60-90 s	5-6	N/A	

Example competition week, intensity-focused training programme

Back Squat	4	3	3-4 min	8-9	2-1	>85%
Jump Squat	4	3	3-4 min	Max intent	N/A	~30-60%
Landmine punch	4	2-3 es	3-4 min	Max intent	N/A	~30-60%
Rotational Med ball throw	4	2-3 es	3-4 min	Max intent	N/A	~30-60%
Seated band row	4	3	3-4 min	8-9	2-1	>85%

RPE = Rating of Perceived Exertion. RIR = Repetitions in Reserve. 1RM = One-repetition maximum. Es = each side. Note: For exercises such as medicine ball throws or jumps, the athlete should be aiming to throw or jump with maximum intent across a range of external loads. This will ensure the athlete is exposed to velocity and force focused power development exercises, therefore RIR is not usually used for these types of exercises.

RPE and RIR relationships adapted from Helms et al. (2016) and Zourdos et al. (2015).

Table 3.2 RPE and RIR relationships

RPE	RPE descriptors (Egan et al., 2006. Borg et al., 1998)	RIR related descriptors for resistance exercise
0	Rest	
1	Very, very easy	Little to no effort
2	Easy	Little to no effort
3	Moderate	Light effort
4	Somewhat Hard	Light effort
5	Hard	4-6 repetitions remaining
6		4-6 repetitions remaining
7	Very Hard	3 repetitions remaining
8		1-2 repetitions remaining
9		1 repetition remaining
*9.5		No repetitions, but could increase load
10	Maximal	Maximum effort

*= 9.5 was not in the original RPE descriptors, but introduced for resistance specific exercise (Zourdos et al., 2015).

Source: adapted from Helms et al., 2016 & Zourdos et al. 2015.

working together again in late 2020. BE turned professional in 2007 having won two Faldo Series events and has played over 300 tournaments across the Challenge Tour, Alps Tour, and European Tour.

AB: **You have been on tour for a long time at various levels from European Tour, through Challenge Tour and Alps Tour. How do you try and plan the season?**

BE: When you say plan I think about doing a lot of hotel reservations and flight bookings, I wouldn't necessarily straight away think about planning my gym stuff. I feel like that would be more short-term, I don't know whether that's just me.

AB: **So how do you plan what tournaments you're going to play in and the structure of the season?**

BE: When the schedule comes out. I don't have a manager, but my dad probably works as my manager and does a lot of the admin. I generally block enter every tournament. You don't want to turn up at a tournament where you're not entered. I would enter every event and then pull out of events that I don't want to play. On the Challenge Tour my category would be good so I could pick and choose what I want to play in. When the schedule comes out, I would look through it and say, "these are the big events I need to play in". On the Challenge Tour the money makes such a big difference, if you have a good week in a big money event it can be the difference between you getting a card and not getting a card in the top 20 on the Order of Merit. Generally, if you play well, you have a good chance of finishing top 20. But if you play well in the wrong week where the money's not very good then it's not as helpful as doing it where the purse is really big.

You can't really control how you play week to week and what events. I've been one of those players that generally played a lot of tournaments in a row. I feel I play better when I've played more in a row. But I think at one point in 2017, I played 11 tournaments in a row, and that wasn't just in Europe. Towards the end I played Dunhill Links in Scotland, did well and then flew to China to play two Challenge Tour events. It ended up only being one week because I got into the Spanish Open on the European Tour so I had to fly home. The Spanish Open was my 11th week in a row.

At the time, you just get on with it. You can't think, "Oh, I'm really tired!" Part of being a professional golfer is that sometimes you have to get up at four o'clock, you've got to get yourself ready for your tee time at seven o'clock. It's just part of it. And getting on a plane, flying somewhere is part of it as well. You have to just suck it up.

AB: **I remember that well. I think Valderrama was your last event and you got off to a really good start as well [Ben was fifth after two rounds before finishing T36].**

BE: yeah, I was doing well. I flew back from China...

AB: **...And then I think the jetlag and the fatigue kicked in! You mentioned you try and play well all year, but you try and focus on particular events?**

BE: On the Challenge Tour I'll go through the season and I'll pick out the top events because I don't know what the prize funds are going to be like. Over the years, events like Kazakhstan have always been one of the bigger events and then a few events in China towards the end of the season. Those are the "majors" really on that tour. They're the ones that you have to be in and your whole year can come down to these events where you have to try and peak. Trying to peak in golf though is tough. There was talk of Tiger trying to peak but I mean, you have to be in pretty good control of your golf ball to be able to be say, "I'm going to peak for this event" or "I'm going to peak for that event". I think just going out there trying to play well every single day and get momentum gets confidence going.

It's interesting on the Challenge Tour. Guys will finish second and then next week they'll win, or they'll win a tournament and then be right up there the following week. Or they might even win two in a row. It's amazing how often that happens on the Challenge Tour. I don't know why? Maybe you hit some good form and then suddenly you can you can be right up there most weeks? I don't know if that is anything to do with planning really? It's probably more to do with confidence and just hitting the ball well, holing putts and your game feeling good.

AB: **Is there anything you do to try to peak the right times? Do you do anything different in your training or your prep? Or do you play a certain number of tournaments beforehand?**

BE: Well, that's interesting. I wouldn't ever go to a big tournament as my first event. I would always like to have a tournament or a couple of tournaments building up to it. Generally, that's how I've played my best golf, in stretches or runs of tournaments, but it can be fairly late in a run as well. I seem to have played better towards the end of the season rather than the start. I don't know if that's getting more golf in? Or I get halfway through the season and I think something's not right and I try and put a few changes in place, and then they start coming into effect towards the end of the season. I don't really know.

But I think where you [S&C coach] would come in is planning my fitness. I really like to try and get into it over the winter and then when the season really starts kicking off, when you play one two three four two in a row I think... I don't know.... I like practising a lot. You don't want to get too tired because energy levels are a huge part of tournament golf and being ready to play. You don't want to burn out.

However, I'm spending quite a bit of time in the gym now [it's the winter and Ben's off-season], and you come out the gym feeling amazing! You feel amazing and that would be quite useful to take to a tournament. Instead of getting back to the hotel room and having a shower and then just checking your phone for two hours, actually the good thing to do is probably go to the gym for an hour and have a shower. You'd probably feel great. Hopefully, you get up in the morning and still feel great, depending on what you've done in the gym, you don't want to feel sore. I think so far, I've always thought I need to save my energy levels rather than trying to work out, but I don't think it really works like that. I think you probably sleep a lot better if you have trained too.

AB: **You mentioned using the winter to do a big block of strength work and that fits well with training theory. However, you don't tend to get much of a winter because you might have your last tournament in September or October and the season might start again in a couple of weeks' time. How do you try an account for having basically no off season?**

BE: Let me go back to what you just said. We started doing some work in November or December [2020], I had a programme and then we went into [COVID] lockdown, January to March. If you were an elite sportsman you could still train and practise if your golf club would let you go. A friend of mine who is also a professional golfer, had an outdoor gym in his mum's garden. I was going there every other day for nine or ten weeks. It wasn't doing stuff with proper gym equipment. We had heavy logs, and we were swinging axes and doing pull ups and press ups and it was really interesting and we built that in to my S&C programme. Towards the end of March, I went to Kenya for two weeks for two tournaments and I don't know whether it was the sun or the heat, but I hit the highest ball speeds I have ever hit. I had a ball speed of 183 [mph]!

Midseason, my strength and speed dropped off so much. When I was warmed up and I was really hitting it hard I could get to 174–5 [mph] and then my average was 169–170 [mph]. I hit one on the golf course with my Quad [a launch monitor that Ben has] at 180 [mph] on the course in Kenya. I was 183 [mph] on the range and 180 [mph] on the course. That's speed that I've never even seen before! It is amazing how quickly it dropped off with me not coming home in season and I stopped training. I wasn't really doing anything, not even your programme. It just completely went, I don't know where it [the speed] went!

AB: **There's a conversation in golf S&C currently around whether just playing tournament golf gives you enough of a training stimulus to keep your fitness up? Sounds like what you're saying is that potentially...**

BE: No! Nowhere near to the level I got to! If you said to me, when you get to Kenya you'll be 183 [mph], I would think 183 [mph] is not even possible for me. Obviously, it's hot, but club speeds of like 120 [mph] something, 123 [mph], 124 [mph]? If I went outside now and swung one I'd probably be like 112–114 [mph]. But also, I think you have to do the right thing. You have to do that kind of fast, fast stuff as well as the just lifting.

AB: **So what are the main barriers to doing your strength work during the season? I would say, in the years I have known you, you have**

had a fluctuating relationship with S&C. Sometimes you get really into it and you get strong and then other times it backs off. What are your main challenges around consistency?

BE: My main challenge is I like practising more than going in the gym, especially when the season starts. I see things in my game I want to work on. I put more time into working on that than I probably do in the gym. The gym always takes a bit of a back foot really. Even now. The time I have to go practise, I probably will be would be better off splitting that to half practise and half gym. At the moment I'm probably doing it 80/20. I think that's the main reason. I think that I can get more improvements on my game on the range or just practising really than going in the gym.

But I also think that's probably quite short-sighted. Over the last 15 years or so I have been a pro, it's not often that you find "it" on the range. It's not often that you're at a tournament and on a Wednesday afternoon, "Oh I've found it! I've got it!" That's probably happened to me twice throughout my whole career. If I use that time better and I spend that time on my body I would be in a much better position and allow me to play better.

I'm trying to say, I feel like all the hours I've spent hitting balls, has that actually helped? I mean, I guess it could, but it's hard to really tell. If I spent a lot more of those hours on my body and myself, and I was 20% stronger than I am now, that would help dramatically on the golf course. I guess I like hitting balls, and I like looking at my swing, and I like being able to improve on a shot that was bad today, or improve if my putting isn't right. I guess it's just easier than going in the gym. This is why I need to do it and this is what I should be doing. I think it's hard.

AB: **When we first started together, you were fairly inexperienced in the gym, but now you've quite experienced. You're probably able to look after yourself a bit more. From a motivation perspective, maybe it's good having an S&C person there to help you plan and I think maybe tell you what you need to do each week?**

BE: I've got to get a squat rack in the gym at home. I'm all set up but I still go in there and I still really need to have my plan. It's a dream to have it in the garage, especially having a little son who is 15 months old. It saves all the travel time to a gym. I still get in the garage gym and I'm like, what do I do? Is this going to help? And I don't know. Maybe it's because I haven't actually seen you for a long time [BE relocated mid-season and face-to-face coaching with AB stopped].

AB: **Do you think that's one of the barriers to you then keeping it going during the season?**

BE: Obviously in the ideal world, let's say I was top 30 on the Order of Merit and I've got a couple of wins on my belt. I could say, "Alex you're going to come to tournaments one week every three". If financially I could do that and I could bring you I feel like it would be a lot easier to train every single week. But I think that shouldn't that shouldn't really be the limiting factor. I should really be able to understand and control it a bit more and do more from my end. Having seen the gains that I can get from this time last year, I think I need to really organise what I'm doing in the gym now.

AB: **Do you try and focus on different things physically at different points in the year?**

BE: Speed and strength in the winter are two huge ones. Generally, when I'm playing, it's probably more mobility. I go through a morning warm-up before I even hit balls, which I guess you'd probably class as mobility but that would mostly be it.

In 2017, when we started working a lot together [AB went to multiple tournaments with BE and had regular face-to-face coaching outside of tournament weeks], I was doing more in the gym at tournaments than in the last few years. When we stopped for a few years, I haven't when the season's got going. I just tailed off. And actually, I can see that in my strength and my speed and probably even some flexibility as well has just gone. I get to the end of the year and I say "this needs to change. My body doesn't feel right and I feel slow or I don't feel very strong". That's why I get fired up over the winter. I think I need to be like that all year round, and that's really where you're going to see loads of benefit.

AB: **I programme a lot for amateurs and I programme for high-level guys like yourself too. That approach is fine for high-level amateurs. If you're playing Challenge Tour you do get a gap but when you're playing European Tour…**

BE: You've got about three weeks. From the middle of December to mid-January, that's it really.

AB: **Trying to find times during the season to get a good block of training in is difficult. Where do you see strength conditioning going in the next few years for golf and particularly on building it into your playing year?**

BE: It's something I really need to focus probably 40% of my time on. I hadn't thought about it when I was younger. But I'm 35, I feel like golf is also about longevity, it's a career that even at 50 you can earn a living on. When I turned pro at 19–20 you don't even think about it. Whereas now, there's still a lot of good golf to play and your body might help you do that. I don't know whether seeing what Bryson has done has woken everyone up a bit. We knew it was important. Lots of golfers do really well and don't ever go in the gym. It's not the be all and end all, but if you want to improve yourself as a golfer, there are gains to be had in the gym.

At the moment, I need to change something in the way I'm working. Not just my golf but my body. If I can keep fit with my mobility and my strength that should really help me during the season, keeping my speed up and hit the ball further, it'll help scoring. I just have to focus on getting the ball in the hole during the season and that means that I have let my S&C slip, but I am going to focus on improving my consistency this year.

Conclusions

Planning the season for golfers is a complex process. The integration of S&C into the playing schedule can be equally complicated, as highlighted in the player's perspective in this chapter. Currently, there is little empirical evidence available on this topic to support players and coaches so S&C coaches will utilise and adapt traditional training theory and periodisation strategy, or infer from other sports when planning. However, particularly at the elite level, golf comprises unique challenges making this difficult. As the golf season is long, and competition is frequent, trying to maintain strength and other physical qualities will necessitate that S&C training takes place during the season. Manipulating training volume, intensity, and frequency will allow for S&C training to take place during competition and still enable golfers to focus on performance on the course. Players and coaches reading this chapter might try to identify periods in the calendar where they can undergo more dense blocks of training, but doing this in the season is not always possible.

Some of the challenges posed by planning the year are articulated in the player interview. While readers will each take different things from the transcript, a few things that stood out are that the thought processes of players may be different to strength coaches. BE mentioned that when thinking about planning the year, S&C isn't one of the first things that comes to mind. S&C coaches must appreciate that we are there to support the player and, particularly in a skill-based sport like golf, S&C will play a small (but arguably important) part of the overall golf plan. BE also articulated an issue that is common in my experience, concerns around the fitness/fatigue trade-off with players being cognisant of "burning out" but also "feeling amazing" when they have performed physical training. BE also discussed how quickly physicality can decrease if not training regularly in-season. The skilled S&C coach can have demonstrable impact here, and plan effectively around competition to ensure that physical fitness is maintained (and even improved) during the season. It is often difficult for the player to do this on their own when away at competition, particularly if inexperienced in the gym, or lacking intrinsic motivation (BE talks about preferring to hit golf balls, for example). To achieve a positive outcome here, a two-way education process is likely required, with the player detailing all of their planning and competition considerations, and the S&C coach outlining what optimal physical training looks like, before a compromise is reached that works for all parties.

Players and coaches who wish to incorporate S&C into their annual plan are encouraged to seek the support of a specialist S&C coach as, through their academic and/or vocational training, will have acquired knowledge of periodisation and planning strategies, and will ensure that training also follows the SPORT principle and will encourage adaptations that benefit golf performance. Lastly, before deciding on how to plan and periodise the year, players are encouraged to work with their S&C coach and golf coach to establish what the key performance determinants are for the individual player that, if targeted and improved, will increase the likelihood of success.

References

Bliss, A., Livingstone, H., & Tallent, J. (2021). Field-based and overspeed potentiated warm-ups increase clubhead speed and drive carry distance in skilled collegiate golfers. *Journal of Sport and Exercise Science.* 5(2): 107–113.

Bompa, T., & Buzzicheli, C. (2019). *Periodization: Theory and Methodology of Training 6th ed.* Champaign, IL: Human Kinetics.

Borg, G. (1998). *Borg's perceived exertion and pain scales.* Champaign IL: Human Kinetics.

Cleather, D. (2018). *The little black book of training wisdom: How to train and improve at any sport.* CreateSpace Independent Publishing Platform.

Cunanan, A., DeWeese, B., Wagle, J., Carroll, K., Sausaman, R., Hornsby, G., Haff, G., Triplett, T., Pierce, K., & Stone, M. (2018). The general adaptation syndrome: a foundation for the concept of periodization. *Sports Medicine.* https://doi.org/10.1007/s40279-017-0855-3

Damas, F., Libardi, C, A., & Urgrinowitsch, C. (2018). The development of skeletal muscle hypertrophy through resistance training: the role of muscle damage and muscle protein synthesis. *European Journal of Applied Physiology.* 118: 485–500.

Ehlert, A. (2020). The effects of strength and conditioning interventions on golf performance: a systematic review. *Journal of Sports Sciences.* https://doi.org/10.1080/02640414.2020.1796470

Ehlert, A. (2021). The correlations between physical attributes and golf clubhead speed: a systematic review with quantitative analyses. *European Journal of Sport Science.* 21(10): 1351–1363.

Farrow, D., & Robertson, S. (2017). Development of a Skill Acquisition Periodisation Framework for High-Performance Sport. *Sports Medicine.* 47(6): 1043–1054. https://doi.org/10.1007/s40279-016-0646-2

Fleck, S. (1999). Periodizes strength training: a critical review. *Journal of Strength and Conditioning Research.* 13(1): 82–89.

Fleck, S., & Kramer, W. (2014). *Designing Resistance Training Programs 4th Ed.* Champaign, IL: Human Kinetics.

Fradkin, A, J., Sherman, C, A., & Finch, C, F. (2004). Improving golf performance with a warm up conditioning programme

French, D. (2016). Chapter 5: Adaptations to anaerobic training programs. In Haff, G., & Triplett, T. *Essentials of Strength Training and Conditioning* (pp. 87–114). Champaign, IL: Human Kinetics.

Godfrey, R. J., Ingham, S. A., Pedlar, C. R., & Whyte, G. P. (2005). The detraining and retraining of an elite rower: a case study. *Journal of Science and Medicine in Sport.* 8(3): 314–320. https://doi.org/10.1016/s1440-2440(05)80042-8

Graham, T., & Cleather, D. J. (2021). Autoregulation by "Repetitions in Reserve" Leads to Greater Improvements in Strength Over a 12-Week Training Program Than Fixed Loading. *Journal of strength and conditioning research.* 35(9): 2451–2456. https://doi.org/10.1519/JSC.0000000000003164

Haff, G. (2016). Chapter 21: Periodization. In Haff, G., & Triplett, T. *Essentials of Strength Training and Conditioning* (pp. 583–604). Champaign, IL: Human Kinetics.

Haff, G. (2021). Chapter 20: The essentials of periodisation. In Jeffreys, I., & Moody, J. *Strength and Conditioning for Sports Performance 2nd Edition* (pp. 394–427). London: Routledge.

Hellström, J., Nilsson, J., & Isberg, L. (2014). Drive for dough. PGA Tour golfers' tee shot functional accuracy, distance and hole score. *Journal of Sports Sciences.* 32(5): 462–9.

Helms, E., Cronin, J., Storey, A., & Zourdos, M. (2016). Application of the repetitions in reserve-based rating of perceived exertion scale for resistance training. *Strength and Conditioning Journal.* 38(4): 42–49.

Joffe, S., Price, P., & Tallent, J. (2021). Maximal isometric force in the start of the first pull exhibits greater correlations with weightlifting performance than in the mid-thigh position in national and international weightlifters. *The Journal of Sport and Exercise Science.* 5(3): 202–211.

Jones, A., & DiMenna, F. (2011). Chapter 3.4: Cardiovascular assessment and aerobic training prescription. In Cardianle, M., Newton, R., & Nosaka, K. *Strength and Conditioning: Biological Principles and Practical Applications* (pp. 291–304). Oxford: Wiley-Blackwell Publishing.

Kiely, J. (2017). Periodization theory: confronting an inconvenient truth. *Sports Medicine.* https://doi.org/10.1007/s40279-017-0823-y

Mujika, I., & Padilla, S. (2000). Detraining: Loss of Training-Induced Physiological and Performance Adaptations. Part I: Short Term Insufficient Training Stimulus. *Sports Medicine.* 30: 79–87. http://dx.doi.org/10.2165/00007256-200030020-00002

Schoenfeld, B., Grgic, J., Ogborn, D., Krieger, J, W. (2017). Strength and hypertrophy adaptations between low- vs. high- load resistance training: a systematic review and meta-analysis. *Journal of Strength and Conditioning Research.* 31(12): 3508–3523.

Selye, H. (1951). The general-adaptation-syndrome. *Annual Review of Medicine,* 2: 327–342. https://doi.org/10.1146/annurev.me.02.020151.001551

Suchomel, T. J., Nimphius, S., Bellon, C. R., Hornsby, W. G., & Stone, M. H. (2021). Training for Muscular Strength: Methods for Monitoring and Adjusting Training Intensity. *Sports Medicine,* *51*(10): 2051–2066. https://doi.org/10.1007/s40 279-021-01488-9

Verkhoshanksky, Y., & Siff, M. (2009). *Supertraining:* 6th Edition – Expanded version. Rome: Verkhoshansky SSTM.

Zourdos, M., Klemp, A., Dolan, C., Quiles, J., Schau, K., Jo, E., Helms, E., Esgro, B., Duncan, S., Garcia Merino, S., & Blanco, R. (2016). Novel resistance training-specific rating of perceived exertion scale measuring repetitions in reserve. *Journal of Strength and Conditioning Research.* 30(1): 267–275.

4 Warming-up for Golf

Jack Wells and Ben Langdown

Introduction

The Impact of Warm-ups on Golf Performance

Within many sports, a well-designed warm-up is seen as a fundamental part of an athlete's routine to prime themself both physically and mentally for performance (Jeffreys, 2007). Benefits include a decrease in muscle and joint stiffness, alterations in the force–velocity relationship, increased transition rates of nerve impulses and improved energy production (Bishop, 2003). From a mechanical standpoint, these physiological responses can increase the rate of force development, strength, power and jump height (Jeffreys, 2007; Perrier et al., 2011). A successful warm-up within golf could be determined from the effects it has on the desired ball flight (i.e. increased distance, and control over direction and curvature). However, this is directly determined by optimising the impact conditions between the clubhead and the ball. While clubhead speed (CHS) accounts for 75% of the variance in determining ball speed (Sweeney et al., 2013), there are several other impact factors, namely centredness of strike, clubface alignment, dynamic loft, club path and angle of attack, that act together to determine the outcome of the shot (Betzler et al., 2014). Golf specific research has evidenced that engaging in a warm-up can lead to a significant improvement in centredness of strike (Moran et al., 2009), straighter swing-paths (in-square-in) (Moran et al., 2009), increased CHS (Bliss et al., 2021; Fradkin et al., 2004; Hébert-Losier & Wardell, 2021; Moran et al., 2009), ball speed (Langdown et al., 2019; Moran et al., 2009) and drive distance (Sorbie et al., 2016; Tilley & Macfarlane, 2012). When considering these findings collectively, a golfer can improve their impact conditions, ball flight, and thus scoring potential simply through engaging in a warm-up.

It is not uncommon for golfers to want to '*increase distance and accuracy*' following physical and technical interventions. Given the aforementioned benefits of warming-up, this presents an opportunity to coaches to enhance both ball flight and impact through the application of a well designed warm-up. Improving distance and accuracy off the tee provides a meaningful impact on performance by allowing a more controlled approach shot to the green, (i.e. when

DOI: 10.4324/9781003099321-4

using a shorter, more lofted club). Research assessing PGA Tour professionals has indicated that golfers who hit the ball further tend to also be straighter hitters (Broadie, 2014). Aside from dispersion, there are also several other noteworthy advantages to increasing driving distance such as navigating the course more effectively. Increasing distance may mean that a golfer can benefit from additional tactical variations. For example, reducing the distance of holes where a dogleg is present by selecting a target line over the corner, or carrying a hazard as opposed to 'laying-up' short. Further still, this could have positive psychological outcomes with regards to increased confidence and advantages in both stroke- and match-play situations when outdriving an opponent.

Despite these benefits, research has highlighted only 29.4% of golfers perform a warm-up (Fradkin et al., 2003). Indeed, 81% of 703 golfers have been observed to spend less than 10 minutes warming-up (Gosheger et al., 2003). Other research indicated that 54.3% of 1040 golfers reported performing a warm-up (Fradkin et al., 2001). Upon further analysis, these warm-ups consisted predominately of air swings on the tee (60.5%) or before the tee (24.0%). This is of great concern given that a warm-up has no associated cost, whereas a golfer will likely invest in the latest driver amidst advertising claims that it will improve drive distance.

Despite suggestions that warming-up is an important factor in reducing the risk of injury, there is currently insufficient evidence to substantiate these claims (Fradkin et al., 2006). In contrast to lesser skilled golfers, better players appear to recognise the importance of warming up, with 86.51% of highly skilled golfers either agreeing or strongly agreeing that engaging in a warm-up protocol will improve their performance (Wells & Langdown, 2020). However, the authors' anecdotal experiences would suggest that most golfers either avoid warming-up or adopt a strategy that may not provide the required stimuli to enhance performance. As such, the purpose of this chapter is to 1) highlight the body of evidence advocating the benefits of warming-up, 2) compare highly skilled and low skilled golfers' perceptions and practices on warming-up and 3) propose effective practical recommendations that can be implemented prior to both play and practice.

Highly Skilled and Elite Golfers

Research has evidenced that PGA Tour players who can increase drive distance by 20 yards are able to save 0.75 strokes per round (Broadie, 2014). In a tournament setting, this could make the difference between making or missing the cut (1.5 shots over two days) or winning or losing an event (3 shots over four days). From applied experience, in recent years there appears to be a far greater demand from golfers to hit the ball further. However, previous research indicates that highly skilled and elite golfers may have not always fully utilised a warm-up to benefit their performance. Bridge et al. (2008) conducted a two-day observational study assessing the warm-ups of Ladies European Tour (LET) players prior to tournament rounds. Observations indicated that, on average, the

LET players spent just 73 and 84 seconds conducting static stretches on day one and two respectively. Additionally, the LET players spent just 27 and 29 seconds performing dynamic stretches on day one and two respectively. These dynamic stretches were only comprised of shoulder rotations and air swings. The study concluded that these golfers spent very little time engaging in a warm-up on the practice range, with their modalities typically focussed on static stretching. However, as the observations were solely conducted on the range, the findings omit any warm-up protocols being undertaken elsewhere (e.g. the locker room). This may, therefore, misrepresent what constituted a warm-up for LET golfers at the time of the research. Organisations such as the European Tour often provide designated areas for players to warm-up (such as the European Tour Performance Institute Unit or gym facilities), which means that the golfers can prepare for an event away from the range area and the public eye.

From the authors' collective experiences of working within the industry, an ever-increasing number of highly skilled and elite players recognise the value in warming-up and are engaging in these as part of their pre-performance preparation. This was reported in a recent survey by Wells & Langdown (2020), which assessed 430 (males $n = 386$, females $n = 44$) highly skilled golfers' (handicap $= 0.42 \pm 2.81$ strokes) perceptions and practices of warming-up prior to a range session, practice round and tournament round. Of these 430 golfers, only eight failed to conduct a warm-up prior to play or practice. The main anatomical foci for the golfers' warm-up were the shoulders (83.0%), quadriceps (74.3%) and hamstrings (71.7%). Less emphasis was placed on the ankles (28.1%) and lower legs (45.8%), which would be a cause for concern given that the downswing is initiated from the ground-up (Nesbit & Serrano, 2005). When comparing the warm-up durations (combined physical and golf protocols) for these highly skilled golfers, Wells & Langdown (2020) reported that there were significant differences between a tournament round warm-up (37 minutes, 50 seconds) compared to a practice round warm-up (26 minutes, 16 seconds). The findings highlighted that highly skilled golfers may not be performing a thorough warm-up in practice conditions where there is 'little consequence' and may place greater emphasis on warming-up for a round of golf that 'matters' (i.e. tournament rounds). The repetition of a warm-up allows the acute adaptations to be validated during practice conditions. Should a golfer decide to engage in this for the first time prior to an important event, they may suffer from significant detrimental impact on performance and therefore scoring. Consequences may include, fatigue going into the round following an inappropriate warm-up intensity or reduced force generating capacity where inadequate preparation or inappropriate static stretching has been employed.

Less Skilled Golfers

Broadie (2014) highlighted that as the skill level of the golfer reduces, the value of hitting the ball 20-yards further exponentially increases (Table 4.1).

Table 4.1 The skill level of the golfer and the strokes each category of player would save if they were to increase their drive distance by 20 yards

Strokes per round (i.e. indicator of skill level)	Strokes saved
PGA Tour average	0.75
80	1.30
90	1.60
100	2.30
115	2.70

Source: Broadie (2014).

Broadie's (2014) work highlights that perhaps there are additional benefits to encouraging lower skilled golfers to warm-up. This presents a valuable opportunity to the S&C practitioner, given that the majority of golfers in the industry would be of a lower skill level (e.g. average handicap for club golfers in England: males = 16.4 strokes, females = 26.9 strokes; England Golf, 2021). Gosheger et al. (2003) reported that golfers who warmed-up for >10 minutes had a lower average handicap (14.3 strokes) than golfers who spent <10 minutes warming-up (22.0 strokes). However, it is important to recognise that these differences in warm-up duration could be due to a number of different factors (e.g. the golfer's individual perceptions and understanding of the benefits of a warm-up, level of knowledge and confidence to perform the exercises, and the environment in which they are warming-up etc.) Fradkin et al. (2003) indicated that of 1040 golfers surveyed, a large proportion either 'never' (48.3%) or 'seldom' (22.3%) warmed-up. This was based on the golfers' perceptions that they 'don't need to' (38.7%), 'don't have enough time' (36.4%), and 'can't be bothered' (33.7%). Fradkin et al. (2001) reported that the number of muscles stretched by the 1040 golfers was as little as three. The primary areas were the shoulders (73.2%), the torso (21.3%) and lower back (5.2%). Given the findings, it appears prudent that practitioners publicise and share the shots saved statistics (Table 4.1) to encourage their golfers to warm-up and to ensure that the protocols employed target the whole body in an appropriate manner.

Static and Dynamic Stretching for Golf

The choice of warm-up modality used is of great importance. Prior to a practice round and tournament round, Wells & Langdown (2020) reported that highly skilled golfers commonly utilised both dynamic (54.65% (practice round) to 61.63% (tournament round)) and static stretches (46.98% (practice round) to 54.42% (tournament round)). With a growing amount of supporting evidence being published in academic research, there are now substantiated performance benefits to encourage golfers to conduct a warm-up that includes dynamic stretching. Therefore, it is important that practitioners and golfers understand the impact that both dynamic and static stretching can have on perform-ance. Research from other domains has highlighted the negative effects static stretching can have on vertical jump performance. For instance, static stretching of the hamstrings, quadriceps and soleus over various intensities (100% [the point of discomfort], 75% and 50%) were all shown to reduce jump height by 2.4 to 8.0% (Behm & Kibele, 2007). Additionally, Haddad et al. (2014) reported a significantly reduced length in 'five jump distance' when comparing the static stretch to the dynamic stretch condition 24 hours post stretch. Given the ground reaction forces required for jumping, the negative impact of static stretching is of concern, especially as all three principal components (anterior to posterior, medial to lateral and vertical force vectors) are significantly related to clubhead speed (Han et al., 2019). Additionally, research has highlighted that countermovement jump positive impulse can predict 39.7% of the variance in CHS (Wells et al., 2019). It is therefore plausible to suggest that static stretching may negatively impact a golfer's performance if conducted within the 24-hour period prior to play and practice.

Golf specific research has compared the differences in performance between a control condition using a golf club warm-up (i.e. hitting shots) and the com-bination of this warm-up with static stretches (Gergley, 2009). When compared to the control condition, the combined static and golf club warm-up resulted in a significant reduction in CHS (-4.19%), distance (-5.62%), accuracy (-31.04%) and perceived ball contact (-16.34%). Given that both warm-up groups utilised the same golf club warm-up, this evidence highlights the negative effects static stretching can have on drive performance. Furthermore, Moran et al. (2009) reported that when compared to both static stretching and no stretching, dynamic stretching resulted in a significant increase in CHS (no stretch = 88.58 mph, static = 88.14 mph, dynamic = 92.39 mph), ball speed (no stretch = 124.37 mph, static = 123.93 mph, dynamic = 131.76 mph), and a straighter swing path (no stretch = 4°, static = 3.9°, dynamic = 3.3°). Straightening a swing path (assuming clubface alignment is square to the target line) will help to reduce the curvature of the ball flight. When the clubface alignment and swing path are square to the target line at impact, this reduces the tilt of the spin axis on the ball, thus reducing the curvature during the flight. Moran et al. (2009) also reported that dynamic stretching resulted in significantly more centred strikes than static stretching (no stretch = -0.5 cm, static = -0.7 cm, dynamic = 0.0 cm), however there were no statistical differences when comparing dynamic stretching with no stretching.

Gergley (2010) compared the acute (0 mins post warm-up) and latent (i.e. 15, 30, 45, and 60 mins post warm-up) effects of an active dynamic warm-up and static stretching warm-up. Following the static stretch protocol, prolonged and significant impairments to drive performance were observed (Table 4.2).

Table 4.2 highlights that static stretching can negatively impact perform-ance for at least 60 minutes, which, in the context of a tournament round, could mean that drive performance and scoring is impacted for up to 6 holes. The collective evidence presented within this section demonstrates that static

Table 4.2 The effects of static stretching on drive performance over prolonged periods of time

Time post stretching (mins)	Speed (%)	Distance (%)	Accuracy (%)	Perceived ball contact (%)
0	–4.92★	–7.26★	61.99★	–31.29★
15	–2.59★	–5.19★	58.78★	–31.29★
30	–2.19★	–5.47★	59.46★	–23.56★
45	–0.95	–3.30★	61.32★	–27.49★
60	–0.99	–3.53★	36.82	–15.70★

Note: ★ indicates statistical significance at $p \leq 0.05$. The greater the value for accuracy, the further the ball is from the target line.

Source: Gergley (2010).

stretching can have detrimental effects on both distance and accuracy. Recent research has, however, suggested that if static stretches are followed by a comprehensive high intensity dynamic warm-up, there are no detrimental effects on performance (Blazevich et al., 2018). It is worth noting that there is currently no evidence supporting this for golf.

Further research has compared static and dynamic stretching protocols to increase the understanding of the warm-up methods golfers should employ. Sorbie et al. (2016) compared the impact of both dynamic and static stretching on carry distance, accuracy, and perceived ball contact. The dynamic stretching group achieved a statistically significant increase of 4.05 yards in carry distance compared to the static stretch group. Additionally, driving accuracy was significantly better in the dynamic stretch group compared to the static stretch group: dispersion of 6.14 yards and 6.98 yards respectively. There were no statistically significant differences in perceived ball contact between the groups: however, the dynamic stretching group tended to have an improved ball contact (78% vs. 70%). Despite a lack of statistical significance, these marginal differences in perceived ball contact may have contributed to the improved accuracy and distance in the dynamic stretch group. The impact between the club and the ball is fundamental to determine the ball flight characteristics. For instance, a one degree change in club path or a 1 cm change in horizontal impact location on the clubface will alter the initial start direction by 0.269° and 0.494° respectively (Betzler et al., 2014). This has subsequent consequences on drive distance and distance away from the intended target. Furthermore, when combined with club face alignment, swing path and horizontal impact location account for 87.9% of the variance in initial start direction (Betzler et al., 2014). Additionally, the further away from a centred strike, the greater the reduction in ball speed. Specifically, for every cm^2 that impact occurs away from the centre of the clubface, there is a reduction of 1.32 mph (0.59 $m \cdot s^{-1}$) in ball speed (Betzler et al., 2014). Therefore, a shot hit 1 cm from the centre of gravity reduces ball speed by 1.32 mph, whereas a shot hit 2 cm away from the centre of gravity reduces ball speed by 4 times this amount, i.e. 5.28 mph (2.36 m·s⁻¹).Warming up appropriately provides the golfer with an ideal opportunity to optimise impact conditions and potentially reduce the likelihood of off-centred strikes.

Practical Recommendations

Before every practice session, workout or competition it is important to prepare the body for the specific activity ahead and to optimise subsequent performance by warming-up. Jeffreys (2007) comments that a needs analysis must consider the physiological, biomechanical and technical requirements of the activity in order for a coach to provide a specific and effective warm-up protocol that will prepare the body for the physical activity ahead (see Chapter 2). The warm-up should gradually raise the temperature of the body, activate and increase blood flow to the working muscles, mobilise the joints and get the body primed and ready (i.e. potentiate) for the sport specific actions of the golf swing. This process can be termed RAMP: Raise, Activate, Mobilise and Potentiate. The RAMP warm-up protocol has been accepted as a valid method of achieving the acute adaptations that are possible to improve performance. RAMP is a method that follows:

Raise – preparing the systems of the body for performance, resulting in raised heart rate, respiration rate, blood flow and joint fluid viscosity (influencing range of movement available at the joints) via low-intensity activities.

Barriers to engagement: This phase, may present a barrier to engagement in golf club contexts. With many golfers lacking access to a gym environment in which to perform a warm-up, it may feel out of place to complete a jog or other aerobic activity (e.g. rope skipping) around the practice facilities at their golf club. For many golfers a brisk walk (e.g. from the car park to the driving range) would act as a suitable activity here. Alternatively, combining the 'raise' element into the 'activate and mobilise' phase of the warm-up protocol may equally work to increase engagement in warming-up for subsequent golf performance. We also believe that the (sometimes strict) regulations around wearing smart golfing attire can contribute to the disengagement as some club golfers may not associate a warm-up with this culture or dress. In contrast when athletes go to play a team sport such as hockey, netball, football, etc. they will be in sports kit and a warm-up will be commonplace and completed as a team prior to any training or match situation. This practice is embedded into the culture of team sports. Spectators also see players physically warming-up in these sports. If a warm-up for golf is done away from public view (e.g. in the locker room) then it will not be seen and therefore not be associated with the game of golf. As previously noted, the lack of warm-up engagement from the golfers surveyed in Fradkin et al. (2003) supports our conclusions here.

Activate and mobilise – Ensuring that the muscles used in performance are activated, ready to produce maximal force, and to mobilise the joints that are to be used in the swing. Specific exercises can be used to target muscle groups that have been identified as important to golf performance based upon a prior needs analysis (see Figure 4.1). Dynamic stretching (activation and mobility exercises) can target an individual's specific limitations to allow acute increases in range of movement of these joints. As Jeffreys (2007) states, this requires a shift from traditional approaches of static stretching or targeting individual muscles towards a movement based warm-up. He continues to state that the advantages to this approach are that 1) the 'raise' element of the warm-up is maintained through this dynamic stage, 2) it focuses on the movements that golfers will use in their sport, and 3) it is time efficient. With the typical poor engagement in golf warm-ups the time efficiency of a RAMP warm-up protocol potentially assists in overcoming one of the barriers, in this regard. Strength and conditioning coaches working with golfers should look to design warm-ups that suit and benefit each individual while keeping in mind the need to address the key biomechanical and physiological requirements of the sport. For instance, there is an inherent importance in mobilising the hips and the thoracic spine due to the rotational requirements of the backswing and follow through (Chu et al., 2010). It is important to consider the muscle activity that is typical in the golf swing and to target movements that will both activate the musculature involved and mobilise the joints that have been cited as important for allowing increased time over which force can act. McHardy & Pollard (2005) highlighted the activation of muscle groups during the swing (Figure 4.1) and practitioners should consider these when designing warm-up protocols. McHardy & Pollard's (2005) report stated that the gluteals on the trail side are 98–100% active and 58% active on the lead side at the point between mid-downswing (club horizontal to the floor) to impact. As such, exercises that include either squat or lunge movement patterns, either in a dynamic bodyweight or resisted form are useful examples here.

Barriers to engagement: The most likely issue with this phase is a lack of understanding around what exercises constitute an activation and mobilisation protocol. There is often a disconnect between academic research (in this case showcasing the benefits to golf warm-up protocols) and applied practice (Bishop, 2008; Eisenmann, 2017; Finch, 2011). This chapter aims to further reduce any disconnect by providing practical recommendations and solutions to barriers to engagement. With Fradkin et al.'s (2003) survey results suggesting an increased likelihood of warming-up would occur when golfers knew how to conduct a suitable protocol, it is clear that further education is required to ensure club golfers have an increased awareness of not only the protocols but also the performance benefits. While this is being addressed within golf coaching education (e.g. through The Professional Golfers' Association's higher education programmes), it is important that these messages are disseminated to golfers of all abilities.

Potentiate – This phase requires the athlete to perform activities that will improve the effectiveness of subsequent performance (Jeffreys, 2007). For golfers, this may simply mean performing their golf swing – building towards full speed drives. However, alternative methods have been proposed, for example, post

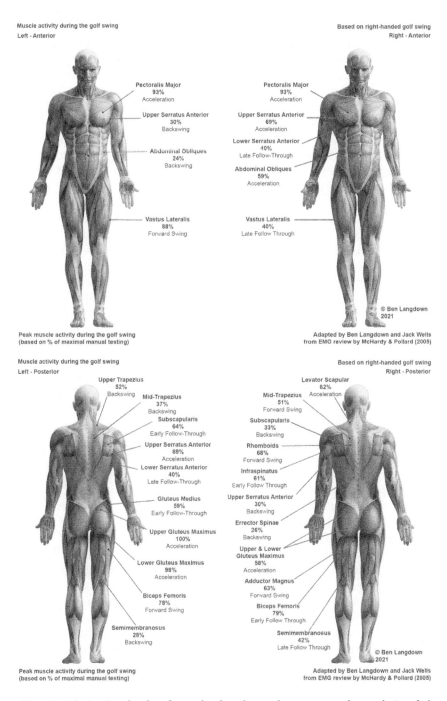

Figure 4.1 Activation levels of muscles based on electromyography analysis of the golf swing
Source: adapted from McHardy & Pollard (2005).

activation potentiation (PAP) research by Read et al. (2013). Their protocol employed a dynamic warm-up prior to three countermovement jumps (CMJ), where the CMJ acted as a potentiation exercise, prior to hitting any golf shots. This protocol led to a 2.2% increase in CHS vs. a control condition of just the dynamic stretching warm-up. As an aside, this also leads to the possibility of using CMJs throughout the round prior to tee shots where distance is of increased importance. Acute potentiation responses may benefit in these circumstances. Recent golf specific research has investigated the effects of overspeed protocols on performance. Hébert-Losier & Wardell (2021) reported that a SuperSpeed Golf™ warm-up acutely increased CHS (2.6 mph) when compared to a control condition (golf swing warm-up using a selection of clubs from sand-wedge to driver). Although SuperSpeed Golf™ claim enhanced performance for 30 mins post warm-up, the results here showed that, following 400m of walking (six mins), the CHS changes were reduced to trivial levels from a statistical standpoint (range 1.5–1.7 mph). Although statistically, this is considered 'trivial', these 1.5–1.7 mph increases may still be important to the golfer, thus providing merit to including potentiation in their warm-up protocol. A note of caution: It is important to recognise that although there were increases in CHS, these failed to transfer to improved ball speed suggesting that centeredness of strike was likely compromised. Further research in this area observed that a bodyweight potentiation protocol (3x10 CMJs and 2x10 plyometric press-ups) elicited similar significant increases in CHS when compared to the use of an overspeed protocol where light, medium and heavy speed sticks where swung at maximal speed (40 reps in total) (Bliss et al., 2021). The addition of CMJs and overspeed training (such as weighted clubs) on top of a dynamic stretching condition can significantly increase CHS. However, the need for overspeed training is questionable since it offers no additional benefits in golf performance when compared to bodyweight exercises. If maximal intent swings are recommended, then it would appear wise to utilise equipment that the golfer will use (i.e. their own driver) as opposed to an implement that may vary in mass and length and therefore presents a different moment of inertia and ultimately 'feel'. At the time of writing, golf research has shown some positive gains from potentiation exercises (Bliss et al., 2021; Hébert-Losier & Wardell, 2021; Read et al., 2013) but further research is required to fully understand the mechanisms, the most effective protocols, and recovery periods required for maximal CHS gains.

Research from sports such as rugby have provided alternative approaches, for example, the use of an 80% 1RM loading in a high hang pull exercise (one set of three reps) (Parr et al., 2017). The authors stated that a gluteal specific, 'activation warm-up may facilitate recruitment of the gluteal musculature by potentiating the glutes in such a way that a smaller neural drive evokes the same or greater force production during movement' (Parr et al., 2017). It is clear that only a minority of golfers will have both the access to a gym facility at their golf club, and the technical competence to complete a warm-up protocol using an exercise like the high hang pull at 80% 1RM (Parr et al., 2017). In the sport of rugby, this may be feasible as the higher skilled athletes may well be engaged in both S&C and regular warm-up protocols prior to training and matches. Strength and conditioning coaches should therefore consider the most relevant protocol for each individual golfer, their access to facilities and equipment, views on and willingness to engage in warm-up protocols and ensure their competency levels are sufficient so that they can demonstrate each exercise safely for use on their own in their golf specific context.

A note of caution: Research highlights that PAP research is not yet complete or conclusive due to many projects failing to confirm the presence of PAP or fatigue (see MacIntosh et al., 2012), and indeed, minimal evidence has been presented that PAP plays a significant role where 'multiple physiological processes have already been upregulated by a preceding, comprehensive, active muscle warm-up' (Blazevich & Babault, 2019). As such, the effects of potentiation during a warm-up should be viewed with caution. Research suggests that beneficial, potentiating effects are only applicable within one to five minutes of completing the potentiating exercises (see MacIntosh et al., 2012), which poses issues for those golfers who are warming-up prior to hitting balls, and then putting before approaching the first tee. It may be necessary to repeat potentiating exercises prior to the first tee shot, and again throughout the round to maximise the acute adaptations and benefits to drive performance. Golfers should also be aware of ensuring reps and sets are kept low (i.e. ~three reps at >80% 1RM if using loaded activities) and allowing sufficient recovery time prior to maximal effort golf swings after the exercise stimulus (Kilduff et al., 2011; MacIntosh et al., 2012).

Barriers to engagement: Due to the potential low engagement of club level golfers in this phase, it's important for coaches to consider which protocols represent the most viable option that will engage golfers in warming-up. The use of three CMJs, albeit in golf attire, presents an effective means of achieving some potentiating practises in a golfer's routine, without the need for resisted exercises to be undertaken. Performing plyometric push-ups (as in the bodyweight potentiation protocol in Bliss et al. (2021)) on a range or beside the first tee is likely to discourage many club golfers from engaging with the warm-up. However, the potential use of overspeed protocols perhaps offers a more inconspicuous route to potentiation. This may be because the overspeed protocol looks like a golf swing, whereas the jumping and press-ups, despite the benefits they provide, look increasingly alien to the sport. However, with 27 and 40 reps being performed in the Hébert-Losier & Wardell (2021) and Bliss et al. (2021) protocols respectively, it is important that golfers adapt their own warm-up to account for fatigue and recovery times to optimise their own drive performance. It is not uncommon for some professional golfers to hit over 300 balls, plus perform practice swings, during each range session (Thériault & Lachance, 1998). Adding a further 27–40 maximal swings through a warm-up substantially increases the volume of shots per session. The additional cumulative load across a week that included 3+ range sessions, not to mention gym-based sessions, means that they will be exposing their body to a potential spike in training volumes. With excessive and rapid increases in training load linked

Table 4.3 Example of a warm-up based on the RAMP protocol

Phase	Modality	Links to research
Raise	Brisk walk or jog	
Activate and Mobilise	Clock lunges (4 reps each leg: Forwards, lateral, reverse, crossed reverse lunge)	(Langdown et al., 2019)
	Overhead squats (10 reps)	
	Scapula wall slides (2 x 30 seconds)	
	Thoracic rotation (6 reps each side)	
	Hip openers (i.e. open and close the gate exercises) (6 reps in each direction on each side)	
Potentiate	Vertical jump (3 reps)	(Bliss et al., 2021; Hébert-Losier & Wardell, 2021; Read et al., 2013)
	Max. intent air swing with a driver (3–5 reps)★	

Note: ★SuperSpeed warm-ups involved 40 swings in total. Given that there are already other modalities utilised within this warm-up template, the authors feel that 3–5 reps should suffice. Warm-up validation should take place to appropriately amend this warm-up.

to greater risk of injury (Gabbett, 2016), we would suggest that, to mitigate risks, a golfer should perform three to five maximum air swings with their own driver. This should suffice as a potentiation protocol to elicit the required acute adaptations.

To guide the reader towards an example of a suitable warm-up protocol, a template has been provided (Table 4.3). Please note, this represents an example guide and this protocol should be adapted for individuals based on their training status, fitness levels, physical requirements and following the completion of a physical activity readiness questionnaire (PAR-Q).

Fostering an Environment to Encourage a Warm-up

With the potentially significant barriers to conducting a warm-up identified, it is crucial that coaches foster an environment that is conducive to encourage warm-ups. Golfers need to appreciate that a time efficient protocol can be implemented that may add distance to their drives. Indeed, this may play a significant role in helping them achieve their performance/outcome goals for the year and that, like purchasing a new driver, it is worth investing in an individualised protocol. Of course, there is not a one-size-fits-all protocol that coaches can apply to every golfer. Golf coaches and S&C coaches must liaise to establish what is feasible given the underpinning health and training status of each individual, the facilities available and the perceptions and current behaviours of the golfer. Warm-up protocols should therefore be adapted to the individual and the environment in which their warm-up is likely to take place.

Demonstrating the Benefits through Dissemination of Relevant Warm-up Research

As Jeffreys (2007) suggested, it is useful for athletes, in this case golfers, to consider a warm-up as 'performance preparation'. By encouraging a shift in attitudes, towards warming-up for performance, a golfer's engagement levels may increase to achieve the acute physiological adaptations that bring about maximal CHS and drive distances. An established protocol should be tried and tested in order to ensure an optimal effect on performance.

In our experience, the act of validating a warm-up protocol provides golfers with an affirmation that performance can be significantly impacted within a short period of time (see Figure 4.2). Validating the protocol through the use of a launch monitor or distance markers can facilitate engagement and provides insight into the 'low-hanging fruit' that a warm-up can provide. Specifically, a launch monitor will provide data into drive performance measures such as CHS, ball speed, carry distance, swing path, centredness of strike etc.

Ratings of Perceived Exertion and Subjective Ratings of Performance

When considering the individual response to a warm-up Langdown et al. (2019) stated that it is important to note that each protocol would need to be adapted to the physical capabilities of each golfer. This can be achieved with a Borg scale (Figure 4.3) to establish the level of physical exertion during each protocol (Borg, 1998). Golfers need to feel that they have completed an effective warm-up and not increased the intensity to an extent that it becomes a training session for them, resulting in undue fatigue on the first tee. Equally, the protocol needs to be of a level that elicits the physiological (and possible psychological) benefits that will lead to enhanced performance. We recommend the application of a Borg scale rating of perceived exertion – aiming for a rating of three (moderate) – four (somewhat hard). It is also recommended that this perception rating is taken 15 minutes after the completion of the warm-up to collect a rating that is not influenced by the last exercise performed.

With a validated protocol and appropriate exertion achieved it is possible for significant gains to be made in drive performance. Langdown et al. (2019) reported that one individual in their study gained 40 yards following a resistance band protocol compared to a control condition and 34 yards when completing a dynamic stretching warm-up protocol. Not every golfer will be fortunate to achieve distance gains to this extent but with every ~ten yards gained comes a reduction in the club required to play an approach shot to the green. As previously stated, this allows a variety of tactical advantages and greater control over the next shot.

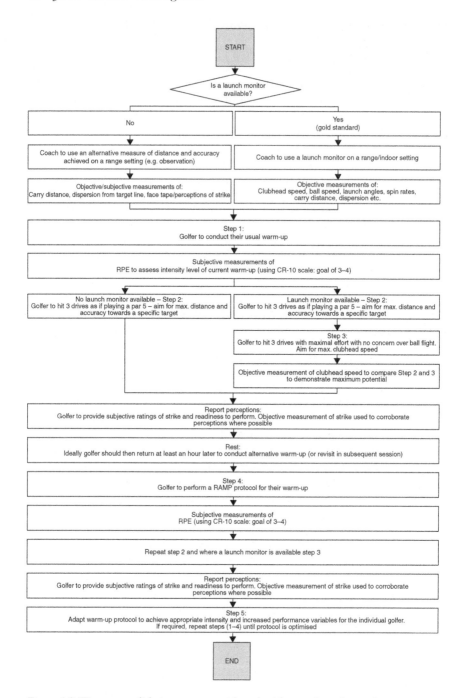

Figure 4.2 Warm-up validation process with and without a launch monitor

Rating	Descriptor
0	Nothing at all
1	Very, Very Easy
2	Easy
3	Moderate
4	Somewhat hard
5	Hard
6	
7	Very hard
8	
9	
10	Maximal

Figure 4.3 Modified category rating of perceived exertion (RPE) scale
Source: Foster et al. (2001).

Additional Coaching Benefits from a Golfer's Warm-Up

In addition to the benefits seen by individual golfers when undertaking a warm-up, there are opportunities for the S&C coach to gain a valuable insight into movement patterns and increased understanding of the golfer's movement competence. It also provides an opportunity to micro-dose S&C exercises that the golfer may otherwise not engage with. The use of dynamic exercises in a warm-up, such as squats, lunges, scapula wall slides and rotation-based dynamic stretches, allows coach observations and assessment of full body mobility, posture, stability through single-leg or split stance exercises, strength in specific areas and the ability to cope with resistance (where bands/weights are incorporated). This can offer an opening to discuss S&C and the impact upon the individual's golf swing or overall performance. If the golfer is already engaged in S&C it offers the opportunity to assess the effectiveness of any systematic interventions and to make amendments as required.

Coaches' Perspectives

Our applied experience provides other methods and practical recommendations and considerations that have supported golfers' engagement in warm-up protocols:

- Sharing high-profile examples of warm-ups – These can be high performing golfers within the club, region or highlighting professional golfers' protocols.
- Create and share programme goals – Within regional and national level programmes there are expectations that young golfers will be competent at performing their own warm-up and be able to adapt this to the context in which they find themselves at tournaments. Club-based programmes can also set warm-up goals for all golfers to achieve.

- Data to prove benefits – An individual validation process is the most effective method of providing evidence on the benefits of a warm-up. However, creating and disseminating case studies may also raise curiosity and motivation to engage in the process.
- Practice what you preach – Coaches are often role models too. It is important that when training or playing golf they are seen to engage in a RAMP protocol and are able to discuss the benefits to golf performance.
- Encourage warm-ups as an expected standard – Coaching the golfer to be autonomous in their warm-up protocol affords them the opportunity to adapt their warm-up to any physical limitations they may experience prior to competing or prior to training and practicing. Discussing and coaching them through various alternatives they can use, given varying contexts, will allow them to utilise the most effective warm-up in each condition (e.g. when away at a tournament with no gym facilities, training in a gym / at home etc.).
- Promote warm-ups using research data and posters around the facilities – Golf manufacturers use promotional materials for the sales strategy of new drivers. In the same way, warm-up benefits can be promoted at your facility/online to raise awareness of the benefits and to upskill golfers through increased understanding of warm-up exercises.
- Stock mini-bands/resistance bands in the gym or pro shop – Making it easy for golfers to apply principles of resisted exercise in their warm-up is critical to engagement. While many golfers will benefit from dynamic stretching in their warm-up, others will want the benefits of resisted exercises that they can do on the range or in the locker room. If coaches are able to competently demonstrate a range of resisted exercises and to provide access to purchase bands, it will allow easy access to engagement. The use of imagery/videos together with the bands will serve as a reminder of how to develop competency in the exercises.
- Insurance – Consideration should be given to making it mandatory to perform a warm-up prior to attending a golf coaching session. This not only benefits the performance of the golfer from the start of their session it also allows the golf coach to assess the movements of the golf swing from a physically prepared condition. From an insurance perspective this may also be a condition of all golf coaching sessions (coaches should check with suppliers of insurance).
- Changing the coaching session culture – Golf coaches would be wise to check that the golfer has warmed-up prior to the lesson (as highlighted above). If the golfer has not engaged in a warm-up, it would be advisable to spend time taking the golfer through a full warm-up protocol. Golfers will most likely want to spend their lesson time refining technical/performance aspects of their game. In this regard, encouragement to conduct the warm-up prior to the lesson will highlight the saving of time for technical and performance coaching. Furthermore, this will help to facilitate a culture shift that will encourage warm-up engagement.

Conclusion

Research has highlighted that warming-up for golf can significantly improve impact factors and ball flight characteristics. However, golfers are yet to fully embrace the benefits that warming-up can bring to their performance. Strength and conditioning practitioners can support golfers and coaches by devising bespoke warm-up routines to enhance performance. It is recommended that a RAMP protocol be followed where possible, however, to support engagement, phases can be combined and manipulated to suit each individual and their specific context. To further encourage golfers' engagement, validation of the warm-up protocols can be undertaken to provide evidence of impact on performance. The inclusion of a launch monitor in this process increases validity and can support the coach to highlight the acute adaptations following a warm-up protocol. While physiological gains are important to clubhead speed, the use of RPE and perceptions of strike can also be critical to the psychological aspects of performance. The application of the evidence presented in this chapter offers both S&C and golf coaches valuable opportunities to encourage a culture shift and increased engagement in warming-up for golf.

References

Behm, D. G., & Kibele, A. (2007). Effects of differing intensities of static stretching on jump performance. *European Journal of Applied Physiology*, *101*(5): 587–594. https://doi.org/10.1007/s00421-007-0533-5

Betzler, N. F., Monk, S. A., Wallace, E. S., & Otto, S. R. (2014). The relationships between driver clubhead presentation characteristics, ball launch conditions and golf shot outcomes. *Proceedings of the Institution of Mechanical Engineers, Part P: Journal of Sports Engineering and Technology*, *228*(4): 242–249. https://doi.org/10.1177/1754337114541884

Bishop, D. (2008). An Applied Research Model for the Sport Sciences. *Journal of Sports Medicine*, *38*(3): 253–263. https://doi.org/10.2165/00007256-200838030-00005

Bishop, David. (2003). Warm up II: Performance changes following active warm up and how to structure the warm up. *Sports Medicine*, *33*(7): 483–498. https://doi.org/10.2165/00007256-200333070-00002

Blazevich, A. J., & Babault, N. (2019). Post-activation Potentiation Versus Post-activation Performance Enhancement in Humans: Historical Perspective, Underlying Mechanisms, and Current Issues. *Frontiers in Physiology*, *10*(November). https://doi.org/10.3389/fphys.2019.01359

Blazevich, A. J., Gill, N. D., Kvorning, T., Kay, A. D., Goh, A. G., Hilton, B., Drinkwater, E. J., & Behm, D. G. (2018). No Effect of Muscle Stretching within a Full, Dynamic Warm-up on Athletic Performance. *Medicine and Science in Sports and Exercise*, *50*(6): 1258–1266. https://doi.org/10.1249/MSS.0000000000001539

Bliss, A., Livingstone, H., & Tallent, J. (2021). Field-based and overspeed potentiated warm-ups increase clubhead speed and drive carry distance in skilled collegiate golfers. *Journal of Sport and Exercise Science*, *5*(2): 107–113.

Borg, G. (1998). *Borg's perceived exertion and pain scales*. Champaign, IL: Human Kinetics.

Bridge, M., Perry, M., & Li, F.-X. (2008). The Warm-up Behaviours of Elite Female Golfers. In D. Crews & R. Lutz (Eds.), *Science and Golf V: Proceedings of the World Scientific Congress of Golf* (pp. 120–127). Florida: LPGA Foundation.

Broadie, M. (2014). *Every Shot Counts*. New York: Avery Publishing Group.

Chu, Y., Sell, T. C., & Lephart, S. M. (2010). The relationship between biomechanical variables and driving performance during the golf swing. *Journal of Sports Sciences, 28*(11): 1251–1259. https://doi.org/10.1080/02640414.2010.507249

Eisenmann, J. (2017). Translational gap between laboratory and playing field: new era to solve old problems in sports science. *Translational Journal of the American College of Sports Medicine, 2*(8): 37–43.

Finch, C. F. (2011). No longer lost in translation: The art and science of sports injury prevention implementation research. *British Journal of Sports Medicine, 45*(16): 1253–1257. https://doi.org/10.1136/bjsports-2011-090230

Foster, C., Florhaug, J. A., Franklin, J., Gottschall, L., Hrovatin, L. A., Parker, S., Doleshal, P., & Dodge, C. (2001). A new approach to monitoring exercise training. *Journal of Strength and Conditioning Research, 15*(1): 109–115.

Fradkin, A. J., Finch, C. F., & Sherman, C. A. (2001). Warm up practices of golfers: Are they adequate? *British Journal of Sports Medicine, 35*(2): 125–127. https://doi.org/10.1136/bjsm.35.2.125

Fradkin, A. J., Finch, C. F., & Sherman, C. A. (2003). Warm-up attitudes and behaviours of amateur golfers. *Journal of Science and Medicine in Sport, 6*(2): 210–215. https://doi.org/10.1016/S1440-2440(03)80256-6

Fradkin, A. J., Gabbe, B. J., & Cameron, P. A. (2006). Does warming up prevent injury in sport?. The evidence from randomised controlled trials? *Journal of Science and Medicine in Sport, 9*(3): 214–220. https://doi.org/10.1016/j.jsams.2006.03.026

Fradkin, A. J., Sherman, C. A., & Finch, C. F. (2004). Improving golf performance with a warm up conditioning programme. *British Journal of Sports Medicine, 38*(6): 762–765. https://doi.org/10.1136/bjsm.2003.009399

Gabbett, T. (2016). The training-injury prevention paradox: should athletes be training smarter and harder? *British Journal of Sports Medicine, 50*: 273–280. https://doi.org/10.1136/bjsports-2016-097249

Gergley, J. (2009). Acute Effects of Passive Static Stretching During Warm-Up on Driver. *Journal of Strength and Conditioning Research, 23*(3): 863–867.

Gergley, J. (2010). Latent effect of passive static stretching on driver clubhead speed, distance, accuracy, and consistent ball contact in young male competitice golfers. *Journal of Strength and Conditioning Research, 24*(12): 3326–3333.

Gosheger, G., Liem, D., Ludwig, K., Greshake, O., & Winkelmann, W. (2003). Injuries and overuse syndromes in golf. *Am J Sports Med, 31*(3): 438–443. https://doi.org/10.1055/s-0031-1277207

Haddad, M., Dridi, A., Chtara, M., Chaouachi, A., Wong, D. P., Behm, D., & Chamari, K. (2014). Static stretching can impair explosive performance for at least 24 hours. *Journal of Strength and Conditioning Research, 28*(1): 140–146. https://doi.org/10.1519/JSC.0b013e3182964836

Han, K. H., Como, C., Kim, J., Lee, S., Kim, J., Kim, D. K., & Kwon, Y. H. (2019). Effects of the golfer–ground interaction on clubhead speed in skilled male golfers. *Sports Biomechanics, 18*(2): 115–134. https://doi.org/10.1080/14763141.2019.1586983

Hébert-Losier, K., & Wardell, G. L. (2021). Acute and persistence of the effects of the SuperSpeed Golf™ weighted-club warm-up on golf driving performance and kinematics. *Sports Biomechanics.* https://doi.org/10.1080/14763141.2021.1887344

Jeffreys, I. (2007). Warm-up revisited: The ramp method of optimizing warm-ups. *Professional Strength and Conditioning, 6:* 12–18.

Kilduff, L, P., Cunningham, D, J., Owen, N, J., West, D, J., Bracken, R, M., & Cook, C, J. (2011). Effect of postactivation potentiation on swimming starts in international sprint swimmers. *Journal of Strength and Conditioning Research, 25*(9): 2418–2423. doi: 10.1519/JSC.0b013e318201bf7a

Langdown, B.L., Wells, J. E. T., Graham, S., & Bridge, M. W. (2019). Acute effects of different warm-up protocols on highly skilled golfers' drive performance. *Journal of Sports Sciences, 37*(6): 656–664. https://doi.org/10.1080/02640 414.2018.1522699

MacIntosh, B. R., Robillard, M. E., & Tomaras, E. K. (2012). Should postactivation potentiation be the goal of your warm-up? *Applied Physiology, Nutrition and Metabolism, 37*(3): 546–550. https://doi.org/10.1139/H2012-016

McHardy, A., & Pollard, H. (2005). Muscle activity during the golf swing. *British Journal of Sports Medicine, 39*(11): 799–804. https://doi.org/10.1136/bjsm.2005.020271

Moran, K. A., McGrath, T., Marshall, B. M., & Wallace, E. S. (2009). Dynamic stretching and golf swing performance. *International Journal of Sports Medicine, 30*(2): 113–118. https://doi.org/10.1055/s-0028-1103303

Nesbit, S. M., & Serrano, M. (2005). Work and power analysis of the golf swing. *Journal of Sports Science & Medicine, 4*(4): 520–533. www.ncbi.nlm.nih.gov/pubmed/24627 666%5Cnhttp://www.pubmedcentral.nih.gov/articlerender.fcgi?artid=PMC 3899668

Parr, M., Price, P. D., & Cleather, D. J. (2017). Effect of a gluteal activation warm-up on explosive exercise performance. *BMJ Open Sport and Exercise Medicine, 3*(1): 1–8. https://doi.org/10.1136/bmjsem-2017-000245

Perrier, E., Pavol, M., & Hoffman, M. (2011). The acute effects of a warm-up including static or dynamic stretching on countermovement jump height, reaction time and flexibility. *Journal of Strength and Conditioning Research, 25*(7): 1925–1931.

Read, P. J., Miller, S. C., & Turner, A. N. (2013). The effects of postactivation potentiation on golf club head speed. *Journal of Strength and Conditioning Research, 27*(6): 1579–1582. https://doi.org/10.1519/JSC.0b013e3182711c60

Sorbie, G. G., Baker, J. S., Gu, Y., & Ugbolue, U. C. (2016). The effect of dynamic and static stretching on golf drive performance. *International Journal of Sports and Exercise Medicine, 2*(1): 1–5.

Sweeney, M., Mills, P., Alderson, J., & Elliott, B. (2013). The influence of club-head kinematics on early ball flight characteristics in the golf drive. *Sports Biomechanics, 12*(3): 247–258. https://doi.org/10.1080/14763141.2013.772225

Thériault, G., & Lachance, P. (1998). Golf injuries: An overview. *Sports Medicine, 26*(1): 43–57. https://doi.org/10.2165/00007256-199826010-00004

Tilley, N. R., & Macfarlane, A. (2012). Effects of different warm-up programs on golf performance in elite male golfers. *International Journal of Sports Physical Therapy, 7*(4): 388–395. www.ncbi.nlm.nih.gov/pubmed/23936749%0Ahttp://www. pubmedcentral.nih.gov/articlerender.fcgi?artid=PMC3735827

Wells, J. E. T., Charalambous, L. H., Mitchell, A. C. S., Coughlan, D., Brearley, S. L., Hawkes, R. A., Murray, A. D., Hillman, R. G., & Fletcher, I. M. (2019). Relationships between Challenge Tour golfers' clubhead velocity and force producing capabilities during a countermovement jump and isometric mid-thigh pull. *Journal of Sports Sciences*, *37*(12): 1381–1386. https://doi.org/10.1080/02640414.2018.1559972

Wells, J. E. T., & Langdown, B. L. (2020). Sports science for golf: A survey of high-skilled golfers' 'perceptions' and 'practices'. *Journal of Sports Sciences*, *00*(00): 1–10. https://doi.org/10.1080/02640414.2020.1737350

5 The Female Golfer

Emma Ross and Fiona Scott

In 2020 The Royal and Ancient Golf Club of St Andrews (R&A), backed by England Golf, unveiled the #FOREeveryone campaign, a long-term drive to bring more women and girls into the game. At the time, only one in four golfers were women, and the golf industry was male dominated (R&A, 2020). In fact, until 2014, for its first 260 years, The R&A had been a men's-only club (Mair, 2016). It's down to sex discrimination and gender inequality being such recent history in the game, combined with a distinct lack of research into women's golf performance, that has created a gender gap when it comes to understanding how to best support, treat and train the female golfer.

We know from other sports like rugby and football, that when women participate in a sport that has been for so long, dominated by men, the approach to training and preparing female athletes for peak performance is often done in ways that have previously been successful for men in that sport, or based on research that has been carried out on men. Training methods transposed from men to women without due consideration for the fact that men and women differ biomechanically, physiologically and psychologically, underserves women in sport. They typically overlook the 'female' part of being a 'female athlete'. Women are different from men. Women have periods and menstrual cycles, they may use hormonal contraception, they may go through pregnancy, they have breasts, they are far more likely to have pelvic floor dysfunction, they have a higher risk of injury, and they manage emotions and derive confidence differently from men. As women continue to pursue optimal performance, from personal achievements to championship successes, we have to think differently about what it takes to allow them to fulfil their potential, because it won't always be the same things that have worked for men.

The gender data gap

Female participation in sport has drastically increased over the past century, as shown by the participation rates of female athletes taking part in the Summer Olympics increasing from 2.2% in 1900 to 48.8% in 2021 (IOC, 2020) and more specifically, within golf, the number of adult female golf club members has increased by around 2000 players since 2017 (England Golf).

DOI: 10.4324/9781003099321-5

Despite this increase in female participation, there is still a void in sport and exercise science and medicine research on the determinants of sports performance, or effectiveness of training programmes, exercise regimes, nutritional interventions, injury prevention or psychological approaches in women (Costello et al., 2014; Cowley et al., 2021). Over a six-year period from 2014 to 2020, only 6% of the research in six sports science and medicine journals was conducted exclusively on women (Cowley et al., 2021). A search for papers on PubMed (an online search engine that comprises more than 32 million citations for biomedical and life science literature) in early 2021, including the search terms 'Women's Golf', 'Ladies Golf', 'Female Golfer' 'Women AND Golf' in the title, show only 11 papers published between 2006 and 2021. In addition to this lack of research, there is poor methodological quality of existing research into female athletes. A meta-analysis of studies looking at the influence of the menstrual cycle on parameters of performance, such as strength, endurance and power, showed 60% of this small body of work was classified as 'low quality' (McNulty et al., 2020). This further compounds our ability to draw conclusions or recommendations on what is best for female athletes from what evidence does exist.

Despite this lack of female specific sport science research, there is enough well-established knowledge of female physiology, practice-based evidence from working with female athletes, and emerging evidence from research, to begin to understand the important considerations for supporting female athlete health and performance. Each topic could be a separate chapter in this book, and for a comprehensive, evidenced-based review of the exercising female, readers are directed to *The Exercising Female: Science and its Application*, edited by Forsyth and Roberts (Forsyth & Roberts, 2019), or *Strength and Conditioning for Female Athletes*, edited by Keith Barker and Debby Sargent (Barker & Sargent, 2018) or to online resources at TheWell-HQ.com. However, it is the ambition of this chapter to introduce these important topics so that considering the female element of being a female athlete becomes an intuitive part of your approach to treating, training, and coaching women.

The female swing

In has been well documented that the key determinants of performance within golf include: greens in regulation (GIR), putts per round (PPR), driving distance (DD) and driving accuracy (DA) (Belkin et., 1994; Moy & Liaw, 1998; Nero, 2001; Dorsel & Rotunda, 2001; Alexander & Kern, 2005). For female players, it has been shown that the percentage of GIR and PPR are important determinants of both scoring average and earnings. On the Ladies Professional Golf Association (LPGA) tour, players with the greatest DD achieve closer proximity to the hole and greater GIR than players with the lowest DD (LPGA, 2018).

Clubhead speed (CHS) is a commonly reported kinematic variable because it accounts for 75% of the variance in ball velocity, which inherently leads to greater DD (Sweeney et al., 2013). External variables such as environmental conditions and centredness of strike can affect DD, but CHS is unaffected by these variables and therefore offers a more robust assessment of performance (Hume et al., 2005; Betzler et al., 2014; Wells et al., 2018). Research indicating significant relationships between lower body strength, explosive strength and CHS (Wells et al., 2018;2019) highlights the importance of training these aspects for increased golf performance. Brearley et al. (2019) states that most amateurs (and many professionals) will benefit from increases in DD secondary to strength training due to their often 'untapped' potential, and this is particularlly true for female players.

Given that women tend to have approximately 25–55% of the upper body strength of men (Zatsiorsky & Kraemer, 2006), and are on average 12 cm shorter and 14 kg lighter than males (Roser et al., 2019; NCD-RiscC, 2020), their power-to-weight ratio is different. Therefore, to achieve the same CHS, it is intuitive that females might need to adopt a different swing technique to their male counterparts to optimise CHS and DD. However, rather than there existing a straightforward sex difference in swing mechanics, swing biomechanical variables seem to be different between individuals (Brown et al., 2011) and it is unlikely that there is a universal swing technique for optimal swing performance in women (Parker et al., 2019). Very little research has been conducted on female swing kinematics, but is has been established that women have a larger range of motion of thorax and pelvis rotation at the top of the backswing (Horan et al., 2011; Zheng et al., 2008) and lower maximum velocity of the wrist and clubhead velocity (Zheng et al. 2008). Lower segmental velocity might be related to women having less muscle mass, reducing absolute force production and reducing the velocity of movement (Horan et al., 2011). Height and arm length also have a strong relationship with CHS, due to the increased distance (radius) between the golfer's centre of rotation and the ball, which generates greater linear velocity at any given angular velocity (Wells et al., 2009).

As evidence from golf is lacking, inference can be taken from other rotational striking sports such as tennis, where, to achieve the same (and sometimes faster) ball speed than their male counterparts (Trolloppe, 2017), elite female players generally use a big sweeping forehand, with a swing path referred to as a 'pendulum', which relies on momentum and gravity rather than muscle and strength (Ward, 2019; Walner, 2019). The same appears to be true in golf, where females adopt a different swing from males to optimise performance. What's important is that this isn't likely to simply be a sex difference, but a physicality difference – there will also be males who are shorter or have less muscle mass who may optimise their swing through different kinematics from taller, stronger peers.

Not only is there considerable evidence showing positive relationships between various strength and power measures and CHS (Wells et al., 2019; Coughlan et al., 2020; Read et al., 2012), but significant CHS improvements have been observed in parallel with improvements in such measures (Coughlan et al., 2019) thus supporting the role of Strength and Conditioning within golf. On occasion these increases in CHS have been attributed to increases in body mass (Brearley et al., 2019) and this provides further insight into the mechanisms by which increased body mass facilitates longer drives, which go beyond the notion that a larger muscle can produce more force. A larger body mass has a dual benefit of both creating a greater anchoring effect, allowing the player to retain more stability at higher swing speeds, as well as providing an increased ability to generate greater angular momentum from the ground up. Many golfers are concerned with their relative strength and power; often tracking progress with measures such as vertical jump height. However, golf doesn't require players to project their body in movements such as sprinting and jumping, and it is in fact their absolute strength and power that matters (Tilley & Brearley, 2020). Since females are on average 14 kg lighter than their male counterparts, it's even more pertinent for female golfers to focus on absolute strength and power as key adaptation qualities in their resistance training programmes.

Other determinants of CHS in female golfers include grip strength and flexibility (Brown et al., 2011). Females are naturally more flexible and mobile than males (Van Herp et al., 2000) and have shown to demonstrate increased rates of hypermobility of the spine and elbow joints (Reuter & Fichthorn, 2019). In golf, females demonstrate a greater range of motion (ROM) at the thorax and pelvis during the golf swing. This enables good separation between the upper and lower body, often called the 'X-Factor', which is important to help generate speed and maintain a stable posture during the golf swing. On one hand this hypermobility can prevent injury caused by lack of mobility exerting excessive lumbar spine rotational forces (which can lead to shoulder overuse injury and decreased swing performance) (Lamb & Pataky, 2018; Rose, 2013). However, on the other hand, an increased ROM at joints can increase the likelihood of injury. Therefore, female golfer's training programmes should aim to strengthen and target the relevant muscles and proprioceptors to improve joint stability while maintaining flexibility.

Training considerations for the female golfer

Resistance training

Women have a similar array of muscle fibre types, but a sex difference does exist in untrained individuals, where women have a larger proportion of slow-twitch than fast-twitch muscle fibres (Hicks et al., 2001). The cause of such a difference is unknown but could, along with the fact that females tend to enter sport less conditioned and with a lower training age, be turned into a potential advantage, with females having a greater potential to see superior results from strength training when they begin their athletic development (Triplett & Stone, 2016; Pitchers & Elliott-Sale, 2019).

This strength potential is seen when females introduce resistance training, albeit there is a brief plateau initially in which fast-twitch muscle fibres need time to 'catch up' with slow-twitch muscle fibre size. The implications for this when training females is that a) females may have to be more patient with the training process, b) the use of relatively heavier resistances is required to stimulate the growth of the fast-twitch fibres in females, and c) if slow-twitch fibres predominate, then a more rapid detraining effect could be seen, implying the importance of training frequency, especially for strength maintenance.

Research shows that muscle hypertrophy (increase in muscle fibre number and size) is similar between the sexes, as well as muscle synthesis rates post exercise and rate of gain of muscle CSA (cross-sectional area) per day (Hunter, 1985; Wernborn et al., 2007). This means that males and females make similar strength gains in response to a well-designed training programme (Triplett & Stone, 2016). If exercises are performed at the same relative percentage of one repetition maximum (1RM), females develop strength equally to males. However, when researchers normalise strength improvements to the entire volume of trained musculature (i.e., absolute muscle power quality) they found, when expressed in this way, women's strength improved by 9% but no change was observed in men's strength (Delmonico et al., 2005). They concluded that improvements in muscle function from strength training result from non-muscle mass adaptations to a greater extent in women than men, possibly down to better coordination of all the muscles involved in the movement and better signalling from the brain to activate the muscle in question. In practise, the prioritised use of compound (multi-muscle, multi-joint), coordinated, sports-specific exercises might take advantage of these superior neuromuscular gains in female athletes.

Research shows that women can perform muscular contractions for longer than men because their muscles are less fatigable (Hunter, 2016). When the load is about 50% 1RM the difference is greatest, with women lasting about 60% longer performing knee extensions than men (Ansdell et al., 2017). This concept holds true for contractions all the way up to 80% 1RM. Interestingly, the level of contractile fatigue at task failure is the same in male and female's muscles, except females perform more muscular work before they reach task-failure. Research has shown this across a number of muscle groups from fingers to elbow flexors to knee extensors (Hunter, 2009; Hunter, 2016). The same body of research also suggests that recovery from neuromuscular fatigue is quicker in females, taking less time to recover and produce maximal strength or power again after performance to fatigue. It is important to build these concepts into training programmes for female athletes so that both programming parameters such as sets, repetitions, tempos, rest periods and load not only suit the desired adaptation, but also take these female specific neuromuscular factors into consideration in order to elicit optimal adaptations for golf performance.

In female golfers, resistance training has been shown to improve driving performance (speed and distance) (Kim, 2010; Hegedus, 2016). For example, Kim (2010) showed that a 12-week core-focussed strength training regime improved back flexion, back extension and squat strength and in this group driver shot performance, CHS and carry distance increased significantly.

In another study, a traditional strength training approach was compared to a golf-specific strength training regime, which focused on strengthening muscles activated throughout the golf swing. Both training programmes increased driver CHS, DD, and 7 iron distance (but not 7 iron CHS) (Hegedus, 2016). In fact, the post training effects were greater in the traditional programme than the golf-specific programme, probably due to the fact that the golf-specific programme replaced many of the traditional compound gym-based exercises with single-limb, balance focused exercises, in an attempt to mimic golf more closely. However, the loading used was likely at inappropriate intensities to elicit strength adaptations. This further supports the scientific principles and theories that have been investigated and illustrated for all to consider when designing golf specific training programmes specifically for the female golfer.

Injury risk and prevention

Golfing injuries

The most prevalent sites of injury in golfers are the lower back, wrist and elbow (Gosheger et al., 2003; McCarroll et al., 1990; Batt, 1992; McCarroll & Gioe, 1982). The lower back, which accounts for 23.7–34.5% of all golfing injuries, is subject to large ranges of motions and forces due to the mechanics of the swing. The forces encountered include: downward compression, side-to-side bending, and back-to-front shearing (Lindsay & Vandervoort, 2014). The most common mechanism of injury is overuse due to the high frequency of practice (both in professionals and amateurs) and poor biomechanics (in amateurs only) (McHardy et al., 2007). Poor mechanics of the golf swing can be seen from swing analysis studies which highlight that amateurs reach 90% of peak muscle activation in comparison with 80% in professionals and although both groups noted the same compressional loads, amateurs incurred 80% more lateral bending and peak shear loads and 50% more torque than their professional counterparts (Hosea et al., 1990). It is thought that these characteristics are due to amateurs trying to hit the ball further by simply swinging harder (McHardy et al., 2006).

Female-specific injury risk

Although the epidemiological data on golf injuries was collected in male golfers, it might be assumed that the mechanism of poor biomechanics could be an even greater problem in female golfers who (with the exception of professionals) usually take up the game later (in one survey participation begun on average, at 42 years (Ashford, 2017), or have long breaks from playing during pregnancy and postnatally.

Active females are, in general, more likely to suffer injury to connective tissue across the body, meaning they are more at risk of joint injury than men (Crossley et al., 2020). The ankle joint is injured about twice as frequently in female athletes, shoulder injuries are more common in women than in men (Wolf et al., 2015) and in particular females are 4.5 times more likely to suffer a non-contact ACL injury than men (Adachi et al., 2008; Chidi-Ogbolu & Baar, 2019; Zumwalt, 2019). For female athletes who suffer an ACL injury, 45% never compete again, 35% do not meet their previous level of athleticism and up to half show signs of osteoarthritis just a decade later (Queen, 2017).

The increased risk in females is thought only to occur after puberty, since equal numbers of ligament sprains occur in girls and boys before adolescence, but girls have higher rates immediately after their growth spurt and into maturity (Wild et al., 2012). Although the reasons why are still being researched, there are some important factors that contribute. The Q angle (the angle from the hip to the knee) is larger in women, in part due to a wider pelvis to accommodate potential childbirth, but primarily due to the fact that men are on average 12 cm taller than women and this longer pelvis–patella distance relative to patella–tuberosity distance, lessens the Q angle in men (Grelsamer et al., 2005). This increased angle in women has been linked to increased knee pain, and to the greater risk of ACL injury because it affects how females land from jumping movements or changes in direction while running. The knee tends to cave inwards, into a valgus position, during impact movements, and this puts a lot of angular stress on the knee joint, at best causing pain and at worst is a contributing factor in injury at the knee joint (Zumwalt, 2019). While running, jumping and landing are not integral movements in golf, they might be integrated into a strength and conditioning programme to condition players for golf, and as such, ensuring good technique and putting increased emphasis on good movement mechanics in females should be prioritised in the coaching process.

More so than anatomical differences, muscle strength and imbalance are important, and modifiable risk factors for joint injury in females. Female athletes demonstrate greater strength in the quadriceps, and preferential activation of this anterior muscle group at the expense of force generation from glutes and hamstring exacerbates this quad dominance. Researchers showed that in sporting tasks such as running, cross-cutting, and side-cutting, women activate their quads more, and hamstrings less compared to men, across all of the tasks (Malinzak et al., 2001). This leads to the anterior muscles developing so that they overpower the posterior muscles of the leg. During movements like running, stable knees require strong quadriceps to straighten the knee and help to flex the foot forward, and strong hamstrings to bend the knee and help to pull the leg backward. If this coordination doesn't exist, because one is strong and one is weak, the knee joint is at greater risk of injury. This is also true when performing the golf swing, as one of the primary muscles involved is the gluteal muscles, therefore highlighting the importance of training the muscles of the posterior chain for optimal CHS, DD and ultimately performance potential. Additionally, increasing the strength of the gluteal muscles, could also help prevent any swing compensations such as knee valgus (when the knee collapses inwards), since the gluteal muscles aid hip abduction and external rotation which are the opposite movements to that of knee valgus (hip adduction and internal rotation).

Phase of the menstrual cycle may also be an additional risk factor for injury in women, since oestrogen decreases stiffness in tendons and ligaments and at times of the cycle when oestrogen levels are high, joints may become more lax or less stable (Chidi-Ogbolu & Baar, 2019). When a joint has increased laxity it is more likely to become injured (Myer et al., 2008). Since oestrogen has been linked to increased knee laxity, and increased knee laxity linked to increased risk of injury, researchers have started to investigate how injury risk in women changes across their cycle, as oestrogen peaks and troughs (Deie et al., 2002). However, there is still no consensus on whether time of the cycle poses a significant risk, and more research is needed to fully understand just how important the menstrual cycle is in influencing injury in athletes.

Interestingly, compressive fractures in older females during the golf swing have been reported in the literature. The fracture sites were confined to the thoracolumbar region and were reported in healthy postmenopausal women who were previously or subsequently diagnosed with osteoporosis (Ekin & Sinaki, 1993). Menopause is associated with an increased risk of musculoskeletal injury, as oestrogen levels decline (Ennus & Tiidus, 2010), and up to 20% of a woman's bone density can be lost as a consequence in the first five years of menopause. This in itself is a very important consideration when training the menopausal female golfer, since regular resistance training is positively correlated with bone mineral density in these women (Pines & Berry, 2007).

Injury risk has been found to be effectively reduced by sports specific, multi-component, strength and conditioning programmes. For example, in football a programme that integrates conditioning exercises into a warm-up for 10–15 minutes prior to training 2–3 times a week has been significant in reducing injury risk in female footballers (FIFA, 2008). A large study with more than 11,000 participants, showed that overall injury rates were reduced by 27% and ACL injury rates by 45% (Crossley et al., 2020). Although these injury prevention programmes have been developed for sports such as netball, rugby and football, no such programme has been developed for golf.

In fact, research has demonstrated that most recreational golfers do not warm up prior to play or practice (Ehlert & Wilson, 2019) despite extensive research highlighting that the incorporation of a warm-up can both improve performance and reduce the risk of injury (Behm & Chaouachi, 2011; McGowan et al., 2015; Woods, Bishop, & Jones, 2007), and that lack of warm up was related to the likelihood of reporting a golfing injury (Fradkin et al., 2007). A systematic review by Ehlert and Wilson (2019) analysed 23 studies investigating the influence of performing a warm-up prior to golf play, but only 12 studies included female participants and on average only 16% of participants across the articles were female. In an observational study, Bridge et al., (2008) evidenced that Ladies European Tour (LET) golfers (n= 25) performed a mixture of static and dynamic stretches which ranged from 27 to 29 seconds over consecutive tournament days (Wells & Langdown, 2018). Static stretching has previously been shown to significantly reduce force production (Power et al., 2004), CHS, DD, DA and centeredness of strike (Gergley, 2009) so it is concerning that it remains as one of the key warm up methods of both LET and highly skilled golfers. This likley reflects a gap in female athlete knowledge, education and coaching.

Injury risk in female players seems to be modifiable by appropriate strength and conditioning interventions to improve muscle balance, strength, coordination and core stability; improved coaching cues for safe technique and movement mechanics; and by prioritising pre-play physical preparation, by incorporating a warm up before play.

Female-specific considerations for health and performance of players

Menstrual cycle

From the onset of periods during puberty (the average age for starting periods in the UK is 13 years) until the menopause a woman's body cycles through hormonal changes. This rhythm of hormonal fluctuation is called the menstrual cycle. In sport we have become accomplished at tuning into and taking advantage of the effects of hormones to inform our practises around priming, training adaptation, nutrition and recovery, but we've failed to really tune in, understand and capitalise on the menstrual cycle hormones in the same way.

The fluctuating levels of hormones across the menstrual cycle create four parts of the cycle where sex hormone levels and ratios are distinctly different from one another (see Figure 5.1). The menstrual cycle is typically described as a 28-day cycle (although only 13% of women actually have a 28-day cycle and anywhere between 23 and 35 days and up to 40 days in teens is considered normal (Bull et al., 2019). The first day of the cycle is the first day of the period. During the period (1), both hormones are at their lowest levels, after which oestrogen starts to rise to its peak in the late follicular phase (2). In the second half of the cycle both hormones rise, with progesterone peaking in the mid luteal phase (3), before both hormones drop down to low levels (4) again if this cycle hadn't resulted in pregnancy.

The hormonal fluctuations, and their influence on a woman's physiology, affects how women feel physically and emotionally. This can differ tremendously amongst women, and every female athlete's experience of her cycle, in relation to her wellbeing, training, recovery, and performance will be different. Importantly, research has shown that determinants of performance, such as VO_{2max}, speed and power are not affected by the changing physiology of the menstrual cycle (McNulty et al., 2020). However, the symptoms that a woman experiences can impact her ability to tap in to her performance potential on any given day of the cycle. When females are being negatively impacted by their cycle symptoms, there are numerous strategies that can be explored to alleviate these symptoms which range from diet, lifestyle, exercise, rest, recovery and stress management through to pharmacological interventions (Panay, 2011).

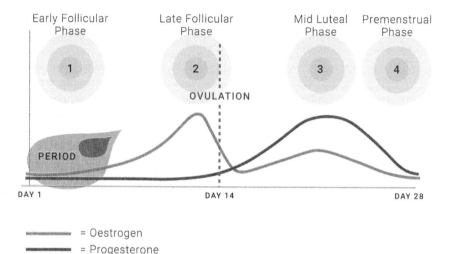

Figure 5.1 A typical menstrual cycle, showing fluctuations of oestrogen and progesterone, and the four points where hormone levels, and/or ratio of oestrogen
and progresterone are distinctly different. Published with permission from
The Well[HQ]

Up to 150 symptoms associated with the menstrual cycle have been reported
(Pizzorno et al., 2015) from gastrointestinal issues, brain fog, migraines, bloating,
abdominal pain, joint inflammation, anxiety, depression, and emotional sensitivity. Most symptoms are reported during the premenstrual phase, as a result of
the rapid withdrawal of both sex hormones at the end of the cycle, and during
the period, when the smooth muscle of the uterus contracts to expel its lining
through the vagina, as a bleed.

Managing heavy periods is also a significant consideration for women
golfers. Heavy menstrual bleeding (HMB) is defined as the perception of
increased bleeding during a period, and women may need frequent period
product changes or experience 'flooding' through clothes (Sheridan & Tarsha,
2018). This can be troublesome for female players, not least because of the
length of time taken for golf matches, often with lack of access to toilets, when
women may need to change their period products every two hours or less.
Athlete's report feeling anxiety if they are unsure of when they can change their
period products and fear leaking menstrual blood through their kit (Lofthouse,
2020). In a survey of female golfers, 33% of players reported experiencing heavy
periods (Ross & Smith, 2021), and this prevalence indicates that due consideration should be given to on-course toilet facilities. HMB also has implications
for health and training adaptation, since women with heavy periods are more
likely to suffer from iron deficiency (Bruinvels et al., 2016) which can compromise aerobic fitness via reduction total haemoglobin mass and therefore
oxygen carrying capacity (Hinton, 2014).

In a survey of over 100 female golfers, 55% experienced menstrual cycle symptoms that negatively affected their training or golf performance (Ross & Smith, 2021). Although tracking of training loads and wellness markers are increasingly popular practise in women's sport, menstrual cycle monitoring has only been reported in around 20% of active women (Heyward et al., 2020). Given the emerging evidence that menstrual cycle phase may influence players health and performance, it is widely recommended that cycle tracking is utilised as standard approach to supporting female athletes (Pitchers & Elliott-Sale, 2019). Menstrual cycle monitoring is a powerful tool for athletes, coaches and support staff alike. It allows an athlete to capture her own experience of the cycle, and how it influences her in the context of her life and her sport. At the very least it can help explain why some days feel better than others; at best it can produce patterns that can be anticipated, exploited, or overcome to optimise training, recovery and performance (Eliott-Sale et al., 2020). Monitoring the cycle requires recording the first day of the period, which indicates day one of the cycle, and over time, tracks cycle length. Physical and emotional changes can be recorded across the cycle, as well as sleep, muscle soreness, motivation to train and any injury or illness. Athletes should note how heavy their flow is during their period, which can help identify HMB. Menstrual cycle can be tracked using a calendar or digital app.

Cycle monitoring also helps women recognise when the cycle is unhealthy. The period is a vital sign of health, and loss of periods (amenorrhea) needs to be investigated. In athletes this is commonly a sign of under-fuelling or low energy availability, and it increases the risk of injury and illness and long-term poor health (Mountjoy et al., 2014; Mountjoy, 2018). Amenorrhea in athletes is often indicative of Relative Energy Deficiency in Sport (RED-S). RED-S still remains poorly recognised by health professionals, coaches and athletes (Curry et al., 2015) despite the significant impact it can have on athlete health. It has been recognised that education on RED-S within coaching qualifications is vital, yet researchers have identified that deficiencies exist in current coach development programmes, and these serve to undermine adequate support of female athlete health and performance (Hamer et al., 2021).

While determinants of performance may be unaffected across the cycle, adaptations to training might be. Oestrogen creates an 'anabolic' environment — one where muscle repair and growth is supported, through influences on antioxidative processes, cell membrane stability and satellite cell proliferation (Mangan et al., 2014). Because of this, researchers have sought to explore whether performing more resistance training in the first half of the cycle, when oestrogen rises to its peak, affects adaptation to resistance training regimes (Reis et al., 1995; Sung et al., 2014). When women 'compressed' strength training sessions into the first two weeks of the cycle, performing it on every other day, and then only performing two strength training sessions in the second half of the cycle, participants saw a 33% increase in muscular strength, compared to a 14% increase when training was scheduled in a more traditional way (Reis et al., 1995) and a 40% vs 28% increase when strength training was compressed in the first half of the cycle vs in the second half of the cycle, respectively (Sung et al., 2014). Consensus in this area is still emerging, yet training mapped to the menstrual cycle may offer another way in which coaches can individualise strength and conditioning programmes to optimise player adaptation.

Hormonal contraception and female athletes

About 50% of 18–30 year-old athletes use hormonal contraception, although for active women in their twenties this can be as high as 66%, dropping to about 11% in the mid-forties (Elflein, 2020). Just like the menstrual cycle, the physiological effects of the synthetic hormones delivered by the pill or other hormonal contraceptives don't just influence the reproductive system but can have consequences throughout the body, that can have positive and negative influences on health and performance of sportswomen, both acutely and chronically.

In addition to its primary purpose of preventing unwanted pregnancies, hormonal contraception can be a very effective strategy to manage severe cycle symptoms, like HMB debilitating period pains (particularly in the case of conditions like endometriosis), or to treat conditions like acne or polycystic ovarian syndrome. Many sportswomen find that using hormonal contraception can counteract the debilitating influences of their symptoms on their training and performance (Martin et al., 2018). However, there is also evidence that the pill can have effects that could be counter-productive for sportswomen, although the research in this area is still emerging (Elliot-Sale et al., 2020).

Women who use hormonal contraception don't have a period to rely on as a window into their health. The bleed that women experience on contraceptives like the pill (called a 'withdrawal bleed') is not the same as that caused by the shedding of the uterine lining, as occurs in a normal menstrual cycle. For players using hormonal contraception there is a risk that it masks RED-S, because, unlike periods which stop, withdrawal bleeds will still occur, even in the presence of prolonged low energy availability (Dudgeon, 2019). As such, greater attention to fuelling which matches the energy requirements for training and playing is needed in players using hormonal contraceptives.

A meta-analysis of performance measures in hormonal contraception athletes vs athletes with a natural menstrual cycle found 'a potentially negative influence' of oral contraceptive pill use on performance (Elliot-Sale et al., 2020). In particular, women whose aerobic capacity, assessed via $VO_{2\,max}$, was not changed across their natural menstrual cycle, saw an 11% decrease when they started taking the pill and peak power during a cycle ergometer test decreased concomitantly by 8%.

Using hormonal contraception is a very individual decision, made in the context of a woman's relationships, life and sport. Knowledge of whether the players you work with are using hormonal contraception gives you an awareness of additional factors that may be influencing health and performance.

Could breasts and bras influence female golf performance?

Since the breast is not actually supported by bone or muscle, it can be described as a wobbling mass situated on a rigid torso (Milligan et al., 2015). A female with a 34D bra size has an approximate additional mass of 460 g per breast, 920 g in total, on the torso (Turner & Dujon, 2005). As a result of this additional mass and the weak intrinsic breast support, the breast moves when a female participates in physical activity (Risius et al., 2017). Research in sporting activities has found breast movement to be linked with increased breast pain, tissue strain and embarrassment for participants. Recent research has also suggested breast displacement could result in performance losses in certain sports (McGhee & Steele, 2020). In particular, the impact of inadequate breast support changes the energy cost of movement and alters gait kinematics (Milligan et al., 2015). While these changes have mainly been observed during running, given the prolonged period of walking during golf match play, it could be postulated that poor breast support in female golfers (via a poorly fitting or unsupportive sports bra) might have similar deleterious effects on performance.

A strong indicator of overall golf ability is performance when hitting a driver, with focus on accuracy but more importantly distance and to improve distance, research suggests that golfers need to increase CHS (Broadie, 2014). Much male golf research has focused on increasing CHS through increasing ground reaction forces, kinematic sequencing (i.e., sequencing of segments) (Han et al., 2019) and increasing hand path length (MacKenzie et al., 2020). Increasing peak vertical forces significantly increases CHS (Han et al., 2019), and interestingly, good breast support has been shown to increase peak vertical ground forces (only tested thus far in running). It could therefore be postulated that a well fitted sports bra could contribute to optimising CHS. Changes to breast placement can also affect torso moment of inertia, which in turn could alter torso rotation and angular acceleration. This too could have significant effects on CHS in golf, where increases in torso range of motion increase hand path length. Further, torso inertia changes can help a player who struggles with segment sequence when the torso rotates and/or accelerates too late. While research in female golfers is still lacking, the available evidence suggests that the kinematics of the golf swing may be impacted by breast movement with a well fitted sports bra, providing optimal support for the breasts, positively influencing swing mechanics. However, in a survey of over 100 female golfers ranging from beginners to professionals (Ross & Smith, 2021), 41% of players reported wearing an everyday bra for golf. Everyday bras are considered low-support, and not do not afford the same reduction in breast movement as sports bras (Milligan et al., 2015). Thus, golfers could benefit, both performance and comfort, by wearing a well-fitted sports bra for training and match play. The University of Portsmouth Breast Health Research Group have established a five-point fit method which gives women the information they need to ensure their sports bra fits well enough to provide high breast support (Figure 5.2).

5 Point Bra fit

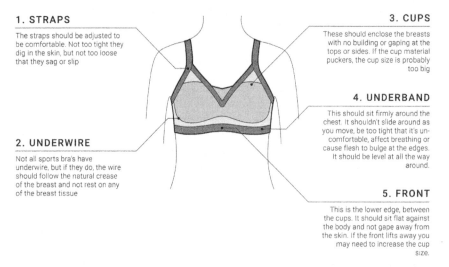

1. STRAPS

The straps should be adjusted to be comfortable. Not too tight they dig in the skin, but not too loose that they sag or slip

3. CUPS

These should enclose the breasts with no building or gaping at the tops or sides. If the cup material puckers, the cup size is probably too big

4. UNDERBAND

This should sit firmly around the chest. It shouldn't slide around as you move, be too tight that it's uncomfortable, affect breathing or cause flesh to bulge at the edges. It should be level at all the way around.

2. UNDERWIRE

Not all sports bra's have underwire, but if they do, the wire should follow the natural crease of the breast and not rest on any of the breast tissue

5. FRONT

This is the lower edge, between the cups. It should sit flat against the body and not gape away from the skin. If the front lifts away you may need to increase the cup size.

Figure 5.2 Rather than focusing on bra size, female golfers should ensure they have a good fit, to optimise breast support and minimise breast movement

Pelvic floor health in female golfers

Pelvic Floor dysfunction can include leaking urine, experiencing anxiety that you might leak or having irresistible urges to empty the bladder or bowels. It is often believed that urinary incontinence (UI) is mainly a problem of elderly and post-natal women. However, recent data shows that female athletes actually have up to three times higher chance of suffering with urinary incontinence than the general population (Bø & Nygaard, 2020; Almeida et al., 2016).

The pelvis is home to organs like the bladder, uterus and rectum, and the pelvic floor muscles are the home's foundation. These muscles act as the support structure keeping everything in place adding support to several organs by wrapping around the pelvic bone. Some of these muscles add more stability by forming a sling around the rectum. The pelvic floor is interconnected to many key structures in the body, and dysfunction here can affect seemingly unrelated parts of the body (Parrotte, 2017). Adequate function of the pelvic floor including the pelvic floor muscles, connective tissue and nervous system, is crucial in counteracting increases in intra-abdominal pressure and ground reaction forces (Bø & Nygaard, 2020) in female golfers. Aside from causing embarrassment and anxiety, dysfunction of the pelvic floor muscles can result pain in the hip, groin or back, and subsequently increase injury risk, or alter gait or swing mechanics (Gill, 2020).

The cause for UI in athletes is still unclear. Young female athletes often experience significant and sudden intra-abdominal pressure increases, especially during high-impact activities such as running and jumping or during a Valsalva manoeuvre during strength training (holding breath while exerting effort), which may play a role in UI. In addition, the cause may be related to female athletes having very strong pelvic floor muscles from continued training of the abdominal muscle, which become overactive leading to an inability to relax or coordinate the pelvic floor muscles effectively.

Female golfers should take a proactive and preventive approach to pelvic floor health, by performing pelvic floor exercises daily. Like every muscle in the body that needs to adapt, the pelvic floor needs to be stimulated, worked and coordinated, mobilised and rested. Many women do not know how to perform pelvic floor exercises correctly, and research has shown that athletes with good knowledge about pelvic floor training are less likely to develop symptoms of dysfunction such as UI (Cardoso et al., 2018). There are also ways that coaches can work with female players to help them manage their intra-abdominal pressure and work with their pelvic floor in training. For example, being mindful of when players are using the breath holding technique to create tension in the core (the Valsalva manoeuvre) during strength training. In women, when there is an increase in pressure above the vagina (intra-abdominal pressure), the pelvic organs are not supported well and there is a risk of prolapse. Our recommendation is to manage core pressure by encouraging players to exhale during the lift when performing sub-maximal and lighter training sets. Saving the breath hold until it's functionally necessary, on the heavier lifts, is an excellent way of supporting the pelvic organs in training.

We must not normalise incontinence as 'just a part of doing sport', but instead work to encourage athletes to seek advice and support if they are experiencing urine leakage at any time. Women's health physiotherapists are experienced at identifying and treating pelvic floor dysfunction. The *Pelvic Obstetric and Gynaecological Physiotherapy network* can be contacted to find local chartered NHS and private practitioners.

Across a player's lifespan

Although every woman's experience of each life stage is unique, there are predictable and inevitable physiological changes across these life stages, which will influence a woman's motivation and ability to exercise and play sport. This section is simply to highlight that women golfers are not a homogenous group, particularly as they go through each life stage – the approach to supporting and coaching them needs to take into account their changing physiology and psychology and seek to understand their needs at each of these times.

Adolescence

This is a time when girls feel especially vulnerable. Their bodies are changing, and they are discovering who they are. They can have real concerns about their body image, and they lack confidence about trying new things. These factors can interfere with a girl's relationship with sport and exercise, or even become a barrier to taking part in sport (Youth Sport Trust, 2017). Dropout rates for girls in sport are much higher than boys and they tend to withdraw at an earlier age (Women in Sport, 2019).

Research into engaging and retaining teenage girls in sport (Women in Sport, 2019) demonstrated that the top three factors in ensuring sport is an environment where girls want to be are:

1. Remove judgement: Take the pressure off performing and give girls a space to simply play and to move.
2. Invoke excitement: Bring a sense of adventure and discovery to sport and training.
3. Develop clear emotional rewards: Don't always make achievement about winning, but about moments of personal achievement, or things that make girls proud of themselves.

The post-natal golfer

Every woman's pregnancy and post-natal experience will be different. As coaches and practitioners supporting active women, we can't anticipate how women will recover from birth, and so really tuning into them and listening is essential. Births rarely go to plan and for a physically capable person, it can be quite a shock and even traumatic. Processing the birth with a skilled professional such as a psychotherapist is really important for someone who wants to return to training regularly. Most importantly, healing and recovery must come first, before training and fitness.

In the weeks after birth, time should be spent restoring the core, mobilising and slowly increasing endurance through walking. These initial steps are fundamental for recovery and to be to able to train at a higher intensity later on. The key points to note with post-natal training are:

1. Pelvic floor work can start straight away – ideally under the guidance of a women's health physiotherapist.
2. The six-week sign-off from the GP or nurse does not indicate training readiness.
3. Running and/or impact work is not recommended to any woman post-natally, regardless of the kind of delivery she had, for twelve weeks.

The reader is signposted to Goom, Donnelly, & Brockwell (2019), an excellent, evidence-based resource for practitioners, therapists and fitness professionals to help return women to training after birth.

Menopause

The menopause is experienced by every female at some point in her life and is when the ovaries stop releasing eggs (and the hormones oestrogen and progesterone) and periods stop. It marks the end of a woman's fertile years. The menopause can be natural, in which case it occurs when a woman hasn't had a period for over a year above the age of 50 or for two years above the age of 45. Or the menopause can be medical (when a woman is given medication to supress her ovaries, say for example with a condition like endometriosis) or surgical (when the ovaries are surgically removed, for example for breast cancer prevention).

Every woman's experience of menopause is unique, but most (about 80%) women will experience some symptoms, the most common ones being hot flushes and night sweats. Other symptoms include insomnia, brain-fog, muscle and joint aches, panic attacks and irritability, weight gain, mood swings, prolapse, urinary incontinence, constipation and vaginal dryness (Bruce & Rymer, 2009). Although these symptoms can become a barrier to exercise for some women, exercise can often improve symptoms (Stojanovska et al., 2014). For its long-term positive effects on cardiac, bone and muscle, and psychological health, exercising beyond menopause has been established as the only non-controversial and beneficial aspect of lifestyle modification (Mishra et al., 2011). Exercise programmes for menopausal women should include weight bearing endurance exercise, strength, and balance training (Mishra et al., 2011).

Coaching the female golfer

While there are more similarities than differences between males and females with regards to sports psychology; differences do occur in goal orientation, sources of confidence, cohesion and preferred coaching styles (Roberts, 2019). About 95% of golf coaches are male (PGA of America, 2010), so it is important to acknowledge that the inability of male coaches to understand how best to engage with female athletes has been recognised as a key barrier to participation, engagement and progression in girls and women in sport (Norman & French, 2013).

Whereas research shows that male coaches prefer an autocratic style of coaching, female players tend to prefer a more democratic approach, where the coaching or training is a joint endeavour, where decisions are made together and the rationale for decisions is explored (Norman, 2016). Female athletes also place more value on being supported as a person, as well as a performer, wanting a good quality personal relationship with their coach or trainer. Females also need enjoyment to be part of their sporting experience, and a sense of enjoyment and adventure has been shown to improve female's motivation in sport and exercise (MacKinnon, 2011).

Since females often have lower feelings of efficacy, lower perception of their athletic ability (Poiss et al., 2004) and lower confidence levels (Krane & Williams, 1994), it is important for coaches and practitioners to understand how to build confidence in female players. While male athletes tend to derive confidence from comparing themselves to others and winning, female athletes tend to derive confidence from their coach's encouragement and positive feedback, and from mastering skills and achieving personal goals (Hays et al., 2009).

The retention rate of women in golf is less favourable than men, 33% versus 53% respectively (PGA of America, 2010). A possible reason as to why women are not continuing to play golf could be that traditional instructional programmes are not meeting women's needs. By focusing on instructional techniques for a gendered perspective, it is possible that guidelines could be developed to improve the way golf is taught to women (MacKinnon, 2011). That is not to say that males cannot successfully teach female athletes, but that more can be done to help educate male professionals on the importance of adequate understanding of gender differences in golf instruction, both physiologically and psychologically. Golf professionals should be encouraged to develop instructional programmes that are tailored to the individual and that male instructional programmes (both physical and psychological) might not be as well suited for the female golfer.

A similar thought process can be utilised when delivering S&C support to female golfers. As the level of female sporting performance and professionalism increases, so too must our understanding of how to optimise a female's athletic performance (Pitchers & Elliott-Sale, 2019). This chapter has touched on the key anatomical, physiological, and psychological differences and considerations and this information and understanding is the first port of call to aid anyone in optimising their delivery of S&C to female athletes. It is even more prudent to ensure that this knowledge is present in the S&C coaching community, since the majority of accredited S&C coaches are male as shown by the statistics in both the UK where 93% of S&C coaches are male (Stewart et al., 2016) and USA where 86.1% of NCAA S&C coaches are male (Lapchick et al., 2019). This gender disparity within S&C coaches highlights the fact that simply understanding through self-experience (as is done in quite a few coaching contexts), cannot be relied upon for these scenarios and instead, education is key.

Conclusion

Female participation in golf is rising, and there is appetite and support from the game's infrastructure to help women's golf realise its potential. However, the current reality is that there is a gender imbalance in golf, and while progress is being made, much more needs to be done. Research shows that golf isn't the most welcoming environment to women, its male-dominated, intimidating culture, often stops women from taking up the game, and causes them to leave (STERF, 2014). Increasing participation and performance in the women's game will depend on a changing culture to ensure that girls and women feel like they belong in the sport, equally. There also needs to be an acknowledgement that equality does not mean doing the same thing for everyone, but that different people will need a different approach to give them an equal opportunity to fulfil their potential in golf. In strength and conditioning, there are important differences between male and female athletes that mean we cannot simply apply the evidence derived from research in male players, on to our practise in female players without careful consideration. Neither can we overlook important female-specific factors such as the menstrual cycle, hormonal contraceptive use, breast health, pelvic health, injury risk and female psychology. There are exciting and rewarding opportunities for coaches of female players to develop their skills and expertise to allow them to support female players fulfil their performance potential and sustain a lifelong enjoyment of the game.

Acknowledgements

With thanks to Lewis Clarke, Tim Exell, Joanna Wakefield-Scurr (University of Portsmouth, Breast Health Research Group) and Baz Moffat (The Well[HQ]) for their contributions to the writing of this chapter.

References

Adachi, N., Nawata, N., Maeta, M., & Kurozawa, Y. (2008). Relationship of the menstrual cycle phase to anterior cruciate ligament injuries in teenaged female athletes. *Arch. Orthop. Trauma Surg., 128*: 473–478.

Alexander, D. L., & Kern, W. (2005). Drive for Show and Putt for Dough?: An Analysis of the Earnings of PGA Tour Golfers. *Journal of Sports Economics, 6*: 46–60.

Almeida, B., Barra, A., & Saltiel, F. (2016). Urinary incontinence and other pelvic floor dysfunction in female athletes in Brazil: A cross-sectional study. *Scandinavian Journal of Medicine and Science in Sports, 26*(9): 1109–1116.

Ansdell, P., Thomas, K., Howatson, G., Hunter, S., & Goodall, S. (2017). Contraction intensity and sex differences in knee-extensor fatigability. *Journal of Electromyography and Kinesiology*, 68–74.

Ashford, J. (2017). *Why Women Love Golf*. Retrieved November 2020, from www.exeter gcc.co.uk/news/why-women-golf/

Bø, K., & Nygaard, I. (2020). Is Physical Activity Good or Bad for the Female Pelvic Floor? A Narrative Review. *Sports Medicine, 50*(3): 471–484.

Barker, K., & Sargent, D. (2018). *Strength and Conditioning for Female Athletes*. Marlborough: Crowood.

Batt, M. E. (1992). A survey of golf injuries in amateur golfers. *Br J Sports Med, 26*(1): 63–65.

Behm, D. G., & Chaouachi, A. (2011). A review of the effects of static and dynamic stretching on performance. *Eur J Appl Physiol, 111*: 2633–2651.

Belkin, D. S., Gansneder, B., Pickens, M., Rotella, R. J., & Striegel, D. (1994). Predictability and Stability of Professional Golf Assocciation Tour Statistics. *Perceptual and Motor Skils, 78*: 1275–1280.

Betzler, N. F., Monk, S. A., Wallace, E. S., & Otto, S. R. (2014). The relationships between driver clubhead presentation characteristics, ball launch conditions and golf shot outcomes. *J Sports Eng Tech, 228*: 242–249.

Brearley, S. L., Coughlan, D., & Tilley, N. (2019). *Training the modern golfer: Jazz Janewattananond*. Retrieved from European Tour: www.europeantour.com/europ ean-tour/news/articles/detail/training-the-modern-golfer-jazz-janewattananond/

Bridge, M., Perry, M., & Li, F. X. (2008). The warm-up behaviours of elite female golfers. In D. Crews, & R. Lutz, *Science and Golf V.* (pp. 120–127). Mesa, AZ: Energy in Motion.

Broadie, M. (2014). *Every Shot Counts*. New York: Avery Publishing Group.

Brown, S. J., Nevill, A. M., Monk, S. A., Otto, S. R., Selbie, W. S., & Wallace, E. S. (2011). Determination of the swing technique characteristics and performance outcome relationship in golf driving for low handicap female golfers. *Journal of sports sciences, 29*(14): 1483–1491. https://doi.org/10.1080/02640414.2011.605161

Bruce, D., & Rymer, J. (2009). Symptoms of the Menopause. *Best Practice & Research Clinical Obstetrics & Gynaecology, 23*(1): 25–32.

Bruinvels, G., Burden, R., Brown, N., Richards, & Pedlar, C. (2016). The Prevalence and Impact of Heavy Menstrual Bleeding (Menorrhagia) in Elite and Non-Elite Athletes. *PloS one, 11*(2): e0149881.

Bull, J. R., Rowland, S. P., Scherwitzl, E. B., Scherwitzl, R., Danielsson, K. G., & Harper, J. (2019). Real-world menstrual cycle characteristics of more than 600,000 menstrual cycles. *Npi Digital Medicine, 2*(83). https://doi.org/10.1038/s41746-019-0152-7

Cardoso, A., Lima, C., & Ferreira, C. (2018). Prevalence of urinary incontinence in high impact sports athletes and their association with knowledge, attitude and practice about this dysfunction. *Sports and Exercise Medicine and Health* (1405–1412).

Chidi-Ogbolu, N., & Baar, K. (2019). Effect of Estrogen on Musculoskeletal Performance and Injury Risk. *Frontiers in physiology, 9*: 1834.

Costello, J., Bieuzen, F., & Bleakley, C. (2014). Where are all the female particpants in sport and exercise medicine research? *European Journal of Sports Science*: 847–851.

Coughlan, D., Taylor, M. J., Jackson, J., Ward, N., & Beardsley, C. (2020). Physical characteristics of youth elite golfers and their relationship with driver clubhead speed. *The Journal of Strength & Conditioning Research, 34*(1): 212–217.

Coughlan, D., Tilley, N., & Brearley, S. L. (2019). *Training Champions with ETPI - Andrea Pavan*. Retrieved from Golf & Health: www.golfandhealth.org/news/training-champions-with-etpi-andrea-pavan/

Cowley, E. S., Olenick, A. A., McNulty, K., & Ross, E. (2021). "Invisible Sportswomen": The Sex Data Gap in Sport and Exercise Science Research. *Women in Sport and Physical Activity Journal, 29*(2): 146–151.

Crossley, Kay, & al., P. e. (2020). Making football safer for women: A systematic review and meta-Analysis of injury prevention programmes in 11 773 female football (soccer) players. *British Journal of Sports Medicine, 54*: 1089–1098.

Curry, E., Logan, C., & Ackerman, K. e. (2015). Female Athlete Triad Awareness Among Multispecialty Physicians. *Sports Med, 38*. https://doi.org/10.1186/s40798-015-0037-5

Deie, M., Sakamaki, Y., Sumen, Y., Urabe, Y., & Ikuta, Y. (2002). Anterior knee laxity in young women varies with their menstrual cycle. *International Orthopedics, 26*(3): 154–156.

Delmonico, M., Kostek, M., Doldo, N., Hand, B., Bailey, J., Rabon-Stith, K., . . . Hurley, B. (2005). Effects of moderate-velocity strength training on peak muscle power and movement velocity: do women respond differently than men? *J Appl Phys*: 1712–1718.

Dorsel, T. N., & Rotunda, R. J. (2001). Low Scores, Top 10 Finishes, and Big Money: An Analysis of Professional Golf Assocciation Tour Statistics and How These Relate to Overall Performance. *Perceptual and Motor Skills, 92*: 575–585.

Dudgeon, E. (2019). *British Journal of Sports Medicine Blog: Relative energy deficiency in sport (RED-S): recognition and next steps*. Retrieved June 2020, from https://blogs.bmj.com/bjsm/2019/04/22/relative-energy-deficiency-in-sport-red-s-recognition-and-next-steps/

Ehlert, A., & Wilson, P. B. (2019). A Systematic Review of Golf Warm-ups: Behaviours, Injury, and Performance. *The Journal of Strength and Conditioning Research*, *33*(12): 3444–3462. https://doi.org/10.1519/JSC.0000000000003329

Ekin, J. A., & Sinaki, M. (1993). Vertebral compression fractures sustained during golfing; report of three cases. *Mayo Clin Proc*, *68*(6): 566–570.

Elflein, J. (2020). *Contraceptive use among women in England 2019/20, by type and ag*. Statista. www.statista.com/statistics/573210/contraceptive-use-among-women-by-type-and-age-in-england/

Eliott Sale, K., Hicks, K., Burden, R., & Ross, E. (2020). The BASES Expert Statement on conducting and implementing female athlete based research, *65*: 6–7)

Elliot-Sale, K., McNulty, K., Andsell, P., Goodall, S., Hicks, K., Thomas, K., Dolean, E. (2020). The Efects of Oral Contraceptives on Exercise Performance in Women. *Sports Medicine*, 50(10): 1785–1812.

Ennus, D. L., & Tiidus, P. M. (2010). The influence of estrogen on skeletal muscle. *Sports Med*, *40*: 41–58.

FIFA. (2008). *FIFA 11+ Manual*. Retrieved 2018, from www.fifamedicalnetwork.com/wp-content/uploads/cdn/11plus_workbook_e.pdf

Forsyth, J., & Roberts, C. (2019). *The Exercising Female: Science and its Application*. Abingdon: Routledge.

Fradkin, A.J., Windley, T.C., Myers, J.B., Sell, T, C., & Lephart, S. (2007) Describing the epidemiology and associated age, gender and handicap comparisons of golfing injuries, International Journal of Injury Control and Safety Promotion, *14*(4): 264–266, DOI: 10.1080/17457300701722585

Gergley, J. (2009). Acute effects of passive static stretching during warm-up on driver clubhead speed, driving distance, accuracy, and consistent ball contact in young male competitive golfers. *The Journal of Strength & Conditioning Research*, *23*(3): 863–867.

Gill, L. (2020). *PGA Tour Active: The Pelvic Powerhouse*. Retrieved June 2021, from www.pgatour.com/active/instruction/golf-fitness-plans-stretching-mobilitiy-exercises-workout-routine-pelvic-powerhouse.html

Goom, T., Donnelly, G., & Brockwell, E. (2019). *Returning to running postnatal – guidelines for medical, health and fitness professionals managing this population*. Retrieved 2019, from https://mailchi.mp/38feb9423b2d/returning-to-running-postnatal-guideline

Gosheger, G., Liem, D., Ludwig, K., Greshake, O., & Winklemann, W. (2003). Injuries and overuse syndromes in golf. *Am J Sports Med*, *31*(3): 438–443.

Grelsamer, R. P., Dubey, A., & Weinstein, C. H. (2005). Men and women have similar Q angles. *The Journal of Bones & Joint Surgery (Br)*, 87, 1498–1501.

Hamer, J., Desbrow, B., & Irwin, C. (2021). Are Coaches of Female Athletes Informed of Relative Energy Deficiency in Sport? A Scoping Review. *Women in Sport and Physical Activity Journal*, *29*(1): 38–46.

Ki Hoon Han, Christopher Como, Jemin Kim, Cheng-Ju Hung, Mohammad Hasan & Young-Hoo Kwon (2019) Effects of pelvis-shoulders torsional separation style on kinematic sequence in golf driving. *Sports Biomechanics*, *18*(6): 663–685, DOI: 10.1080/14763141.2019.1629617

Hays, K., Thomas, I., Maynard, I., & Bawden, M. (2009). The role of confidence in world-class sport performance. *Journal of Sports Sciences*, *27*(11): 1185–1199.

Hegedus, E. J., Hardesty, K. W., Sunderland, K. L., Hegedus, R. J., & Smoliga, J. M. (2016). A randomized trial of traditional and golf-specific resistance training in amateur female golfers: Benefits beyond golf performance. *Physical therapy in sport: official journal of the Association of Chartered Physiotherapists in Sports Medicine*, *22*: 41–53. https://doi.org/10.1016/j.ptsp.2016.04.005

Heyward, O., Nicholson, B., S, E., G, R., & B, J. (2020). Physical Preparation in Female Rugby Codes: An Investigation of Current Practices . *Frontiers in Sports and Active Living*, 2: 177.

Hicks, A., Kent-Braun, J., & Ditor, D. (2001). Sex differences in human skeletal muscle fatigue. *Exercise Sport and Science Review*, *29*, 109–112.

Hinton, P. (2014). Iron and the endurance athlete. *Appl Physiol Nutr Metab, 39*: 1012–1018.

Horan, S. A., Evans, K., & Kavanagh, J. J. (2011). Movement variability in the golf swing of male and female skilled golfers. *Medicine and science in sports and exercise*, *43*(8): 1474–1483. https://doi.org/10.1249/MSS.0b013e318210fe03

Hosea, T. M., Gatt, C. J., & Langrana, N. A. (1990). Biomechanical analysis of the golfer's back. In A. J. Cochran, *Science and Golf I: Proceedings of the World Scientific Congress of Golf* (pp. 43–48). London: E & FN Spon.

Hume, P. A., Keogh, J., & Reid, D. (2005). The role of biomechanics in maximising distance and accuracy of golf shots. *Sports Med, 35*: 429–449.

Hunter, G. R. (1985). Changes in body composition, body build and performance associated with different weight training frequencies in males and females. *Strength and Conditioning Journal*, 7(1): 26–28.

Hunter, S. (2009). Sex differences and mechanisms of task-specific muscle fatigue. *Exercise and Sport Science Reviews*: 113–22.

Hunter, S. (2016). Sex differences in fatigability of dynamic contractions. *Experimental physiology*: 250–255.

IOC. (2020). *Statistics*. Retrieved from International Olympic Committee: www.olympic.org/women-in-sport/background/statistics

Kim, K.J. (2010). Effects of Core Muscle Strengthening Training on Flexibility, Muscular Strength and Driver Shot Performance in Female Professional Golfers. *International Journal of Applied Sports Sciences*, *22*(1): 111–127

Krane, V., & Williams, J. M. (1994). Cognitive anxiety, somatic anxiety, and confidence in track and field athletes: The impact of gender, competitive level and task characteristics. *International Journal of Sport Psychology*, *25*(2): 203–217.

Lamb, P. F., & Pataky, T. C. (2018). The role of pelvis-thorax coupling in controlling within-golf club swing speed. *Journal of Sports Sciences*, *36*(19): 2164–2171.

Lapchick, R., Ariza, P., Ellis, C., Gladney, D., Hudson, I., Mali, M., & Vasquez, A. (2019). *The 2019 racial and gender report card: College sport*.

Lindsay, D. M., & Vandervoort, A. A. (2014). Golf-Related Low Back Pain: A Review of Causative Factors and Prevention Strategies. *Asian J Sports Med, 5*(4): e24289. https://doi.org/10.5812/asjsm.24289

Lofthouse, A. (2020). *BBC Elite SportsWoman survey*. Retrieved August 2020, from www.bbc.co.uk/sport/53705777

MacKinnon, V. (2011). Techniques for instructing female athletes in traditionally male sports: A case study of LPGA teaching professionals. *The International Journal of Sport and Society*, *2*(1): 75–87.

Mair, L. (2016). *Gentlemen Only, Ladies Forbidden – a history*. Retrieved from Womans Golf Journal: https://womensgolfjournal.com/golf/no-women-allowed/

Malinzak, R., Colby, S., Kirkendall, D., Bing, Y., & William, G. (2001). A comparison of knee joint motion patterns between men and women in selected athletic tasks. *Clinical Biomechanics*, *10*(16): 438–445.

Mangan, G., Bombardier, E., Mitchell, A., Quadrilatero, J., & Tiidus, P. (2014). Oestrogen-dependent satellite cell activation and proliferation following a running exercise occurs via the PI3K signalling pathway and not IGF-1. . *Acta Physiol (Oxf)*, *212*(1): 75–85.

Martin, D., Sale, C., Cooper, S. B., & & Elliott-Sale, K. J. (2018). Period Prevalence and Perceived Side Effects of Hormonal Contraceptive Use and the Menstrual Cycle in Elite Athletes. *International Journal of Sports Physiology and Performance*, *13*(7): 926.

McCarroll, J. R., & Gioe, T. J. (1982). Professional golfers and the price they pay. *Phys Sportsmed*, *10*(7): 64–70.

McCarroll, J. R., Retting, A. C., & Shelbourne, K. D. (1990). Injuries in the amateur golfer. *Phys Sportsmed*, *18*(3): 122–126.

McGhee, D. E., & Steele, J. R. (2020). Biomechanics of Breast Support for Active Women. *Exercise and sport sciences reviews*, *48*(3): 99–109. https://doi.org/10.1249/ JES.0000000000000221

McGowan, C. J., Pyne, D. B., Thompson, K. G., & Rattray, B. (2015). Warm-up strategies for sport and exercise: MEchanisms and applications. *Sports Med*, *45*: 1523–1546.

McHardy, A., Pollard, H., & Luo, K. (2006). Golf injuries; A review of the literature. *Sports Med*, *36*(2): 171–187.

McHardy, A., Pollard, H., & Luo, K. (2007). Golf-related lower back injuries: an epidemiological survey. *J Chiropr Med*, *6*(1): 20–26.

MacKenzie, S., McCourt, M., & Champoux, L. (2020). How Amateur Golfers Deliver Energy to the Driver. *International Journal of Golf Science*, *8*(1): 12640.

McNulty, K., Elliott-Sale, K., Dolan, E., Swinton, P., Ansdell, P., Goodall, S., Thomas, K., & Hicks, K.M. (2020). The Effects of Menstrual Cycle Phase on Exercise Performance in Eumenorrheic Women: A Systematic Review and Meta-Analysis. *Sports Medicine*, 1813–1827.

Milligan, A., Mills, C., Corbett, J., & Scurr, J. (2015). The influence of breast support on torso, pelvis and arm kinematics during a five kilometer treadmill run. *Human Movement Science*, *42*: 246–260.

Mishra, N., Mishra, V., & Devanshi, V. (2011). Exercise beyond menopause: Dos and Don'ts. *Journal of Midlife Health*, *2*(2): 51–56.

Mountjoy, M. (2018). IOC consensus statement on relative energy deficiency in sport (RED-S). *British Journal of Sports Medicine*, 52: 687–697.

Mountjoy, M., Sundgot-Borgen, J., & Burke, L. e. (2014). The IOC consensus statement: beyond the Female Athlete Triad – relative energy deficiency in sport (RED-S). *British Journal of Sports Medicine*, 48(7): 491–497.

Moy, R. L., & Liaw, T. (1998). Determinants of Professional Golf Tournament Earnings. *The American Economist*, *42*: 65–70.

Myer, G., Ford, K., P. M., N. T., & ., H. E. (2008). The effects of generalized joint laxity on risk of anterior cruciate ligament injury in young female athletes. *Am. J. Sports Med*, *36*: 1073–1080.

NCD-RiscC. (2020, Nov 7). Height and body-mass index trajectories of school-aged children and adolescents from 1985 to 2019 in 200 countries and territories: a pooled analysis of 2181 population-based studies with 65 million participants. *The Lancet*, *396*(10261). Retrieved from World Data.

Nero, P. (2001). Relative Salary Efficiency of PGA Tour Golfers. *The American Economist*, *45*: 51–56.

Norman, L. (2016). Is there a need for coaches to be gender responsive? A review of the evidence. *International Sports Coaching Journal*, *3*(2): 192–196.

Norman, L., & French, J. (2013). Understanding how high performance women athletes experience coach-athlete relationship. *International Journal of Coaching Science*, 7: 3–24.

Panay, N. (2011). Managment of premenstrual syndrome: evidence-based guidleines. *Ostetrics, Gynaecology and Reproductive Medicine*, 8(2): 221–228.

Parker, J., Hellström, J., Olsson, C. (2019) Differences in kinematics and driver performance in elite female and male golfers, Sports Biomechanics, DOI: 10.1080/14763141.2019.1683221

Parrotte, K. (2017). *It's all connected: How pelvic floor dysfunction can contribute to hip pain*. Retrieved November 2020, from https://beyondbasicsphysicaltherapy.com/blogs/blog/it-s-all-connected-how-pelvic-floor-dysfunction-can-contribute-to-hip-pain

Pitchers, G., & Elliott-Sale, K. (2019). Considerations for coaches training female athletes. *Professional Strength and Conditioning* (55): 19–30.

Pines, A., & Berry, E, M. (2007) Exercise in the menopause – an update. *Climacteric*, 10(sup2): 42–46, DOI: 10.1080/13697130701600153

Pizzorno, J., Murray, M., & Joiner-Be, H. (2015). Premenstrual Syndrome. In J. Pizzorno, M. Murray, & H. Joiner-Be (Eds.): *The Clinician's Handbook of Natural Medicine* (3rd ed., p. 830). London: Churchill Livingstone.

Poiss, C. C., Sullivan, P. A., Paup, D. C., & Westerman, B. J. (2004). Perceived importance of weight training to selected NCAA Division III men and women student-athletes. *Strength and Conditioning Research*, 18: 108–114, DOI:10.1519/00124278-200402000-00016.

Power, K., Behm, D., Cahill, F., Carroll, M., & Young, W. (2004). An acute bout of static stretching: effects on force and jumping performance. *Medicine & Science in Sports & Exercise*, 36(8): 1389–1369.

Professional Golfers' Association of America. (2010). *The research deck: The consumer marketing department: Women in golf*. Retrieved from Professional Golfers' Association of America.

Queen, R. (2017). Infographic: ACL injury reconstruction and recovery. *Bone & joint research*, 6(11): 621–622.

R&A. (2020). *Women in Golf Charter*. Retrieved November 2020, from www.englandgolf.org/wp-content/uploads/2020/10/RA_003_FOREeveryone_Toolkit_EnglandGolf.pdf

Read, P. J., Lloyd, R., De Ste Croix, M., & Oliver, J. (2012). Relationship between field-based measure of strength and power and golf club head speed. *The Journal of Strength & Conditioning Research*, 27: 2708–2713.

Reis, E., Frick, U., & Schmidtbleicher, D. (1995). Frequency variations of strength training sessions triggered by the phases of the menstrual cycle. *Int J Sports Med.*, 16(8): 545–550.

Reuter, P. R., & Fichthorn, K. R. (2019). Prevalence of generalized joint hypermobility, musculoskeletal injuries, and chronic musculoskeletal pain among American university students. *PeerJ*, 7: e7625. https://doi.org/10.7717/peerj.7625

Risius, D., Milligan, A., Berns, J., Brown, N., & Scurr, J. (2017) Understanding key performance indicators for breast support: An analysis of breast support effects on biomechanical, physiological and subjective measures during running, Journal of Sports Sciences, 35(9): 842–851, DOI: 10.1080/02640414.2016.1194523

Roberts, C. -M. (2019). The psychology of female sport performance. In &. C.-M. J. Forsyth, *The exercising Female: Science and its application* (pp. 175–186). Abingdon: Routledge.

Rose, G. (2013, May 28). *My TPI.* Retrieved from Improve My Game - Articles: www.mytpi.com/articles/screening/the_seated_trunk_rotation_test

Roser, M. R., Appel, C., & Ritchie, H. (2019, May). *Human Height.* Retrieved from Our World In Data: https://ourworldindata.org/human-height#how-has-height-chan ged-globally

Ross, E., & Smith, F. (2021). *Female Golfer Survey.* Retrieved September 2021

Sheridan, T., & Tarsha, S. (2018). *British Journal of Sport Medicine Blog: Heavy menstrual bleeding (HMB) in female athletes [Part 1: Recognition and diagnosis].* Retrieved June 2021, from https://blogs.bmj.com/bjsm/2018/12/31/heavy-menstrual-bleeding- hmb-in-female-athletes-part-1-recognition-and-diagnosis/

STERF. (2014). *The Opportunity to Grow Golf: Female Particpation.* Retrieved July 2021, from www.sterf.org/Media/Get/1741/the-opportunity-to-grow-golf-female- participation.pdf

Stewart, P., Maughan, P., & Turner, A. (2016). A review of strength and conditioning internships: The UKSCA's state of the nation survey. *Professional Strength & Conditioning* (43): 27–33.

Stojanovska, L., Apostolopoulos, V., Polman, R., & Borkoles, E. (2014). To exercise, or, not to exercise, during menopause and beyond,. *Maturitas*, 77(4): 318–323.

Sung, E., Han, A., Hinrichs, T., Vorgerd, M., Manchado, C., & Platen, P. (2014). Effects of follicular versus luteal phase-based strength training in young women. *SpringerPlus*, 3: 668. https://doi.org/10.1186/2193-1801-3-668

Sweeney, M., Mills, P., Alderson, J., & Elliott, B. (2013). The influence of club-head kine- matics on early ball flight characteristics in the golf drive. *Sports Biomech*, 12: 247–258.

Tilley, N., & Brearley, S. (2020, Aug 12). *How the best golfers in the world are using Strength & Conditioning to elevate their performance.* Retrieved from BMJ Blogs: https://blogs. bmj.com/bjsm/2020/08/12/how-the-best-golfers-in-the-world-are-using-stren gth-conditioning-to-elevate-their-performance/

Triplett, N. T., & Stone, M. (2016). The female athlete. In D. Joyce, & D. Lewingdon, *Sport injury prevention and rehabilitation* (pp. 429–435). Abington: Routledge.

Trolloppe, M. (2017). *Men's and Women's Tennis: As Different as Believed?* Retrieved February 2021. https://tennismash.com/2017/02/16/mens-womens-tennis-differ ent-seem/

Turner, A. J., & Dujon, D. G. (2005). Predicting cup size after reduction mammaplasty. *British journal of plastic surgery*, 58(3): 290–298. https://doi.org/ 10.1016/j.bjps.2004.11.008

Van Herp, G., Rowe, P. J., & Salter, P. M. (2000). Range of Motion in the Lumbar Spine and the Effects of Age and Gender. *Physiotherapy*, 86(1): 42.

Walner, C. (2019). *ATP vs WTA: Anatomy Of Great Groundstrokes.* Retrieved Jan 2020, from https://serveandvolleytennis.com/atp-vs-wta-anatomy-of-great-ground strokes/

Ward, J. (2019). *Using Evidence Based Practises to Keep More Women in Tennis.* Retrieved February 2021, from https://wctatennis.org/using-evidence-based-practices-to- keep-more-women-in-tennis-jo-ward/

Wells, G. D., Elmi, M., & Thomas, S. (2009). Physiological correlates of golf perform- ance. *Journal of strength and conditioning research*, 23(3): 741–750. https://doi.org/ 10.1519/JSC.0b013e3181a07970

Wells, J. E., & Langdown, B. L. (2018). Warm-Up Habits Of Highly-Skilled Golfers Prior To Practice And Tournament Conditions. *World Scientific Scientific Congress of Golf.* Abbotsford, BC, Canada.

Wells, J. E., Charalambous, L. H., Mitchell, A. C., Coughlan, D., Brearley, S. L., Hawkes, R. A., . . . Fletcher, I. M. (2019). Relationships between Challenge Tour golfer's clubhead velocity and force producing capacbilities during a countermovement jump and isometric mid-thigh pull. *Journal of Sports Sciences, 37*(12): 1381–1386.

Wells, J. E., Mitchell, A. C., Charalambous, L. H., & Fletcher, I. M. (2018). Relationships between highly skilled golfers' clubhead velocity and force producing capabilities during vertical jumps and isometric mid-thigh pull. *Journal of Sport Sciences, 36*(16): 1847–1851.

Wernborn, M., Augustsson, J., & Thomee, R. (2007). The influence of frequency, intensity, volume and mode of strength training on whole muscle cross-sectional area in humans. *Sports Medicine, 37*(3): 225–264.

Wild, C., Steele, J., & Munro, B. (2012). Why Do Girls Sustain More Anterior Cruciate Ligament Injuries Than Boys? *Sports Medicine, 42*: 733–749.

Wolf, J., Cannada, L., Van Heest, A., O'Connor, M., & Ladd, A. (2015). Male and Female Differences in Musculoskeletal Disease. *Journal of the American Academy of Orthopaedic Surgeons, 23*(6): 339–347. https://doi.org/10.5435/JAAOS-D-14-00020

Women in Sport. (2019). *Reframing Sport for Teenage Girls.* Retrieved June 2020, from www.womeninsport.org/wp-content/uploads/2019/04/Reframing-Sport-for-Teenage-Girls-small.pdf

Woods, K., Bishop, P., & Jones, E. (2007). Warm-up and stretching in the prevention of muscular injury. *Sports Med, 37*: 1089–1099.

Youth Sport Trust. (2017). *Key Findings from the Girls Active Survey.* Retrieved June 2020, from www.womeninsport.org/wp-content/uploads/2017/11/Girls-Active-statistics-1.pdf

Zatsiorsky, V. M., & Kraemer, W. J. (2006). *Science and Practice of Strength Training.* Leeds: Human Kinetics.

Zheng, N., Barrentine, S. W., Fleisig, G. S., & Andrews, J. R. (2008). Kinematic analysis of swing in pro and amateur golfers. *International journal of sports medicine, 29*(6): 487–493. https://doi.org/10.1055/s-2007-989229

Zumwalt, M. (2019). Musculoskeletal injury and the exercising female. In J. &.-M. Forsyth (Ed.), *The Exercising Female: Science and its application* (pp. 142–159). Abingdon: Routledge.

Survey Data: www.linkedin.com/pulse/women-golf-understanding-womens-experiences-thewellhq

6 The Junior Golfer

Ben Langdown

Introduction

A note on terminology: When used throughout this chapter, the terms 'children' or 'junior golfer' refers to all phases of growth from 'early childhood' (0–5 years), through 'middle childhood' (boys 5–12 years, girls 5–10 years) and into 'adolescence' (i.e. boys 12–21 years, girls 10–20 years) before reaching adulthood. Where a specific age range focus is required, the appropriate terminology will be used. The term 'athlete' represents any child who is engaging in strength and conditioning/physical activity/the sport of golf as they all have the potential to develop physical competencies through athletic development (i.e. the process of developing all physical characteristics throughout childhood).

In recent years, there has been an increasing body of research to help guide the coaching of children in sport and physical activity. In 2019, some 35,000 children took part in school golf competitions across the United Kingdom (HSBC, 2020), and there were more than 300,000 registered junior golfers in Europe, accounting for 7.5% of total golfers (The R&A & The EGA, 2019). Despite participation levels, there remains a paucity of research into the training of junior golfers, limiting the influence on applied practice and interventions. This chapter draws on case studies, the author's experiences in applied settings, and supporting research from both golf and other sports. Evidence is provided to support coaches' understanding of key physiological concepts, considerations required when coaching junior golfers in strength and conditioning (S&C) environments and when discussing these areas with parents, coaches, and junior golfers themselves.

Early specialisation refers to selecting and intensely training for a single sport at the exclusion of others, all year-round, at a young age and focussing training and practice towards improving performance (Read et al., 2016). Early specialisation in children's sport has been under scrutiny in recent times due to the consequences it can have on a child's longevity in a sport. This, however, has not deterred the rise of various junior golf tours (e.g. U.S. Kids Golf, with the World Championships attracting more than 1600 children with

DOI: 10.4324/9781003099321-6

categories starting for children aged <6 years (US Kids Golf, n.d.)) and many children focusing their attention to golf at an increasingly early age. In golf, this may affect the total volume of practice, training and competition undertaken by children and, if not carefully managed, result in overuse injuries, overtraining and burnout. Research has shown that these injuries are more likely in children who early specialise compared to those who engage in a diverse selection of sport and fitness activities (Hall et al., 2015; Jayanthi et al., 2015), because of the high workload and repetition of similar movements involved in the one sport. The causes of overuse injuries can be multifaceted, with training volume, early specialisation, and maturation status all having been shown as risk factors (Myer et al., 2015). Indeed, Lloyd et al. (2016) strengthen the argument for junior golfers to be engaged in regular and progressive S&C sessions, highlighting that this approach can reduce the risk of overtraining and enhance physiological adaptations and performance. This is especially so where children may be physically underprepared and at risk of overuse injury because of high workloads associated with practice and competition and an absence of preparatory conditioning (Lloyd et al., 2016; Myer et al., 2011).

In late specialisation, a child will continue to engage in numerous sports or fitness activities until they are at least in the adolescent phase. Late specialisation allows children to develop many different physical competencies beneficial to golf. Motivation towards participation can often be higher, and their chances of injury reduced due to the child developing a resilience through physical literacy and many physical qualities (e.g. strength) to protect them against the demands of their sport (Blagrove et al., 2017), in this case golf. Regardless of a child's existing engagement in sport, all junior golfers should be encouraged to engage in regular physical activity and 'afforded the opportunity to enhance athleticism in an individualized, holistic, and child-centered manner' (Lloyd et al., 2016, p. 1491).

Coach's perspective

From an applied perspective, junior golfers and parents are often keen to suggest that they are 100% focused on golf as they believe that's what club, county or regional coaches want to hear. This is an immediate opportunity to begin the education and relationship with the golfer and parent(s) to work towards a common goal of creating an athlete before, or alongside, becoming a golfer. A discussion around the benefits of engaging in a multisport approach during early- and middle-childhood for improved golf performance can encourage time away from the sport and allow children to continue their passion for other sports without the guilt or perceived pressure of 'needing' to solely focus on golf.

Benefits of early engagement in S&C

Engaging junior golfers in S&C programmes from an early age affords many benefits. For example, in order to ensure junior golfers are able to self-manage their programmes and adapt their training to suit the context/environment in which they find themselves (e.g. when travelling, where it can be difficult to maintain consistent training and nutrition routines), these goals should be built into a systematic S&C programme. This self-management extends to the understanding of nutrition and hydration to both fuel their training and performance and provide adequate recovery post S&C sessions and on course play. S&C coaches are often responsible for establishing appropriate habits in the areas of physical preparation, fuelling and refuelling pre/during training and golf, and effective recovery strategies to include physical modalities, nutrition, hydration and sleep hygiene (e.g. discussing sleep hygiene packs for tournaments away from home – pillow, earplugs, eye-mask, blackout-blind etc.). With younger golfers relying on the input and support of parents, it is crucial that this education and habit formation is systematically disseminated wider than just the squad or individual golfers. Parents should be involved in the process as they can ensure resources are in place, where appropriate, and help with habit formation away from supervised sessions.

How well do you know me?

How well coaches know and monitor junior golfers and how they then adapt S&C interventions and coaching to respond to the child's particular wants, needs, training age and maturational status can ultimately impact on the golfer's acute performance, chronic adaptations and engagement in the sport. There is no single optimal solution to training children, and knowledge of biological as well as chronological age can help coaches develop personalised programmes. As Ehlert (2020) suggested, owing to the inter-individual differences in training responses between golfers, practitioners should ensure that individualised programmes are underpinned by testing and monitoring of the physical capacities of each junior golfer. This allows adjustments to be made through the monitoring of the psychophysiological response to any prescribed external load (see Chapter 2).

Considerations of the junior golfer's global cumulative workloads (i.e. training, golf and other physical activity loads; arbitrary units) are required to adapt S&C programming to suit the individual. Within this, it is important to consider Physical Education sessions in school, additional school and external sports training/competition, leisure time physical activity, golf practice (on and off-course) and tournaments. It is also critical to understand what rest days are built in and what the junior golfer and their parents/coaches perceive 'rest days' to mean. Applied, anecdotal experience tells us that a rest day can be perceived as 'just hitting balls on the range for an hour'. From a needs analysis and workload perspective it is a useful exercise to ask junior golfers to document a typical week of physical activity. This can highlight those that are either specialising on golf and those who are undertaking greater volumes/intensities and may find completing multiple S&C sessions each week a difficult proposition. It is important to align this information to the goals and expectations of the parents, coach, and junior golfer. This may involve careful negotiations around workloads associated with S&C sessions and those external to a set programme. Allowing the junior golfer the opportunities to take ownership of this is important with regards motivation and adherence to their long-term engagement with the S&C programme. Where sport is a key focus within their education setting there can be many demands placed on the child which need to be managed carefully and discussed with other coaches (both within golf and other sports) with regards to cumulative workloads and taking an integrative approach (Myer et al., 2011). Academic pressures can also take a toll on adherence to training and attendance at sessions. Around exam times, solutions to keep young golfers engaged can take the form of education around the benefits of physical activity in memory recall and retention of information (e.g. Mavilidi et al., 2016) – this can be an effective way of balancing continued S&C maintenance work with academic revision pressures. The minimal effective dose strategy (i.e. the minimum amount of training that is required to prevent reversibility – the loss of previously gained adaptations) can be applied in these situations to ensure that the golfer is able to perform well in their academic setting without entering a reversibility phase of training.

Given the unique variety of demands placed on junior golfers, an effective solution to understanding a junior golfer's total workload (and more specific session training loads) can be to use an athlete monitoring system (Williams et al., 2018). This may be in the form of a mobile application which shares data to both the golfer, parents and coaches, or a log with athlete self-report measures completed prior to sessions and post-session calculated training load using Session Rating of Perceived Exertion (sRPE; see Bourdon et al. (2017)):

Training load (au) = sRPE x Session Duration

Ideally, monitoring of junior golfers' practice, competition and S&C would be conducted live (e.g. logging alongside their sessions as and when each shot is played with sRPE completed post-session). However, if the tools are not available then retrospective recall can be used as Hayman et al. (2012) have shown this to be a reliable method of monitoring in golf. In addition to session-based workloads, the inclusion of athlete self-report measures will allow the junior golfer and S&C coach to adjust programmes in line with the moderators of internal load (i.e. the psychophysiological response to training loads; see Chapter 2). Measures may include, but not limited to:

- Fatigue & energy levels
- Stress (non-golf)
- Motivation

- Sleep duration and quality
- Perceived recovery from previous activities/training
- Muscle soreness

There is a paucity of empirical research demonstrating the amount of practice and training junior golfers conduct on a session to session, weekly, monthly, seasonal, or annual basis and the impact this can have on performance and risk of injury. In the only study to date, Langdown et al. (2018) highlighted that there were significant variations in junior golfers' practice and tournament volumes from month-to-month. In particular, spikes in volumes occurred around the holiday periods (Easter and summer). This is unsurprising as these periods represent improved weather, and an increase in the number of tournaments and daylight hours available to them to practice and compete without any academic attendance requirements. Langdown et al. (2018) also stated that there were significant variations across the sample of 111 junior golfers from England Golf regional and national programmes (e.g. average monthly long-game shots ranged from 146 to 4,108 for those that logged practice sessions). With results revealing that the volume of long-game practice junior golfers undertake is a small significant predictor of changes in handicap (Langdown et al., 2018) it is feasible to suggest that S&C programmes need to protect them against the effects of this volume and in particular, the significant changes in volumes (and workload) in a short duration. In many countries, the winter months lead to increasing use of range mats by juniors when practicing (and for some, this continues year-round). Cabri et al. (2009) stated that counterforces (i.e. the force of the impact between club and ball) are transmitted by the clubhead and shaft to the hands and arms. With practice mats being less forgiving than playing from the turf in spring and summer months, these impact forces may be increasingly damaging for the wrist, elbow, and shoulder. Floor surfaces aside, the volume of long game shots played may also play a role in increased injuries to other areas of the body, and subsequently, longer term overuse injuries. As an example, with lower back pain being a prevalent injury within golf, Edwards, Dickin, & Wang (2020) argue that adequate physical preparation through S&C adaptations can allow the body to manage the stresses of the golf swing. However, without clear evidence from longitudinal data collection it is challenging to argue a case for the impact of certain volumes of practice and tournament play (or to suggest guidelines to set individual limits), and also to define the role that S&C can play in protecting junior golfers long term. Practitioners must, therefore, draw on other research which demonstrates the case for S&C's protective benefits and use it to educate and promote the benefits of integrative training to suit the various demands and goals of each child (Myer et al., 2011).

Growth and maturation

Children grow at different rates with some children developing earlier or later than the 'average'. This can mean that, if two children are born on the same day, and share the same *chronological age*, they may be at very different stages of physical development and maturational status, i.e. their *biological age*. This inevitably creates gaps between individual children in terms of their potential athletic development and key golf metrics such as clubhead speed (CHS) and drive distance. In addition to potential variations in biological age, coaches should be aware of dates of birth when coaching a group of children formed based on chronological age (e.g. U14s). This can be explained by the 'relative age effect' (RAE; Andronikos et al., 2016) and can be a factor in athletic development pathways or squad selections (see RAE example: part 1). The RAE refers to the consequence of cut-off dates being used in sport and indeed in other walks of life, such as education, to classify age groups and therefore training squads. This can have a significant impact upon children on both sides of the equation (early/late developers) and mean that late developers often miss out on S&C coaching opportunities when not selected for squads (Lloyd et al., 2014).

Relative age effect example: Part 1

Dina and Sara are in the same school year and both are club golfers aspiring towards future county squad selection. Today is the 2nd September. Both girls are 10 years of age with their birthdays separated by just under a year. Dina was born on the 3rd September and Sara on the 30th August. This puts the girls almost one year apart in terms of chronological age. Add in biological age differences and it could go either way. However, in this example Dina is an early developer and Sara is a late developer.

Next day: 3rd September (Dina's birthday)

Dina – 11 years of age, but +2 years for biological age = 13 years of age biologically

Sara – still 10 years of age, but minus one year for biological age = nine years of age biologically

The girls have a biological age difference of four years due to their chronological age and their maturation status. If the cut-off date to play in the U11 squad is 1 September, then Dina will effectively have a four-year biological advantage over Sara.

If Sara does not get selected for the county's junior squad, she may find herself feeling rejected and demotivated towards golf. This may lead to her dropping out of the setting. Conversely, it may drive her to face the additional challenges, continue golf outside the county pathway, and come back to performance pathways/senior squads later in her adolescent years. Developing this resilience and returning later to, perhaps, be even more successful than Dina, is known as 'relative age reversal' (McCarthy et al., 2016).

Andronikos et al. (2016) explain that, based on the influence of additional challenges experienced throughout the development journey, children can close the RAE gap as they progress towards adulthood (see RAE example: part 2). It is important S&C coaches assess the maturation of children (every three to four months; Lloyd et al. (2014); Lloyd et al. (2016)) and their training age as additional components to provide insight into the growth and development of each individual child and set appropriate interventions (Lloyd et al., 2014). These assessments can be used to highlight periods of rapid growth, to align with levels of fitness, strength, motor skill performance, and technical proficiency that we can expect from those individuals (Lloyd et al., 2016) and to help build interventions that increase resilience and motivation towards training (McCarthy et al., 2016). This also ensures that S&C interventions, from structure and priority perspectives, are matched to their maturational status and individual needs analysis while helping to nullify any impact of RAE on training and coaching opportunities.

Relative age effect example: Part 2

Building on the example of Dina and Sara – fast forward eight years, they are now 18 years of age and Dina has caught up with Sara in terms of biological age. Recently, Dina has found herself struggling to win compared to in the past when she would have many physical advantages over opposition.

Sara: she has faced many physical and development challenges due to being a late developer. This has encouraged her to solve problems, hone her skills (e.g. using her short game to help her compete in early years) and wait for the physical advantages to come. Psychologically this may have been tough, but research shows that this can build resilience as she progresses into adulthood and higher levels of sport (McCarthy et al., 2016). Sara was most vulnerable to dropout in the earlier years where she was faced with the biggest challenges of competing against earlier developers.

Dina: The physical advantage that she may well have relied upon during her childhood has been removed. She may have become complacent as she was growing and not faced as many challenges. Not winning so easily, or as frequently, in comparison to her peers may affect her motivation, confidence, and enjoyment of golf and training. She is more likely to drop out as an adolescent or young adult as she finds it harder to compete.

There are various methods used to assess maturation including x-rays or radiographs (considered gold standard), the Tanner criteria (Tanner, 1962) (which should not be used by coaches due to its invasive nature), somatic age assessment using longitudinal growth curve analysis and predictions of age from peak height velocity (PHV). The most applicable for S&C coaches is to use

Table 6.1 Method of predicting age from peak height velocity and maturity status

---

Average age of maturity (see Lloyd & Oliver, 2012; Malina et al., 2020)

Maturity	~Age at PHV (years; male)	~Age at PHV (years; female)
Early	<13.00	<11.00
Average	13.00–15.00	11.00–13.00
Late	>15.0	>13.0

A worked example of predicting years from PHV for a male

Maturity Offset = −9.236 + (0.0002708 * Leg Length & Sitting Height interaction) + (-0.001663 * Age & Leg Length interaction) + (0.007216 * Age & Sitting Height interaction) + (0.02292 * Weight by Height Ratio)

Male/Female	Male
Age (years)	11.253 years
Height (cm)	149.40
Weight (kg)	40
Leg Length (cm)	70.40
Sitting Height (cm)	79.00
Leg Length & Sitting Height interaction	70.40 * 79.00 = 5561.60
Age & Leg Length interaction	11.253 * 70.40 = 792.21
Age & Sitting Height interaction	11.253 * 79.00 = 888.99
Weight by Height Ratio	(40.00/149.40) * 100 = 26.77

Maturity offset = −9.236 + (0.0002708 * 5561.60) + (−0.001663 * 792.21) + (0.007216 * 888.99) + (0.02292 * 26.77) = −2.02 years from PHV

Age at PHV = current age − maturation offset

11.25 years − (−2.02) = 13.27 years (Average Male Maturer)

Source: Adapted from Sherar et al. (2015).

the latter two methods. These are non-invasive, easy to gather the required assessment data and can be regularly analysed in a spreadsheet with the appropriate equations used (Table 6.1).

PHV is the maximum rate of growth that will occur to all children between the ages of 12–16 for boys (Abbassi (1998) reported a rate of ~9.5cm per year) and 10–14 for girls (Lloyd & Oliver, 2012) (Abbassi (1998) reported a rate of ~8.3cm per year). Monitoring how far away from PHV each child is (see Table 6.1) provides valuable information to better influence assessments, training priorities and structures that coaches apply in coaching settings. Using the Youth Physical Development Model (YPDM; Lloyd & Oliver (2012)) as a basis for training priorities, coaches can align interventions more effectively if they can accurately predict the maturational status of the junior golfer. S&C coaches must then adapt coaching sessions to consider each athlete's needs, reflected by their position on the YPDM and their biological age (maturation status) rather than just focussing on chronological age expectations.

Implications of PHV

As children progress through the prepubertal, PHV and post-pubertal stages of growth, coaches of both S&C and golf need to be aware of the specific implications this may have on performance, competence and psychological characteristics, such as motivation, confidence etc. As Lloyd et al. (2014) state, it is important that coaches understand how growth and training interact to ensure training programmes are designed to develop children's strength to protect them from injury. With mismatched, rapid growth in the long bones relative to muscular lengthening, young golfers may experience disruption to their previously demonstrated range of movement, neuro-muscular function, and physical performance (Lloyd et al., 2014) (e.g. their ability to lift competently in the gym or swing the golf club to produce effective and desired ball flights). Practitioners may need to revise the com-plexity of S&C programmes during phases of rapid growth and reassure junior golfers, parents, and coaches that lower performance levels are to be expected. Additional coaching observations (e.g. through increased fre-quency of supervised sessions) may be appropriate and effective during this phase to ensure form and technique are maintained, therefore ensuring safety, and reducing injury risk. It is also important from an applied per-spective that any decreases in flexibility during a period of rapid growth is (in most cases) attributed to the mismatch between the long bones and the muscles (Mills et al., 2017) and the differential timing of adolescent spurts in leg and trunk length, with acknowledgments made that the mus-cular lengthening and trunk growth will eventually address this imbalance (Philippaerts et al., 2006).

Typical traits of junior golfers

Various sports have evidenced that, while more frequent involvement in a sport increases risk of injury, it is those adolescents that are new to a sport, or have underdeveloped techniques, that have the greatest need for S&C intervention to reduce subsequent injury risk (e.g. volleyball (Wasser et al., 2020), football (Dvorak et al., 2000), golf (Cabri et al., 2009; Meira & Brumitt, 2010) etc.). This notion, combined with the understanding that positive impulse (PI) (i.e. the force exerted to change momentum over a given time, [force x time]) in the counter movement jump test is a significant predictor of CHS in golfers (Wells et al., 2019), means that it is important to note some typical traits from young golfers that enter a performance programme that may influence their injury risk and PI test results. These traits, albeit in anecdotal form, are presented from over a decade of experience and with obvious caution around individual variation and highlighting the need for one-to-one observation and needs analysis. From those with a low training age it is common to see limited lower limb and gluteal strength, and lower PI from the CMJ testing prior to S&C interventions (e.g. see Coughlan et al., 2020). Research highlights that lower limb injuries account for 29–89% of all injuries in high-school sports each year (sport dependent) and that identifying those at risk remains critical to continuing participation and improved performance (Rechel et al., 2008).

Smith et al. (2014) reported lower pre-intervention test results for unilateral lower limb, core, and functional hip strength for junior golfers, using a progressive single leg squat test (SLS). Additionally, Agresta et al. (2017) reported a significant improvement in SLS performance with chronological age but stated that there may be underlying biological reasons for this and highlighting that programme interventions could target single leg stability in order to improve overall functional performance. In young golfers there are often hamstrings and gastrocnemius/soleus flexibility/ankle mobility issues (anecdotally, more males present with this restriction) that may impact upon their ability to competently perform squatting patterns and generate impulse (e.g. see Panoutsakopoulos et al. (2021)) which may, in turn, contribute to ineffective posture and performance during the swing (see Langdown, 2015).

With decreased scapula upward rotation, reduced posterior tilting, and excessive scapula internal rotation all highlighted in shoulder conditions (Struyf et al., 2011) it is important to note that scapula instability is often presented by young golfers. Research states that a high incidence of shoulder protraction is normal during child development and that the prevalence of scapula instability can be as much as 70% of children from 7–12 years of age (Penha et al., 2005), but, that it will improve as part of growth. The instability of the scapula may impact upon the ability to externally rotate the shoulders (Ebaugh et al., 2006) which is required in the downswing (trail-side) and follow-through (lead-side).

VandenBerg et al. (2017) reported that restricted internal (medial) hip rotation is associated with increased risk of an anterior cruciate ligament (ACL) injury and with young golfers being encouraged to engage in other sports, a limitation here should raise concerns. Anecdotally, restricted internal hip rotation is more prevalent with adolescent male golfers and when compared to measures of external hip rotation. Research shows that limitations in the lead hip passive and active internal rotation can be a cause of lower back pain for golfers (Murray et al., 2009). Additionally, although there is less prevalence of hip rotation restrictions in young female golfers, those with low 'training ages' often show increased levels of knee valgus, both during squatting or lunging based exercises and jump testing, again linked to increased ACL injury risk. The use of CMJ impulse testing provides an immediate coaching opportunity to discuss the increased risk of ACL injuries and the implementation of strength-based training interventions. With this type of injury most likely to occur during adolescent years (Dai et al., 2012) it is in the junior golfer population that careful coaching observation and intervention needs to be applied. To help prevent knee valgus, especially during single leg ballistic tasks, it is important to strengthen the muscles surrounding the hip – the hamstrings and the gluteals, which play an important role in stabilising the knee over the line of the foot during pivoting, jumping and landing (Dix et al., 2019).

While the sport of golf does not specifically require these particular fundamental movement skills (FMS; foundation/basic locomotion, manipulation and stabilisation skills used in play and everyday life) to compete, the other sports and training that the junior golfer undertakes may require inclusion of explosive movements, such as jumping. The cueing of knee alignment during lunging and squatting patterns can help to form initial understanding of safe movement during training and help when progressing to more explosive activities (Westbrook et al., 2020). Teaching young athletes how to correctly pivot, land from jumps with greater knee flexion (with control) and with the knees facing straight ahead, over the toe line, is critical in injury prevention. The increased evidence supporting the relationship between lower body force production (e.g. impulse) and CHS (e.g. Wells et al., 2019) reinforces work from Suchomel, Nimphius and Stone (2016), who stated that it is important for a foundation of muscular strength to be established, with increased technical competence (i.e. control over jumping and landing mechanics), prior to a greater emphasis being placed upon development of power, rate of force development and velocity-based training. This includes plyometric or ballistic exercises, which as Ehlert (2020) suggests, may elicit further performance gains in golf.

With all these common traits, it is important to reflect on the athlete's training age and participation in other sports.

> *Training age* is defined as the amount of time accumulated from both periodic and longitudinal participation in training programs and sport related activities that foster the development of musculoskeletal health, basic movement patterns and overall physical fitness.
>
> (Myer et al., 2013; p.15)

Based on the quotation, a 10-year-old child who has been training with a suitably qualified coach since they were eight would have a training age of two years. We know from research that maturity-related differences in body size and motor skill performance begin to emerge around the ages of six–seven years (Malina et al., 2005). These developmental differences in height and motor skill can make programming for children based on chronological age contentious (Myer et al., 2013) and highlight the need to establish specific needs and priorities for each individual child's S&C intervention.

Managing the training programme for a child who is new to golf but has competed at a high level in another sport presents an interesting situation. The child may have a training age of several years for the other sport and will, therefore, not be zero years for the sport of golf. Initial assessment of the physical characteristics and S&C related competence is required here to understand their status in terms of FMS, strength, mobility, agility, endurance etc. in line with both the YPDM, their needs analysis for golf and individual goals.

Children are not miniature adults

When training children, it can be an easy option to replicate programmes that adults complete. However, because children's physiology is in a constant state of change (e.g. fluctuations in hormones such as testosterone, growth hormone, and insulin-like growth factors associated with growth spurts (Lloyd & Oliver, 2012)), practitioners should not view or coach children as miniature-adults (Lloyd et al., 2016). There are many physiological differences that should impact on the design of S&C interventions. We know that a child's $VO_{2\,Max}$ (i.e. the volume of oxygen that can be used by the body for energy production kg^{-1}. min^{-1}) is lower than an adult's, but that it increases progressively with age. With golf being a relatively low-intensity sport, training to increase $VO_{2\,Max}$ and cardiac output may be considered lower priorities when attempting to improve golf performance. However, from a youth physical development perspective, increasing overall fitness allows greater physical capacity and health benefits to potentially influence longevity in the sport.

Hydration for children

Hydration factors play a role in the quality of training that is achieved in each session and performance on the golf course. Indeed, research has shown that dehydration accounts for reduced cognitive function in various athletic populations (Grandjean & Grandjean, 2007; Wittbrodt & Millard-Stafford, 2018). However, there is currently no evidence to support differences in heat dispersal rates between adults and children and no evidence to suggest there are maturational differences in thermal balance or endurance performance during exercise in the heat. Research does show, however, that children have lower sweat rates due to smaller sweat glands with a lower sensitivity to ambient temperatures and less heat being produced by less muscle mass (Rowland, 2008). The heat generated increases as adolescents gain muscle mass and the greater force with which the muscles then contract during exercise (Falk & Dotan, 2008; Rowland, 2008). Establishing effective individualised hydration strategies around training with young golfers may help to engage them in monitoring processes and minimise any negative effects dehydrated states can have on both their training and golf performance. On the golf course, research points towards decreased performance with those starting the round dehydrated playing significantly more shots that those starting in a euhydrated state (Magee et al., 2017). Mild dehydration (i.e. a loss of 1.5% of body mass) has also been shown to reduce shot distance, decrease accuracy, and impair judgement of shot distance compared to euhydration (Smith et al., 2012).

Practical applications

As discussed, developing physical competence, and preparing children for golf performance (at whatever level) across the lifecourse, is not, and should not be, the same as when training adults. Additional considerations include attention spans, peer group socialisation, physical capabilities, and maturation status (both biological and psychological). The process of effectively supporting children in resistance training programmes, to benefit their golf, has been summarised well by Faigenbaum and McFarland (2016), who introduce seven fundamental principles as the 'PROCESS' of youth resistance training. They highlight, that it is not just about meeting the priorities specified on the YPDM or in line with the PHV predictions, elements of creativity, socialisation and, importantly, enjoyment, all need building into training sessions, whether coaching elite or novice junior golfers.

The following 'PROCESS' points are applied and adapted from suggestions of Faigenbaum and McFarland (2016):

(a) Progression

The stress/workload expectations placed on the growing body must be progressed gradually. This does not mean increasing the load used each session, but that training stress and challenges (e.g. novel movement patterns or exercises) should progressively and consistently stimulate adaptations while maintaining engagement in the S&C programme.

(b) Regularity

The frequency of training will depend on the junior golfer's training age, external workload to the S&C sessions and their individual needs. Two-three sessions per week is adequate for most youth athletes (Faigenbaum & McFarland, 2016). In applied settings, it has been a typical behaviour of junior golfers that S&C priorities and training regularity decreases during the summer months due to increased workload contributions from practice (on and off course) and tournament play. It is important to assist junior golfers to adapt training programmes to compliment the increased golf workloads and to avoid the principle of reversibility through the minimal effective dose.

(c) Overload

It is well known that to elicit adaptation the body needs to be stressed beyond the level to which the body is accustomed. Research has shown that gains of ~30–40% are typical in pre-adolescent children following 8–20 weeks of resistance training (Faigenbaum et al., 2009; Lloyd et al., 2014) and that initially bodyweight/free-weights are effective training modalities to improve measures of muscle strength (e.g. maximum voluntary contraction) in untrained children and adolescents (Peitz et al., 2018). To elicit such adaptations, progressive overload must take place through the alteration of training frequency, intensity, time (or volume), and exercise selection. Faigenbaum and McFarland (2016) suggest guidelines to ensure children are progressed in an appropriate manner (Table 6.2).

Athlete self-report measures are a useful tool to inform intervention adjustments to ensure appropriate overload. As junior golfers increase their training age and become familiar and competent in and around a gym

Table 6.2 Youth resistance training progressions based on the golfer's training skill competence and muscular strength

	Low	Resistance Training Skill Competency	High
Sets	1–2	2–4	Multiple
Repetitions	Varied	6–12	≤6
Intensity	≤60%1RM*	≤80%1RM	≥85%1RM
Exercise complexity	Basic – introduce single and multi-joint exercises using a combination of body weight and free weights*	Intermediate – Introduction to more complex lifts (e.g. variations of Olympic lifts)	Advanced – Use of multi-joint exercises such as Olympic lift variations may be incorporated, provided the technical proficiency remains high
Frequency	2/wk	2–3/wk	2–4/wk
	Low	**Muscular Strength**	**High**

Note. There are no fixed boundaries between low and high competency/strength. These are continuums on which the coach and junior golfer must use coaching, observations, assessments, and progressive overload to determine when to increase each component. Where other training priorities are the focus (e.g. hypertrophy) the reps, sets and intensity may vary from these suggestions for strength.

*Progress training competence to sufficient level to allow accurate 1RM to be established through testing (use predictive methods, e.g. calculating 1RM from ≤10RM).

Source: Adapted from Faigenbaum & McFarland (2016).

environment their levels of responsibility, to monitor their own global workload and adjust accordingly, should be increased. This will ultimately benefit them when away at tournaments and in any unsupervised sessions.

(d) Creativity

Getting young golfers to 'buy in' to S&C programmes can mean overcoming barriers, myth busting education and igniting their imagination to overcome preconceived perceptions of what S&C or 'training for golf' looks like. The creativity of the coach to use appropriate exercises, equipment, and programming to meet the needs of each individual requires ingenuity and a flexible, innovative approach. Fostering an environment in which the junior golfer feels comfortable and supported to achieve adaptations through S&C will ultimately increase exercise adherence, thus contributing to the previous factors of progressive overload and regularity. Agans et al. (2013) propose that young people need positive movement experiences (PME) and to be behaviourally, cognitively, and emotionally engaged to benefit from participation. It should be noted that this does not mean using different exercises each session, or indeed recreating golf specific movements in the gym. Simply promoting the benefits of S&C to young golfers and using role models can be enough to stimulate initial engagement with the programme. Bailey et al. (2013) state that it is vital that coaches' behaviours and practices match the needs of the young athlete. Fostering autonomy and choice through challenges posed to the children will further engage them in the sessions and help focus them towards their goals. Creativity is also valuable when it comes to designing S&C programmes for those junior golfers training at home (when unsupervised), and those who have disabilities and require modifications to exercises in order to continue to achieve their training goals.

(e) Enjoyment

The training age of the junior golfer is important here. Matching the programme's skill demand to their level of competence in the gym will ensure they perceive their sessions and programme to be appropriate and enjoyable. As alluded to by Agans et al. (2013) and Bailey et al. (2013), the goal with junior golfer S&C programmes in the first instance has to be adherence through PME, enjoyment and perceived competence through skill development. Many junior golfers enter regional development programmes having very young training ages and low competence in a gym environment, therefore the use of positive coaching behaviours, athlete choice and potentially inspirational role models, in the sport of golf, can offer benefits to motivation, engagement and enjoyment in sessions (see Bailey et al. (2013).

(f) Socialisation

Although golf is, in the main, an individual sport there are still squads and opportunities to engage junior golfers through common S&C goals across groups. Faigenbaum and McFarland (2016) argue that, increases in muscular strength can be maximised when socialisation is prioritised by the S&C coach and juniors can work towards common goals. They also state that socialisation can increase adherence and enjoyment which, ultimately, will allow S&C coaches to achieve progressive overload through regular attendance at sessions and adaptations achieved through training. Group training sessions may foster an element of healthy competition, that as long as technique and form is not compromised, can allow junior golfers to appreciate where they are in line with their own and others' expectations.

(g) Supervision

Despite lots of recent research into youth physical development, some myths still exist surrounding the use of resistance when children train for fitness or sport (see Benjamin & Glow (2003); Lloyd et al. (2016)). As coaches we need to understand that although there is no minimum age to lifting weights, the child must be ready to enter and engage safely in a training environment that is suitably supervised. The supervision principle is crucial here. Coaches need to ensure they are appropriately qualified to be coaching children in resistance-based training (or S&C) sessions. Equally, parents of a junior golfer who is looking to engage in S&C, should seek out those with appropriate qualifications (e.g. United Kingdom Strength and Conditioning Association (UKSCA) or National Strength and Conditioning Association (NSCA) accredited S&C coach) and experience of working in the sport of golf (i.e. demonstrable understanding of the demands of golf and has an appreciation for research in the field).

Case studies from applied work have highlighted occasions where a junior golfer is being supported by a 'trainer' with limited understanding of testing or programming for children, or more specifically, junior golfers. While it is commendable and encouraged for fitness instructors/golf coaches to expand their knowledge of S&C techniques, applied to golf, S&C interventions should be provided by a qualified and experienced coach. Without an in-depth understanding of the science underpinning physiological adaptations (elicited through S&C) and the demands of the sport, it is difficult to maximise the gains a junior golfer can make towards their goals. Injury risks can be reduced and skill based competence (especially those with young training ages) can be maximised by having S&C sessions/programmes and by adhering to this supervision principle (Faigenbaum & McFarland, 2016). Building effective communication channels and establishing relationships with parents allows education and awareness to be raised allowing them to make informed decisions and also support their child's training.

When supervising sessions, it is important the S&C coach considers the level of expectation they place on each junior golfer and how this is shown. This will be very subjective in nature and possibly different for each child. However, coach expectations for each child should remain high enough to ensure a ceiling is not placed on the child's perceived potential. Keeping expectations above where the child currently is (albeit at an appropriate level above), can maintain their self-belief and positive attitude. This is, again, important for parents and other coaches to provide aligned messaging to maximise the gains that supervised and unsupervised sessions can have.

While the 'PROCESS' (Faigenbaum & McFarland, 2016) is there to guide S&C coaches it is essential to listen and communicate with the junior golfer and their support network. Communication, in this regard, is vital to resolve potentially conflicting demands being placed on the junior golfer. At each moment in time consideration must be given to what the overarching priorities are for the child and their parents. These will often shift throughout the academic year, and especially so during exam seasons, with greater expectations coming from academic influences compared to golf and training. As previously mentioned, being able to adapt their programme and frequency of supervised sessions will be important to help maintain focus on key academic priorities without negating the positive impacts that training can have on stress, cognitive function, memory recall etc., during busy periods of revision (Lambourne & Tomporowski, 2010). The junior golfer's training needs during these periods may simply be to act as a distraction from other demands. Communication, an understanding approach, and adaptability are positive coaching behaviours required to ensuring achievement of goals in all areas.

Conclusion

To influence the design of systematic programmes, S&C coaches of junior golfers should prioritise the considerations discussed within this chapter, ensuring the needs of each individual are met. Specifically, S&C coaches should ensure the seven 'PROCESS' principles, suggested by Faigenbaum and McFarland (2016) allow training to be gradually developed while promoting sustained engagement and positive movement experiences. It is vital for coaches to use evidence-based education to dispel myths around a minimal age for children to lift weights, while ensuring each child is mature enough to remain safe in the training environment. Children are not miniature adults; they respond differently to exercise compared to adults and this should be evident in programme design and education around the moderators of internal load. Coaches should provide programmes that protect children from the increased risk of overuse injuries through greater rest and recovery and consider that training age will dictate the frequency of training, with young training ages starting at two to three sessions per week. Training should also prioritise movement (FMS) and resistance training in relation to each golfer's maturation status, while monitoring of load and athlete self-report measures should provide insight to optimise programme amendments. Above all, coaches should endeavour to promote sustained S&C engagement through sessions that develop autonomy and are creative and enjoyable for all young golfers.

References

Abbassi, V. (1998). Growth and normal puberty. *Pediatrics, 102*(S3), 507–511.

Agans, J. P., Säfvenbom, R., Davis, J. L., Bowers, E. P., & Lerner, R. M. (2013). Positive movement experiences: Approaching the study of athletic participation, exercise, and leisure activity through relational developmental systems theory and the concept of embodiment. *Advances in Child Development and Behavior, 45*, 261–286. https://doi.org/10.1016/B978-0-12-397946-9.00010-5

Agresta, C., Church, C., Henley, J., Duer, T., & O'Brien, K. (2017). Single-leg squat performance in active adolescents aged 8–17 years. *Journal of Strength and Conditioning Research, 31*(5), 1187–1191. https://doi.org/10.1519/JSC.0000000000001617

Andronikos, G., Elumaro, A. I., Westbury, T., & Martindale, R. J. J. (2016). Relative age effect: implications for effective practice. *Journal of Sports Sciences, 34*(12), 1124–1131. https://doi.org/10.1080/02640414.2015.1093647

Bailey, R., Cope, E. J., & Pearce, G. (2013). Why do children take part in, and remain involved in sport? A literature review and discussion of implications for sports coaches. *International Journal of Coaching Science, 7*(1), 56–75. http://search.ebscohost.com/login.aspx?direct=true&AuthType=ip,shib&db=s3h&AN=85448465&site=eds-live&scope=site&custid=s1123095

Benjamin, H. J., & Glow, K. M. (2003). Strength training for children and adolescents. *The Physician and Sportsmedicine, 31*(9), 19–26.

Blagrove, R. C., Bruinvels, G., & Read, P. (2017). Early sport specialization and intensive training in adolescent female athletes: Risks and recommendations. *Strength and Conditioning Journal, 39*(5), 14–23. https://doi.org/10.1519/SSC.0000000000000315

Bourdon, P. C., Cardinale, M., Murray, A., Gastin, P., Kellmann, M., Varley, M. C., Gabbett, T. J., Coutts, A. J., Burgess, D. J., Gregson, W., & Cable, N. T. (2017). Monitoring athlete training loads: Consensus statement. *International Journal of Sports Physiology and Performance, 12*, 161–170. https://doi.org/10.1123/IJSPP.2017-0208

Cabri, J., Sousa, J. P., Kots, M., & Barreiros, J. (2009). Golf-related injuries: A systematic review. In *European Journal of Sport Science, 9*(6), 353–366. Taylor and Francis Ltd. https://doi.org/10.1080/17461390903009141

Coughlan, D., Taylor, M. J. D., Wayland, W., Brooks, D., & Jackson, J. (2020). The effect of a 12-week strength and conditioning programme on youth golf performance. *International Journal of Golf Science, 8*(1).

Dai, B., Herman, D., Liu, H., Garrett, W. E., & Yu, B. (2012). Prevention of ACL injury, part I: Injury characteristics, risk factors, and loading mechanism. *Research in Sports Medicine, 20*(3–4), 180–197. https://doi.org/10.1080/15438627.2012.680990

Dix, J., Marsh, S., Dingenen, B., & Malliaras, P. (2019). The relationship between hip muscle strength and dynamic knee valgus in asymptomatic females: A systematic review. *Physical Therapy in Sport, 37*, 197–209. https://doi.org/10.1016/j.ptsp.2018.05.015

Dvorak, J., Junge, A., Chomiak, J., Graf-Baumann, T., Peterson, L., Rösch, D., & Hodgson, R. (2000). Risk factor analysis for injuries in football players: Possibilities for a prevention program. *American Journal of Sports Medicine, 28*(S5). https://doi.org/10.1177/28.suppl_5.s-69

Ebaugh, D. D., McClure, P. W., & Karduna, A. R. (2006). Scapulothoracic and glenohumeral kinematics following an external rotation fatigue protocol. *Journal of Orthopaedic and Sports Physical Therapy, 36*(8), 557–571. https://doi.org/10.2519/jospt.2006.2189

Edwards, N., Dickin, C., & Wang, H. (2020). Low Back Pain and Golf: A Review of Biomechanical Risk Factors. *Sports Medicine and Health Science.* https://doi.org/10.1016/j.smhs.2020.03.002

Ehlert, A. (2020). The effects of strength and conditioning interventions on golf performance: A systematic review. *Journal of Sports Sciences, 38*(23), 2720–2731. https://doi.org/10.1080/02640414.2020.1796470

Faigenbaum, A.D., Kraemer, W. J., Blimkie, C. J., Jeffreys, I., Micheli, L. J., Nitka, M., & Rowland, T. W. (2009). Youth Resistance Training: Updated Position Statement Paper From the National Strength and Conditioning Association. *Journal of Strength and Conditioning Research, 23*(S5), S60–S79.

Faigenbaum, Avery D., & McFarland, J. E. (2016). Resistance training for kids: Right from the Start. *ACSM's Health and Fitness Journal, 20*(5), 16–22. https://doi.org/10.1249/FIT.0000000000000236

Falk, B., & Dotan, R. (2008). Children's thermoregulation during exercise in the heat - A revisit. *Applied Physiology, Nutrition and Metabolism, 33*(2), 420–427. https://doi.org/10.1139/H07-185

Grandjean, A. C., & Grandjean, N. R. (2007). Dehydration and cognitive performance. *Journal of the American College of Nutrition, 26*(S5), 549S–554S.

Hall, R., Foss, K. B., Hewett, T. E., & Myer, G. D. (2015). Sport specialization's association with an increased risk of developing anterior knee pain in adolescent female athletes. *Journal of Sport Rehabilitation, 24*(1), 31–35. https://doi.org/10.1123/jsr.2013-0101

Hayman, R., Polman, R., & Taylor, J. (2012). The validity of retrospective recall in assessing practice regimes in golf. *International Journal of Sport and Exercise Psychology, 10*(4), 329–337. https://doi.org/10.1080/1612197X.2012.705511

HSBC. (2020). *State of Play 2020: HSBC Golf Report.*

Jayanthi, N. A., Labella, C. R., Fischer, D., Pasulka, J., & Dugas, L. R. (2015). Sports-specialized intensive training and the risk of injury in young athletes: A clinical case-control study. *American Journal of Sports Medicine, 43*(4), 794–801. https://doi.org/10.1177/0363546514567298

Lambourne, K., & Tomporowski, P. (2010). The effect of exercise-induced arousal on cognitive task performance: A meta-regression analysis. *Brain Research, 1341*, 12–24. https://doi.org/10.1016/j.brainres.2010.03.091

Langdown, B. L. (2015). *Movement Variability and Strength and Conditioning in Golf* [University of Birmingham]. https://etheses.bham.ac.uk//id/eprint/6164/

Langdown, B. L., Burnett, S., Jones, N., & Coughlan, D. (2018). Practice And Tournament Volumes Of Young Golfers In Regional And National Squads. *World Scientific Congress of Golf.* http://oro.open.ac.uk/id/eprint/55982

Lloyd, R. S., Cronin, J. B., Faigenbaum, A. D., Haff, G. G., Howard, R., Kraemer, W. J., Micheli, L. J., Myer, G. D., & Oliver, J. L. (2016). National Strength and Conditioning Association Position Statement on Long-Term Athletic Development. *Journal of Strength and Conditioning Research, 30*(6), 1491–1509. https://doi.org/10.1519/JSC.0000000000001387

Lloyd, R. S., Faigenbaum, A. D., Stone, M. H., Oliver, J. L., Jeffreys, I., Moody, J. A., Brewer, C., Pierce, K. C., Mccambridge, T. M., Howard, R., Herrington, L., Hainline, B., Micheli, L. J., Jaques, R., Kraemer, W. J., Mcbride, M. G., Best, T. M., Chu, D. A., Alvar, B. A., & Myer, G. D. (2014). Position statement on youth resistance training: The 2014 International Consensus. *British Journal of Sports Medicine, 48*, 498–505. https://doi.org/10.1136/bjsports-2013-092952

Lloyd, R. S., & Oliver, J. L. (2012). The youth physical development model: A new approach to long-term athletic development. *Strength and Conditioning Journal, 34*(3), 61–72.

Lloyd, Rhodri S., & Oliver, J. L. (2012). The youth physical development model: A new approach to long-term athletic development. *Strength and Conditioning Journal, 34*(3), 61–72. https://doi.org/10.1519/SSC.0b013e31825760ea

Magee, P. J., Gallagher, A. M., & McCormack, J. M. (2017). High prevalence of dehydration and inadequate nutritional knowledge among university and club level athletes. *International Journal of Sport Nutrition and Exercise Metabolism, 27*(2), 158–168. https://doi.org/10.1123/ijsnem.2016-0053

Malina, R. M., Cumming, S. P., Morano, P. J., Barron, M., & Miller, S. J. (2005). Maturity status of youth football players: A noninvasive estimate. *Medicine and Science in Sports and Exercise, 37*(6), 1044–1052. https://doi.org/10.1249/01.mss.0000171622.45134.cb

Malina, R. M., Kozieł, S. M., Králik, M., Chrzanowska, M., & Suder, A. (2020). Prediction of maturity offset and age at peak height velocity in a longitudinal series of boys and girls. *American Journal of Human Biology*, November, 1–15. https://doi.org/10.1002/ajhb.23551

Mavilidi, M. F., Okely, A. D., Chandler, P., & Paas, F. (2016). Infusing Physical Activities Into the Classroom: Effects on Preschool Children's Geography Learning. *Mind, Brain, and Education*, *10*(4), 256–263. https://doi.org/10.1111/mbe.12131

McCarthy, N., Collins, D., & Court, D. (2016). Start hard, finish better: Further evidence for the reversal of the RAE advantage. *Journal of Sports Sciences*, *34*(15), 1461–1465. https://doi.org/10.1080/02640414.2015.1119297

Meira, E. P., & Brumitt, J. (2010). Minimizing injuries and enhancing performance in golf through training programs. *Sports Health*, *2*(4), 337–344. https://doi.org/10.1177/1941738110365129

Mills, K., Baker, D., Pacey, V., Wollin, M., & Drew, M. K. (2017). What is the most accurate and reliable methodological approach for predicting peak height velocity in adolescents? A systematic review. *Journal of Science and Medicine in Sport*, *20*(6), 572–577. https://doi.org/10.1016/j.jsams.2016.10.012

Murray, E., Birley, E., Twycross-Lewis, R., & Morrissey, D. (2009). The relationship between hip rotation range of movement and low back pain prevalence in amateur golfers: An observational study. *Physical Therapy in Sport*, *10*(4), 131–135. https://doi.org/10.1016/j.ptsp.2009.08.002

Myer, G. D., Faigenbaum, A. D., Chu, D. A., Falkel, J., Ford, K. R., Best, T. M., & Hewett, T. E. (2011). Integrative training for children and adolescents: techniques and practices for reducing sports-related injuries and enhancing athletic performance. *The Physician and Sportsmedicine*, *39*(1), 74–84. https://doi.org/10.3810/psm.2011.02.1864

Myer, G. D., Jayanthi, N., Difiori, J. P., Faigenbaum, A. D., Kiefer, A. W., Logerstedt, D., & Micheli, L. J. (2015). Sport Specialization, Part I: Does Early Sports Specialization Increase Negative Outcomes and Reduce the Opportunity for Success in Young Athletes? *Sports Health*, *7*(5), 437–442. https://doi.org/10.1177/1941738115598747

Myer, G. D., Lloyd, R. S., Brent, J. L., & Faigenbaum, A. D. (2013). How young is too young to start training? *ACSM's Health and Fitness Journal*, *17*(5), 14–23. https://doi.org/10.1249/FIT.0b013e3182a06c59

Panoutsakopoulos, V., Kotzamanidou, M. C., Papaiakovou, G., & Kollias, I. A. (2021). The Ankle Joint Range of Motion and Its Effect on Squat Jump Performance with and without Arm Swing in Adolescent Female Volleyball Players. *Journal of Functional Morphology and Kinesiology*, *6*(1), 14. https://doi.org/10.3390/jfmk6010014

Peitz, M., Behringer, M., & Granacher, U. (2018). Correction: A systematic review on the effects of resistance and plyometric training on physical fitness in youth- What do comparative studies tell us? *PLOS ONE*, *13*(11), e0207641. https://doi.org/10.1371/journal.pone.0207641

Penha, P. J., João, S. M. A., Casarotto, R. A., Amino, C. J., & Penteado, D. C. (2005). Postural assessment of girls between 7 and 10 years of age. *Clinics (São Paulo, Brazil)*, *60*(1), 9–16. https://doi.org/10.1590/S1807-59322005000100004

Philippaerts, R. M., Vaeyens, R., Janssens, M., Van Renterghem, B., Matthys, D., Craen, R., Bourgois, J., Vrijens, J., Beunen, G., & Malina, R. M. (2006). The relationship between peak height velocity and physical performance in youth soccer players. *Journal of Sports Sciences*, *24*(3), 221–230. https://doi.org/10.1080/02640410500189371

Read, P. J., Oliver, J. L., De Ste Croix, M. B. A., Myer, G. D., & Lloyd, R. S. (2016). The scientific foundations and associated injury risks of early soccer specialisation.

Journal of Sports Sciences, 34(24), 2295–2302. https://doi.org/10.1080/02640 414.2016.1173221

Rechel, J. A., Yard, E. E., & Comstock, R. D. (2008). An epidemiologic comparison of high school sports injuries sustained in practice and competition. *Journal of Athletic Training, 43*(2), 197–204. https://doi.org/10.4085/1062-6050-43.2.197

Rowland, T. (2008). Thermoregulation during exercise in the heat in children: Old concepts revisited. *Journal of Applied Physiology, 105*(2), 718–724. https://doi.org/ 10.1152/japplphysiol.01196.2007

Sherar, L. B., Mirwald, R. L., Baxter-Jones, A. D. G., & Thomis, M. (2015). Prediction of adult height using maturity- based camulative height velocity curves. *Journal of Sports Sciences, 14*(4), 1–9.

Smith, C. J., Lubans, D. R., & Callister, R. (2014). The Effects of Resistance Training on Junior Golfers' Strength and On-Course Performance. *International Journal of Golf Science, 3*(2), 128–144. https://doi.org/10.1123/ijgs.2014-0023

Smith, M. F., Newell, A. J., & Baker, M. R. (2012). Effect of acute mild dehydration on cognitive-motor performance in golf. *The Journal of Strength & Conditioning Research, 26*(11), 3075–3080.

Struyf, F., Nijs, J., Horsten, S., Mottram, S., Truijen, S., & Meeusen, R. (2011). Scapular positioning and motor control in children and adults: A laboratory study using clinical measures. *Manual Therapy, 16*(2), 155–160. https://doi.org/10.1016/ j.math.2010.09.002

Suchomel, T. J., Nimphius, S., & Stone, M. H. (2016). The Importance of Muscular Strength in Athletic Performance. *Sports Medicine, 46*(10), 1419–1449. https://doi. org/10.1007/s40279-016-0486-0

Tanner, J. (1962). *Growth at Adolescence* (2nd ed.). Blackwell Publishing Ltd.

The R&A & The EGA. (2019). *European Golf Participation.* www.randa.org/en/thera nda/initiatives/golf-research

US Kids Golf. (n.d.). *Tournaments.* Retrieved 19 October 2020, from https://foundat ion.uskidsgolf.com/tournaments

VandenBerg, C., Crawford, E. A., Sibilsky Enselman, E., Robbins, C. B., Wojtys, E. M., & Bedi, A. (2017). Restricted Hip Rotation Is Correlated With an Increased Risk for Anterior Cruciate Ligament Injury. *Arthroscopy - Journal of Arthroscopic and Related Surgery, 33*(2), 317–325. https://doi.org/10.1016/j.arthro.2016.08.014

Wasser, J. G., Tripp, B., Bruner, M. L., Bailey, D. R., Leitz, R. S., Zaremski, J. L., & Vincent, H. K. (2020). Volleyball-related injuries in adolescent female players: an initial report. *Physician and Sportsmedicine,* 1–8. Advance online publication https://doi. org/10.1080/00913847.2020.1826284

Wells, J. E. T., Charalambous, L. H., Mitchell, A. C. S., Coughlan, D., Brearley, S. L., Hawkes, R. A., Murray, A. D., Hillman, R. G., & Fletcher, I. M. (2019). Relationships between Challenge Tour golfers' clubhead velocity and force producing capabilities during a countermovement jump and isometric mid-thigh pull. *Journal of Sports Sciences, 37*(12), 1381–1386. https://doi.org/10.1080/02640414.2018.1559972

Westbrook, A. E., Taylor, J. B., Nguyen, A. D., Paterno, M. V., & Ford, K. R. (2020). Effects of maturation on knee biomechanics during cutting and landing in young female soccer players. *PLoS ONE, 15*(5), 1–11. https://doi.org/10.1371/journal. pone.0233701

Williams, S. B., Gastin, P. B., Saw, A. E., & Robertson, S. (2018). Development of a golf-specific load monitoring tool: Content validity and feasibility. *European Journal of Sport Science*, *18*(4), 458–472. https://doi.org/10.1080/17461391.2018.1434239

Wittbrodt, M. T., & Millard-Stafford, M. (2018). Dehydration Impairs Cognitive Performance: A Meta-analysis. *Medicine and Science in Sports and Exercise*, *50*(11), 2360–2368. https://doi.org/10.1249/MSS.0000000000001682

7   The Senior Golfer

Orlaith Buckley and Nicholas Jones

Preface

It was a normal day at the Senior Open Championship, the players coming and going from the Performance Unit preparing for their round of golf. Over the course of the week, one player's preparation had repeatedly caught our eye. He came into the truck, very politely said hello to all present, and with no fuss, began a simple, well-structured and robust warm-up. Its execution simply flowed from one exercise to the next. It contained all of the elements of a good warm-up (Jeffreys, 2007); it got the heart rate up, mobilised all necessary joints, activated the muscles and there was some nice explosiveness built in to fire the nervous system too. The way in which this player moved from one exercise to another made it clear that it was ingrained in him. On this particular day, the Unit was quiet and towards the end of the programme, I approached the player and asked. "Do you do this before every round of golf?" His response. "No, Ma'am. I do this every single day". "Every day! Why?" I asked. "Because I'm afraid that if I don't, I won't ever be able to play golf again". The player in question was Mr Tom Kite, at the time he was in his mid-sixties and his warm-up was as thorough as any elite athlete or competitor would perform. He is by no means an exception to how Senior professional golfers conduct themselves. Robust, comprehensive workouts are part and parcel of many senior players programmes. While such attention to strength and conditioning (S&C) may be less the case for club golfers, this chapter aims to present the need for good-quality strength and conditioning for all senior golfers from club to elite level.

Introduction

Senior Golf is played by those aged 50 and above, with the category of Super Senior referring to players above the age of 65 years. A recent, large-scale survey commissioned by The R&A of the impact of Covid on golf participation showed that of the 19,501 responders, ~75% were over 51 years of age, with the sub category (n= 17,567) of avid golfers (those who played golf once

DOI: 10.4324/9781003099321-7

or more per week prior to Covid-19) consisting of 77% over 51s (Post Covid Opportunity Research- Research for The R&A. Sports Marketing Surveys. 2021. www.sportsmarketingsurveys.com). Indeed, in Great Britain, of the 5.2 million golfers on a full-length course, the average age of these golfers was 41 years (source www.randa.org/News/2021/05/GBandI-Golf-Participation-Report), meaning there is a substantial number of senior golfers playing the game and therefore, a specific chapter on how S&C can support senior golfers is warranted.

From an elite senior golf perspective, the senior professional golf circuit is well represented worldwide, with players competing on several continents. The senior tours worldwide are: The Champions Tour in USA, The Legends Tour in Europe, PGA Seniors in Japan, The Sunshine Senior Tour in South Africa and The Legends Tour in Australia. Competitions vary from one-day events to four-day events, with the major events of The US Senior Open, The US Senior PGA and The Senior Open Championship being played over four rounds, with a cut after two rounds, as per main tour formats. On both The Legends tour and The Champions Tour the majority of tournaments are played over three days, with the addition of a pro-am day, being a precursor to each competition.

Professional golfers are migratory, due to the nature of the tours. On The Legends Tour in Europe, for example, in the 2019 season over 50% of the Top 50 players, played across two to four international tours per year e.g., Peter Fowler, who hails from New Zealand has, in his senior career, held status in Australia, New Zealand, Japan, Europe and America. Players hold a Category on their respective tours. The categories represent the player's rank, the top category going to previous tournament winner(s), major senior champions and subsequent categories being filled according to rank, as per main tour. This means players in the highest categories will automatically qualify for one or more tours, on turning 50. For a player on The Legends Tour, they can play approximately 16–20 events a year. This is the minimum that many of the players participate in, as they would also have local pro-am and mini tours that are played off-season. As per the main tour, senior professional golf can be played year-round.

Whether amateur or professional, many of the approaches, topics and ideas detailed throughout the other chapters in this book will be applicable to senior golfers. However, there are a number of physical and physiological considerations for senior golfers that require further detail here. A number of physiological processes or conditions are more present in senior golfers and an exploration of some of these underlying processes, how they impact the golfer, but crucially how S&C can help to support the senior golfer may be useful for senior players who are considering adopting S&C to support their golf. The role of S&C for senior golfers in context is discussed below and we will end the chapter with a case study of a senior golfer undertaking regular S&C.

Special Considerations for Senior Golfers

The Ageing Process

Earth's human population is ageing. In 2020, the population was 7.79 billion and of those, 24.2% (1.88 billion) were 50 years old, or older (United Nations, Department of Economic and Social Affairs, Population Division. Source: https://population.un.org/wpp/DataQuery/ accessed 17/10/2021). The number of people aged 65 years or older is projected to increase from 254 million in 2010 to approximately 1.5 billion in 2050 (Geard et al., 2017; Jenkin et al., 2017).

With both an increasing and ageing population more generally, there will be an increasing number of people who are "senior" with regards golf. The challenge from a S&C perspective is not only to keep golfers participating in the game for as long as possible, but to allow them to do so in as peak a physical condition as possible. Additionally, it is crucial to understand what "peak" physical condition means for each individual, whether professional or amateur. In order to achieve this, we must understand the physical ageing process and how it can be influenced. Some pertinent conditions associated with the ageing process are outlined below.

Osteoarthritis

As life expectancy is increasing the number of people living for prolonged periods with severe osteoarthritis (OA) is expected to grow (Fernandes et al., 2013). OA is a chronic disorder of synovial joints, in which there is progressive softening and disintegration of articular cartilage accompanied by the growth of osteophytes (Vaishya et al., 2016). So, what does that mean? The role of cartilage is, grossly, to protect the bony surfaces of the joint and allow for friction-free movement. Ageing causes a number of changes to occur naturally in our joints. The cartilage reduces in depth and gradually breaks down. In advanced cases, as the cartilage is eroded, the underlying bone can be exposed, leading to bone-on-bone contact. The body responds to these changes by thickening the bone beneath the cartilage and growing extra bone around the affected joint surface margins. These bony outcrops are called osteophytes. They are the body's reaction to the demand being placed on the affected joint (Fernandes et al., 2013; Vaishya et al., 2016). The most commonly affected peripheral joints are the hip, hands and knees (in that order) (Gay et al., 2016).

It must be noted that OA is the everyday wearing/degrading of the skeleton. We will all have these changes, to some degree or other, in our joints throughout our lifespan. Our lifestyle in terms of fitness, diet and weight, may all play a role in the level of wear and tear in our joints, however, genetic and epigenetic factors appear to have an underpinning role in OA (Reynard & Barter, 2020).

While many people will live a full and active life regardless of the wear and tear in their joints, OA can result in pain, stiffness, loss of movement and function for the person affected by it. How OA manifests itself, though, is as individual as the person in front of you. It is important that the advice we give be tailored, therefore, to the client.

Take, for example, the following two cases. In the first case, on x-ray, OA may appear quite advanced, with a loss of joint space, loss of cartilage, bone on bone contact and osteophyte formation. However, the person may only complain of joint stiffness or a loss of function e.g. an inability to bend down to read a putt or unable to climb out of a bunker. Likewise, a person's x-ray may show mild changes to the cartilage and the joint space being intact. However, this person presents with an inflamed joint and severe pain resulting in an inability to walk the course and requesting a buggy in order to play even a few holes of golf. So, our choice and prescription of exercise will be tailored to the player and how OA affects them, rather than the severity of their disease.

As regards the management of OA, research has shown that while the joint changes cannot be reversed, the affected joint can be supported with exercise (Fernandes et al., 2013; Goh et al., 2018). The mainstays of researched treatment are in exercise, education and weight loss. While the evidence to support exercise in OA knee is of excellent quality, the research is not quite as good for other joints (Fernandes et al., 2013; Goh et al., 2018; Lefèvre-Colau et al., 2016; Wallis et al., 2013). Overall, research reports generically about strengthening the legs, or in the case of the knee joint, many of the studies refer solely to strengthening the quadriceps. However, EULAR, (European Alliance of Associations for Rheumatology) have gone a little further and included information about intensity suggesting that loading the "moderate to vigorous 60–80% of 1RM for 8–12 repetitions produced results in the management of OA" (Source: www.eular.org/index.cfm). The general consensus is that exercise is beneficial and consistent exercise is to be encouraged (Fernandes et al., 2013).

It is important when working with patients with OA that their fear of exercise is addressed (Gay et al., 2016). Research reports that many patients fear that overloading the affected joint will increase pain and cause more damage. Many older golfers have never taken part in S&C or structured gym-based exercise and if they do start, due to their beliefs around pain and potential further damage to the affected joint, adherence to programmes can be poor. If isolated and not given adequate support, clients will avoid exercise or grossly underload and fail to progress. Educating the player on the importance of improving overall strength to support the affected joint is crucial to keeping them engaged for long enough to allow them to feel the benefit.

Osteoporosis

Osteoporosis is the loss of bone density as a result of the ageing process. While age is the main predictor of osteoporosis, other issues that may accelerate it include early onset of the menopause, a maternal history of hip fracture, a fracture after 40 years of age, low body weight, or specific diseases and treatments (e.g. prolonged use of corticosteroids increase susceptibility to fractures (Reginster & Burlet, 2006). Due to the connection between osteoporosis and the menopause we must ask female clients if they are perimenopausal or menopausal and suggest to and support them in getting tested for osteoporosis and osteopenia. We need to promote this as a normal test and debunk the fear associated with it as a diagnosis. As with the other conditions, this is and will continue to be, more prevalent due to the improved life expectancy of the general population. The indication is that the numbers of people with osteoporosis worldwide, are high at over 200 million, with around 1.2 million Australians, 10.2 million Americans and 15 million European men and women over 50 years of age being affected (Harding et al., 2017).

Medication and exercise form the mainstay of treatment for these patients. However, the advice around exercise and its dosage varies. This is reflected in anecdotal evidence from patients who, on diagnosis, are advised to walk more frequently and avoid lifting heavy weights, without any guidelines as to what exactly a heavy weight is. In our experience, there is a lot of fear amongst the newly diagnosed who feel very vulnerable even with activities of daily living. As practitioners we must use the research to debunk these negative beliefs towards resistance training. Harding et al. (2017) and Watson et al. (2015) have challenged the current perceptions of avoiding heavy lifting through their own research and suggested that the optimal exercise choice for osteoporosis and osteopenia would impose dynamic, high-magnitude loads applied at a rapid rate. Indeed, there is a growing body of evidence to support that high velocity resistance training is safe and effective intervention for improving muscle power, functional performance and mobility in older individuals (Schaun et al., 2021). For example, a previous study by Watson et al. (2015) also investigated the effect of strength training in women with osteoporosis. They used a high-intensity progressive resistance training programme including deadlifts, back squats and overhead press in their research. While this is part of a larger study, their initial results were promising, in so far as their early findings showed a reversal of osteoporosis in people with low to very low bone density.

Sarcopenia

Sarcopenia is a disease which results in the loss of lean muscle mass and muscle strength as we age (Cruz-Jentoft et al., 2019). This loss of muscle results in decreased strength, metabolic rate, aerobic capacity and thus, functional capacity (Fielding et al., 2011). In 2018, a consensus was made on the definition and diagnosis of sarcopenia. While originally, a consensus in 2010 had focused on the loss of muscle mass and an increase in visceral fat, in addition to this, a more recent consensus agreed that loss of muscle strength was a principal determinant (Cruz-Jentoft et al., 2019). Ultimately, sarcopenia is problematic in older people as it results in the increased risk of falls, fractures and physical disability. While the effect of sarcopenia is most obvious in advanced old age, it begins in a much younger cohort. A progressive loss of muscle mass occurs from approximately 40 years of age (Cruz-Jentoft et al., 2019). This loss has been estimated at about 8% per decade until the age of 70 years, after which the loss increases to 15% per decade. Furthermore, in the lower limb, a 10–15 % loss of leg strength, per decade, is observed until age 70, after which a faster loss, ranging from 25% to 40% per decade is reported (Cruz-Jentoft et al., 2019). Other research papers have estimated that over the age of 50, there is a loss of between 1–2% muscle mass per year and a loss muscle strength of 1.5%–5% per year (Papa et al., 2017). In particular, studies have reported that Type II, fast-twitch muscle fibres are more affected by sarcopenia than Type I, slow-twitch fibres. This is due to a reduction in high-intensity activities that recruit Type II fibres as people age, while Type I fibres are used for most activities of daily living and during submaximal exercise and thus are more frequently stimulated (e.g. walking) (Fielding et al., 2011; Foster et al., 2007). However, it should also be noted that sarcopenia occurs regardless of a person's ability to train or otherwise. A related example of this is illustrated by the dramatic age-associated decline in the world weightlifting records. These records decline by 30% in men and over 50% in women between the ages of 30 to 60 years (Huebner et al., 2019; 2020).

The cause of sarcopenia remains unknown. It is hypothesised that neuron loss (neuromuscular ageing), age related changes in hormone production and sensitivity, poor or inadequate nutrition, chronic illness and physical inactivity all play a role in its occurrence (Dhillon & Hasni, 2017). While there may be many triggers for sarcopenia, research shows that improving nutrition and exercise can slow the rate of deterioration (Dhillon & Hasni, 2017). Again, weight training is identified as an essential part of the exercise regime for patients with sarcopenia. Research by, Hunter et al, 2004, also investigated the existing evidence-base on strength training in older adults (over 60 years of age). They identified that women responded best to bi-weekly resistance training sessions. This was supported by the work of Hunter et al. (2004) that showed bi-weekly resistance training in women resulted in more hypertrophy than that of their male counterparts. For men, a more frequent loading session was needed to gain the same hypertrophic response. It is worth noting that women in the older age bracket appear to require a longer recovery period between high intensity sessions to maximise the benefits from the sessions.

In terms of golf, the authors are only aware of limited research that has investigated the effect of golf on sarcopenia directly (Herrick et al., 2017, Stockdale et al., 2017). As golf has a wide age span, and much of the research to date has been on the under-50 population, there is further scope to look specifically at the effect that playing golf and training for golf, has on sarcopenia in the older golfing population.

Summary

What we can take from this is, that while age is not a factor that prevents a player enjoying golf, ageing is. Therefore, as coaches and clinicians we should be as proactive as possible in promoting strength and conditioning to all of our clients and club members over the age of 40. There is an abundance of opportunity for strength and conditioning coaches to link in with their local clubs and club professionals to promote strength and conditioning for club members. The influence they can have can vary from keeping older club members involved for longer, to delaying or even reversing the onset of the ageing process in the middle aged and younger age groups in the senior category improving their enjoyment of the game. In line with this, clubs can accommodate the older members of clubs by adapting the course to accommodate them, simple changes such as the 9-hole competition, ratified by The R&A, allows senior and super senior members to remain competitive. As a further example, while some course design strategies, such as taking bunkers out of play, can adapt a course to suit seniors, a potentially more golfer-centred approach would be to improve their fitness to such an extent where movements such as climbing into and out of bunkers are not seen as barriers to play.

Case Study

A number of professionals demonstrate the effect ageing has on the body and the important role exercise plays in both recovery from surgery or injury and keeping them competitive in their senior careers. This is the story of one such player. The player is (at the time of writing) 62 years old, turned pro in 1977 and has played competitively, around the world since. He played on the European Tour from 1983 until losing his card in 1996. At the time he recalls that his lack of fitness was resulting in his being over par for the last four holes of many tournaments. In 1999, he regained his tour card and made a decision that winter (off season) to rebuild his game and his fitness. He was 40 years old. He maintained his card on European Tour until he joined the ranks of the European Senior tour in 2009 and has gone on to win seven tournaments (2011–2019) and took part in an additional 2 playoffs. Pre-Covid, he played 30–35 weeks of the year, with 18 of those in either Europe and the USA, and 17 in either Australia and New Zealand. Nine of the tournaments were played prior to 1 June and the remaining 16 tournaments were played from June to December. In his Senior career, he has played on the Australian PGA Tour, the Australian/New Zealand Legends Tour, European Legends Tour, USA Champions Tour (Open events) and in 2016/17 season, he played tournaments on all of these tours and on the Japanese Senior Tour.

In discussing life on tour, we discussed his "non-negotiables". These were good sleep and regular exercise. He finds long-haul travel takes a toll on his body. He needs seven to ten days to adjust to local time, when flying to Europe from the Southern Hemisphere. As a result, flying to and fro was not an option. He based himself in the UK for the European Tour season, thereby mitigating the potential jet lag of multiple return trips. However, in the 2016/17 season, he was unable to avoid long-haul flights, as the European, US and Japanese Tours overlapped. He found that season to be particularly gruelling. His calendar necessitated that he travel to Japan for one or two tournaments and return to Europe for another event. This meant flying overnight from Japan to the event in Europe, arriving on Monday and being ready to compete again on Friday of the same week. In order to deal with the jet lag, he would go to bed at 7pm, as he was invariably awake again by midnight. This allowed him a minimum of five hours' sleep plus or minus a short nap, prior to his tournament round. He considers sleep as paramount to his ability to recover from each round and each tournament. He commented that a good night's sleep helped him feel physically strong and ready for the rigours of his game.

The other non-negotiable was exercise. This player has had numerous joint issues over the years and Table 7.1 shows the medical interventions he has required to treat them. He also has to work continuously on his right shoulder for a longstanding and ongoing issue.

Regarding exercise, he has a daily timetable of exercise and he is diligent in following it. During the season, Monday is gym-based and includes a weight-training programme. When there is no gym available, this is adapted to bodyweight and resistance bands. Tuesday focuses on mobility work. Wednesday is a bike ride or swim followed by a stretching programme. (I remember arriving at an event in Germany and as the car I was travelling in slowed down, on approach to the tournament venue, I spotted this player emerge from a lake across the road! He has always found a body of water for his biweekly swims.) Thursday is a combination of mobility exercises, stretches and a bike ride. In tournament weeks, this is also pro-am day, which would involve a five-hour round of golf.

Tournament days include a thorough warm up and cool down. Pre- and post- round exercises include dynamic body weight exercises and loading with resistance bands. He carries a mobile gym of resistance bands, foam roller and massage ball to all events. If there are gym facilities onsite, he will use weights during tournament weeks also. Due to the effect the multiple surgeries have had on him, flexibility and mobility are key parts of his routine, when he is on the road. Travelling between tournaments, hours spent practising, length of time spent playing a competitive round all contribute to players stiffening up (or feeling as though they are stiffening up) over time. As a result, their focus is on maintaining mobility (range of movement throughout all the joints in the body) and flexibility, as much as and in some cases more so, than on power and strength.

Table 7.1 Medical interventions

Year	Intervention
2007, 2015, 2016	Injections into cervical spine (neck)
2009	Lumbar spine (lower back) disc surgery
2009, 2010, 2016	Right hip arthroscopy
2018	Right hip replacement
2020	Right knee arthroscopy

Training Programmes

Historically, for the senior golfer, S&C has not been associated with golf. In the professional game until the late 1990s, functional movement, aerobic golf specific exercises were the prevailing methods of training. From club player to professional, lifting weights was considered of detriment to the swing and in our experience, this belief remains the case in senior golf both in amateur and professional ranks today. It was also poorly understood by golf coaches and there were very mixed messages and opinions regarding the use of S&C for golfers. However, research would support resistance training is not only of benefit to sport in an ageing population, as discussed earlier, it may also influence the ageing process itself (Hunter et al., 2004; Papa et al., 2017).

In order for players to want to engage in exercise, it is important to induct them into exercise at a level that they are comfortable with, while still being challenged. Tables 7.2 to 7.4 show examples of how this can be achieved. Initially, we encourage the players to begin moving. Each row represents a different movement and each column represents a level of difficulty. For example, the easiest exercise for glute strength is a glute squeeze and the most difficult, a supported stork stand. The aim is to pick six exercises, one from each row and do each for a minute. The level of difficulty can be asserted by picking an exercise that while challenging, allows good form to be maintained for the one-minute duration.

For each of the rows, the player may choose a different level of difficulty for each movement, they are not confined to picking all exercise from the same column. While a player may have good strength and choose an exercise from the right-side columns for leg and glute strength. They may have poor mobility and therefore choose an exercise from the left for Upper body rotation and posture, for example. Over time, the aim is to progress all six exercises to Level +3 at which point the player can progress to the next level of training.

The progressions in each Table and from one Table to another, serve another purpose. If a player is injured and if complete rest is deemed unnecessary, they can choose an easier form of an exercise to allow them to continue to train or play. There have been times, on tour, when players have over trained or overexerted themselves on the practice ground and have gone home without seeking advice, as they perceive rest to be their only option. Their fear being that to play into pain or with pain, is a sign of causing damage and that is not necessarily the case. For example, an osteoarthritic joint can be uncomfortable or painful when aggravated and may need relative and not complete rest, to settle it down. Once reassured that "hurt does not equal harm", they can be allowed return to a suitable level of training. Finding the correct level of movement for each player, can keep them competitive and build their confidence in their ability to return to play quickly following an actual or a perceived injury. The loading in the exercise in Tables 7.2 to 7.4 can be modified to maintain movement, while offloading an affected joint or limb and allowing a more productive recovery.

Table 7.2 Physical Development Programme – Phase One – How Much?

Physical Development Programme
Phase One ~ How Much
Six exercises in six minutes

-3	-2	-1	Movement	+1	+2	+3
Glute squeeze (lying down and standing)	Hip bridge	Hip bridge on bench	**Glute Strength**	Hip bridge, single leg	Hip bridge, single leg on bench	Supported stork stand with rotation and push into floor
Side lying with arms opening	Four point kneeling chicken wings	Four point kneeling reach through	**Upper Body Rotation**	Bent over knee push with one arm rotations	Supported wall rotation	Star hold rotations
Upper body dissociation	Lower body dissociation	Pelvic tilt	**Posture**	Hip hinge with club from kneeling	Hip hinge with club from standing	RDL
Front plank	Side plank left and right	Press up hold with arms moving	**Core**	Kneeling overhead band press	Standing overhead band press	Single arm standing overhead band press
½ squat hold for 10 seconds	Full squat	Overhead squat with club	**Leg Strength**	Single leg ¼ squat with knee up	Forward, side & reverse lunge	Supported single leg squat to ¼
Box plank	Long arm plank	Farmers walk with golf bag	**Trunk Stability**	Suitcase carry with golf bag	Suitcase carry in front of body	Single hand overhead carry

Table 7.3 Physical Development Programme – Phase Two – How Well?

Physical Development Programme
Phase Two ~ How Well
Fundamental Movement Patterns

-3	-2	-1	Movement	+1	+2	+3
Band-assisted OHS	Broomstick OHS	Sumo squat weight transfer	**Squat**	DB goblet squat	Hex bar deadlift	Back/front squat
Wall push up	Band assisted push up	DB bridge/floor press	**Push**	BW or suspended push up	BB bench press	BB push press
Bear crawls	Band Pallof variants	Asymmetric band-kneeling overhead raise	**Brace / AntiRotation**	Dish sit	DB plank row	Loaded carries
Band rows	45 degree suspended row	Inverted row (calf on bench)	**Pull**	Horizontal suspended row	DB single arm row	Chin up
Barbell RDL	KB RDL	Band pull through	**Hinge**	Single leg RDL rear foot supported	Single leg RDL (loaded contralaterally)	Good morning
1-leg bridge	BW reverse lunge	Step up variants	**Single Leg Stability**	Sit to stand	Pistol squat	BB rear foot elevated split squat
MB kneeling throw	MB overhead toss	MB shot throw	**Explosive Strength**	BB squat jump	MB lying throw	MB slam

Table 7.4 Physical Development Programme Phase Three, How Strong?

Physical Development Programme
Phase Three ~ How Strong

Upper body push vertical	Upper body push horizontal	Lower body anterior chain	Strength training style	Lower body posterior chain	Upper body pull horizontal	Upper body pull vertical
Standing press	DB flat press	Forward lunge	**Stage 1 ~ Negative pyramids 10/8/6**	Reverse lunge	Standing row	Pulldowns
Seated press	DB incline press	Front squat to ½	**Stage 2 ~ 5 rep max**	Trap bar deadlift	Bent over row	Chin ups
Kneeling press	DB flat press one arm	Step up medium box	**Stage 3 ~ Positive pyramids 4/5/6**	Forward and backward lunge	One arm bench row	One arm pulldowns
DB seated press one arm	DB incline press one arm	Front squat ½	**Stage 4 ~ 3 rep max**	Deadlift	Bent over row	Chin ups
DB kneeling press one arm	DB bridge press	Single leg ½ squat to box	**Stage 5 ~ Waves 5/3/5**	Reverse lunge	Standing row one arm	Pull ups neutral grip
DB seated press lowering only	DB incline press lowering only	Back squat ½ lowering only	**Stage 6 ~ Eccentric fives**	Romanian deadlift	Seated row lowering only	Pull ups lowering only
Standing press	Bench press flat	Back squat to ½	**Stage 7 ~ Clusters threes**	Trap bar deadlift	Decline pulls	Pull up

Once a player has become competent at basic movements, they progress to Table 7.3 and Fundamental Movement Patterns. The concept remains the same, each row is a different movement pattern and the column are the varying degrees of difficulty. Again, the exercises can be adapted to training both on and off the road or for club golfers, they can be done either at home or in the gym. For those training at home or on the road, dumbbells can be replaced with any weighted item such as a loaded backpack or golf bag. The weight can be incrementally increased as the player gets stronger.

Difficulty is based on the ability to maintain good form and can be progressed or regressed according to how the player feels on a given training day. These training sessions can also be continued in tournament and for the Senior Players, like their counterparts in the Main Tour and Challenge Tour or younger age categories, training all year round is essential. Again, this is a concept that challenges many of our players, who would still be of the belief that training is for off season only, although the tide is slowly turning towards the benefits of year-round training.

Finally, when all of the movement skills in Table 7.3 are mastered, the player can progress to Table 7.4 which focuses on the development of a player's strength through the use seven different training styles. Players can perform each stage for a number of weeks to progressively challenge the body to increase in strength. In the professional rankings, there are a growing number of players that begin their senior career with a well-established training age and the use of these training styles also accommodates these players. The player in this case study has made steady and consistent progress through these exercise Tables and continues to work on their S&C to support their golf.

Review of S&C Support for the Player

In relation to our case study, he started in the gym at the age of 40 and has adhered to a daily workout schedule since. This year the player is aged 62 (at the time of writing) and he has added more explosive work and heavier sessions in the early part of the week and tapering to lighter, maintenance sessions during tournament days as was previously discussed.

The athlete has reported to us that aged 40 he could hit a ball 250 yards and that was hitting it as hard as he could, every shot. Now, at the age of 62, he is hitting the ball 270 yards and in the optimum conditions he can hit it 300 yards. While some improvement may be related to equipment design, he also reports that he suffers less pain now, than when he was 40 despite his injuries and surgeries and he attributes this success to his consistency and dedication to his S&C programme.

Conclusions

As was noted at the beginning of this chapter, we are an ageing population and in order to keep golfers active for as long as possible, resistance training must be considered as an important factor for senior golfers going forward. Although evidence is lacking as to the precise effect it has on the individual's game, research fully supports exercise and resistance training as an important tool in the prevention of diseases and the effects of ageing. Encouraging this population to begin such training as early as possible and to being consistent is key in gaining the maximum potential later in life. We can incentivise this population to train effectively by promoting the ability to play for longer but also by promoting the fact that exercise can slow down and, in some cases, reverse, diseases such as osteoporosis, sarcopenia and osteoarthritis.

As of late 2021, the oldest professional golfer registered to play and still competing on Champions Tour is Hale Irwin at 76 years old. He repeatedly scored better than his age in the 2020 season. With an active and ageing population, Hale and his Senior and Super Senior counterparts are an example of our ability to play and preform at a very competitive level regardless of age. We must strive to use our platform in strength and conditioning and associated therapies to promote resistance training in the over-50 golfing population and in so doing improve the depth and quality of research which is currently lacking in this area.

References

Cruz-Jentoft, A. J., Bahat, G., Bauer, J., Boirie, Y., Bruyère, O., Cederholm, T., Cooper, C., Landi, F., Rolland, Y., Sayer, A. A., Schneider, S. M., Sieber, C. C., Topinkova, E., Vandewoude, M., Visser, M., Zamboni, M., Bautmans, I., Baeyens, J. P., Cesari, M., Schols, J. (2019). Sarcopenia: Revised European consensus on definition and diagnosis. In *Age and Ageing* (Vol. 48, Issue 1, pp. 16–31). Oxford University Press. https://doi.org/10.1093/ageing/afy169

Dhillon, R. J. S., & Hasni, S. (2017). Pathogenesis and Management of Sarcopenia. In *Clinics in Geriatric Medicine* (Vol. 33, Issue 1, pp. 17–26). W.B. Saunders. https://doi.org/10.1016/j.cger.2016.08.002

Fernandes, L., Hagen, K. B., Bijlsma, J. W. J., Andreassen, O., Christensen, P., Conaghan, P. G., Doherty, M., Geenen, R., Hammond, A., Kjeken, I., Lohmander, L. S., Lund, H., Mallen, C. D., Nava, T., Oliver, S., Pavelka, K., Pitsillidou, I., da Silva, J. A., de La Torre, J., Vliet Vlieland, T. P. M. (2013). EULAR recommendations for the non-pharmacological core management of hip and knee osteoarthritis. In *Annals of the Rheumatic Diseases* (Vol. 72, Issue 7, pp. 1125–1135). https://doi.org/10.1136/annrheumdis-2012-202745

Fielding, R. A., Vellas, B., Evans, W. J., Bhasin, S., Morley, J. E., Newman, A. B., Abellan van Kan, G., Andrieu, S., Bauer, J., Breuille, D., Cederholm, T., Chandler, J., de Meynard, C., Donini, L., Harris, T., Kannt, A., Keime Guibert, F., Onder, G., Papanicolaou, D., Zamboni, M. (2011). Sarcopenia: An Undiagnosed Condition in Older Adults. Current Consensus Definition: Prevalence, Etiology, and Consequences. International Working Group on Sarcopenia. *Journal of the American Medical Directors Association*, 12(4), 249–256. https://doi.org/10.1016/j.jamda.2011.01.003

Foster, C., Wright, G., Battista, R. A., & Porcari, J. P. (2007). Training in the aging athlete. In *Current Sports Medicine Reports* (Vol. 6, Issue 3, pp. 200–206). https://doi.org/10.1007/s11932-007-0029-4

Gay, C., Chabaud, A., Guilley, E., & Coudeyre, E. (2016). Educating patients about the benefits of physical activity and exercise for their hip and knee osteoarthritis. Systematic literature review. In *Annals of Physical and Rehabilitation Medicine* (Vol. 59, Issue 3, pp. 174–183). Elsevier Masson SAS. https://doi.org/10.1016/j.rehab.2016.02.005

Geard, D., Reaburn, P. R. J., Rebar, A. L., & Dionigi, R. A. (2017). Masters athletes: Exemplars of successful aging? In *Journal of Aging and Physical Activity* (Vol. 25, Issue 3, pp. 490–500). Human Kinetics Publishers Inc. https://doi.org/10.1123/japa.2016-0050

Goh, S. L., Persson, M. S. M., Stocks, J., Hou, Y. F., Lin, J. H., Hall, M., Doherty, M., & Zhang, W. (2018). *FRI0546 Relative efficacy of different exercises in knee and hip osteoarthritis, 798*, 1–798. https://doi.org/10.1136/annrheumdis-2018-eular.3370

Harding, A. T., Weeks, B. K., Watson, S. L., & Beck, B. R. (2017). The LIFTMOR-M (Lifting Intervention for Training Muscle and Osteoporosis Rehabilitation for Men) trial: Protocol for a semirandomised controlled trial of supervised targeted exercise to reduce risk of osteoporotic fracture in older men with low bone mass. *BMJ Open, 7*(6). https://doi.org/10.1136/bmjopen-2016-014951

Herrick, I., Brown, S., Agyapong-Badu, S., Warner, M., Ewings, S., Samuel, D., & Stokes, M. (2017). Anterior Thigh Tissue Thickness Measured Using Ultrasound Imaging in Older Recreational Female Golfers and Sedentary Controls. *Geriatrics (Basel, Switzerland), 2*(1), 10. https://doi.org/10.3390/geriatrics2010010

Huebner, M., Meltzer, D. E., & Perperoglou, A. (2019). Age-associated Performance Decline and Sex Differences in Olympic Weightlifting. *Medicine and Science in Sports and Exercise, 51*(11), 2302–2308. https://doi.org/10.1249/MSS.0000000000002037

Huebner, M., Meltzer, D., Ma, W., & Arrow, H. (2020). The Masters athlete in Olympic weightlifting: Training, lifestyle, health challenges, and gender differences. *PLoS ONE, 15*(12 December). https://doi.org/10.1371/journal.pone.0243652

Hunter, G. R., McCarthy, J. P., & Bamman, M. M. (2004). Effects of resistance training on older adults. In *Sports Medicine* (Vol. 34, Issue 5, pp. 329–348). https://doi.org/10.2165/00007256-200434050-00005

Jeffreys, I. (2007). *UK STRENGTH AND CONDITIONING ASSOCIATION Warm up revisited-the "ramp" method of optimising performance preparation.* www.uksca.org. uke:info@uksca.org.uk15

Jenkin, C. R., Eime, R. M., Westerbeek, H., O'Sullivan, G., & van Uffelen, J. G. Z. (2017). Sport and ageing: A systematic review of the determinants and trends of participation in sport for older adults. *BMC Public Health, 17*(1). https://doi.org/10.1186/s12889-017-4970-8

Lefèvre-Colau, M. M., Nguyen, C., Haddad, R., Delamarche, P., Paris, G., Palazzo, C., Poiraudeau, S., Rannou, F., & Roren, A. (2016). Is physical activity, practiced as recommended for health benefit, a risk factor for osteoarthritis? In *Annals of Physical and Rehabilitation Medicine* (Vol. 59, Issue 3, pp. 196–206). Elsevier Masson SAS. https://doi.org/10.1016/j.rehab.2016.02.007

Papa, E. V., Dong, X., & Hassan, M. (2017). Resistance training for activity limitations in older adults with skeletal muscle function deficits: a systematic review. *Clinical interventions in aging, 12*, 955–961. https://doi.org/10.2147/CIA.S104674

Reyard, L. N. and Barter, M.J. (2020) Osteoarthritis year in review 2019: genetics, genomics and epigenetics. *Osteoarthritis and Cartilage* (Vol 28, Issue 3, pp. 275–284). https://doi.org/10.1016/j.joca.2019.11.010

Reginster, J. Y., & Burlet, N. (2006). Osteoporosis: A still increasing prevalence. *Bone,* *38*(2 SUPPL. 1), 4–9. https://doi.org/10.1016/j.bone.2005.11.024

Schaun, G. Z., Bamman, M. M., and Alberton, C. L. (2021) High-velocity resistance training as a tool to improve functional performance and muscle power in older adults. *Experimental Gerontology,* Vol. 156. https://doi.org/10.1016/j.exger.2021.111593

Stockdale, A., Webb, N., Wootton, J., Drennan, J., Brown, S., & Stokes, M. (2017). Muscle Strength and Functional Ability in Recreational Female Golfers and Less Active Non-Golfers over the Age of 80 Years. *Geriatrics (Basel, Switzerland),* *2*(1), 12. https://doi.org/10.3390/geriatrics2010012

Vaishya, R., Pariyo, G. B., Agarwal, A. K., & Vijay, V. (2016). Non-operative management of osteoarthritis of the knee joint. In *Journal of Clinical Orthopaedics and Trauma* (Vol. 7, Issue 3, pp. 170–176). Elsevier B.V. https://doi.org/10.1016/j.jcot.2016.05.005

Wallis, J. A., Webster, K. E., Levinger, P., & Taylor, N. F. (2013). What proportion of people with hip and knee osteoarthritis meet physical activity guidelines? A systematic review and meta-analysis. In *Osteoarthritis and Cartilage* (Vol. 21, Issue 11, pp. 1648–1659). https://doi.org/10.1016/j.joca.2013.08.003

Watson, S. L., Weeks, B. K., Weis, L. J., Horan, S. A., & Beck, B. R. (2015). Heavy resistance training is safe and improves bone, function, and stature in postmenopausal women with low to very low bone mass: novel early findings from the LIFTMOR trial. *Osteoporosis International,* *26*(12), 2889–2894. https://doi.org/10.1007/s00198-015-3263-2

8 The Elite Golfer

Simon Brearley, Dan Coughlan, and Alex Bliss

Introduction: How Can S&C Support and/or Improve Golf Performance? A Philosophy for Strategising Performance Impact

Few players have sustained championship winning performances over an extended period of time in the history of the game, which is reflected in the very exclusive "career grand slam" club (a winner of all four major tournaments). For the majority of players, high performance is elusive and fleeting, which is indicative of the complexities of golf performance, which is subject to both the non-linearity of human movement control and the vagaries of human cognitions and behaviour. Consequently, this makes prediction fraught with challenge and specific training interventions difficult to justify with any great confidence. Indeed, players often produce performances which are at odds with, for example, their disrupted preparations or recent playing level. Conversely, they might underperform when the supporting evidence (e.g. data and coaching insight) suggests they should be succeeding.

The above is particularly true from a physical preparation standpoint, which we have to accept for golf is not as intertwined with the performance outcome as it is in physiology-dominated sports such as cycling or rowing. Naturally, this is intuitive to most support staff working in golf and one of the reasons clubhead speed (CHS) has become a major focus of S&C programmes. This measure is one that has been heavily researched and allows us to apply the scientific "cause and effect" method, reduce uncertainty, and evidence our potential to impact performance. For example, it is possible to work to a deterministic model of CHS to reverse engineer a performance impact strategy. This approach will likely produce greater impacts than generically applied programmes built on ideology. However, "big picture thinking" will also help us compliment this reductionist approach by considering the ways physical preparation can accumulate into an equal or greater performance impact. This approach is depicted by a previously published "Probability of Performance Impact model" (Figure 8.1) which acts as an overarching philosophy to how the European Tour Performance Institute (ETPI) support players on the European Tour. Working to this model adds clarity to how we can change performance,

DOI: 10.4324/9781003099321-8

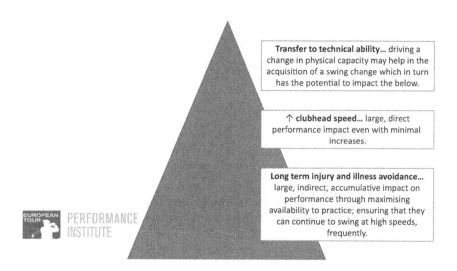

Figure 8.1 Probability of Performance Impact Model from Brearley et al. (2019). The model demonstrates higher probability towards the bottom of the pyramid and less probability towards the peak

and helps ensure we "ask the right questions" with respect to each avenue for potential impact:

- **Availability:** Given the technical nature of the sport, one metric almost certainly related to success will be availability to practice and compete. It has been demonstrated that individuals with superior strength levels are less susceptible to overuse injury (Lauersen et al., 2014) and those with better cardio-respiratory fitness are more resilient to, and recover quicker from bouts of illness. Therefore, a good question to pose as a starting point when tackling the individual player performance puzzle is: Q1. *Can the player tolerate the training they need to do to get to, and remain at, the top level in the sport?*
- **Durability & Readiness:** Just because a player is available to play (i.e. not injured or ill) doesn't necessarily mean they are ready to perform week after week. Given the stressors and psycho-physiological burden associated with being a tour professional, another important question to consider and monitor is: Q2. *Can the player tolerate the lifestyle/schedule and have the durability to sustain performance at the highest level?*
- **Movement:** The third obvious avenue for impact is to change how players move. This could be with a view to increasing CHS, improving consistency of strike, or moving more efficiently. Any intervention directed towards changing movement should be formulated with the entire support team so it can be built around a shared understanding of what technical changes

are desired. Each practitioner can then have a clear understanding of what their relative contributions are, while crucially respecting this as an optimisation problem, navigating the complex inter-relationship of technical variables and physical qualities. The reader is referred to Chapter 10 for greater detail around the challenges and opportunities faced by the S&C coach in this space. However, the questions for the support team to ponder here are: Q3. *Why is the player self-selecting their existing movement strategy? Q4. Is their existing movement "healthy" or attritional? Q5. Are there any physical constraints that may be limiting future movement options?*

As discussed above, the ability to measure changes in CHS (together with the growing body of research around how to improve it) makes it easy to become blinkered by this single metric when designing training programmes to impact golf performance. However, any doubt over Q1, Q2, or Q4 above arguably indicates an orientation of training and tracking measures towards resilience and readiness. As practitioners we should keep in mind the words of Albert Einstein, which are very apt in this regard:

> "Not everything that can be counted counts, and not everything that counts can be counted."

Readiness and resilience are hard to gauge and quantify, but this shouldn't mean we overlook these critical qualities in the process of training programme design. Future research may offer greater clarity on the physiological predictors of durability and help us design better training plans. In the meantime, we should strive to engineer the training process so that insight is gained into the individual response of players, thereby affording us greater certainty in our future training planning and programming decisions. We should embrace our creativity and not be afraid to make the design of these training programmes aligned to these outcomes and the player's preferences, as opposed to industry ideologies.

Practical Applications

Considerations for the Elite Touring Golfer. Individual S&C Coach? Or a Tour/NGB-Provided S&C Coach?

An elite touring athlete's life can be both enriched and complicated by the necessity of international travel (Pipe, 2011). On the PGA Tour, there is frequent interstate travel, and occasional tournaments outside of the mainland United States, or in neighbouring countries such as Mexico. On the European Tour, there is frequent intercontinental travel. In 2020, the European Tour held tournaments as far East as Australia, as well as in the Middle East, Asia, Africa, and across Europe and therefore the notion of a "European Tour" is arguably an incongruity. For the elite, touring golfer, an important area of consideration is where they choose to "base" themselves during the season. Golfers may choose to follow the tour and reside wherever the next tournament is being held. High-profile, high-earning golfers may choose this approach, or have multiple properties to allow them to achieve a semblance of normality to their schedules when away from their main home. However, for the majority of tour golfers, available finance will be a major constraint to this approach and therefore they will likely base themselves in their home country when not competing.

The requirement for frequent interstate or international travel may prove problematic if the elite golfer requires support staff to attend events. High-earning golfers may have the financial resources to appoint an S&C coach to travel with them and provide support throughout the season. This is a recognised approach in other individual sports such as tennis. However, to counter these constraints, the ETPI provide a support service for players that is based at most tournaments throughout the year. The ETPI has been successful and popular with players, with most players utilising various aspects of the service in the 2021 season. However, there are players who choose to have their own individual S&C coach. It is advisable for the home or individual S&C coach, if they cannot travel to events, to liaise with the player about availability of gyms or training facilities in those weeks. If maintaining strength during the season is a focus of the S&C programme, then having multiple weeks where the athlete is left to find their own training space and conduct their own sessions could be problematic (see Chapter 3), particularly if the player has low S&C training experience or motivation. If the home S&C coach is unable to work with their player face-to-face while the player is travelling, then digital/remote coaching is also a possibility, particularly with improvements with online conferencing and video call software. Additionally, the home S&C coach could choose to collaborate with certified service providers (if available) on the player's tour to ensure exercise habits are maintained and programmed sessions are able to be conducted.

Travelling Player

The interstate or international touring elite golfer is exposed to frequent travel demands, usually across time zones. In addition to maintaining high sport performance levels throughout the season, the athlete must ensure that they maintain their health in order to maximise playing opportunities, and by extension, opportunities to earn money, points, and win tournaments. It is known that regular long-distance travel results in fatigue and the effects can be cumulative in nature, with jet-lag (which can occur where athletes cover more than three time zones in a journey) being a primary cause (van Rensburg et al., 2020; 2021). This is particularly so in west–east travel, which has been shown to impair performance in a range of physical assessments, as well as sleep onset, duration, and motivation in athletes (Fowler et al., 2017). Players will experience (as a rule of thumb guide) jet lag symptoms that last for 24 hours for each time zone crossed in an easterly direction, and 12 hours for westbound travel (Leatherwood & Dragoo, 2013). A player's natural body clock has profound effects on their biological function (Vitale et al., 2019) and disruptions to the athlete's circadian rhythms can result in a range of physical, physiological, and psychological issues. Commonly reported issues are effects on sleep quality and quantity and gastro-intestinal disruptions which will ultimately impact on the ability of that athlete to perform during competition (van Rensburg et al., 2020; 2021).

To mitigate the effects of extensive travel, particularly where west–east travel is required across multiple time zones, research has suggested that players should reset their watches and mobile phones to the destination time when flying, avoid blue light from electronic devices at night, and also bring objects with them from home such as their own pillows or bed sheets to encourage nat-ural sleep and alleviate the "first-night effect" where poor sleep is particularly common (Vitale et al., 2019). These "lifestyle" factors, in our opinion, should be attempted first and, if unsuccessful, then the player may seek medicinal intervention, if required, under recommendation from a qualified healthcare practitioner.

In-Season and Tournament S&C Considerations

A major consideration for the S&C coach supporting elite players is the main-tenance of physical qualities during the competitive season. The competitive golf season at elite level is as long as the player chooses it to be. On the European Tour for example, there are tournaments scheduled from November to October and a player with sufficient ranking points and those who qualify for major championships and end of season Race to Dubai tournaments *could* choose to play year-round. For the majority of players though who are lower ranked and do not have the necessary invites or qualification to play all scheduled tournaments will likely need to have a more reactive approach to their tourna-ment and therefore S&C schedule.

While this is discussed in greater detail in the Chapter 3, Figure 8.2 below shows an example of a typical week, and how this could vary depending on tee time and whether the player makes the cut for a standard 72-hole stroke play tournament. This Figure was devised for an article for the *PGA Magazine* (Bliss, 2018) and shows a real-world example of a support strategy for a European Tour professional. The aim of the Figure is to highlight how the structure of the week can adapt to allow the player to continue to train in competition weeks. It is contingent on the golf athlete having a willingness to train regardless of whether they make the cut or not. Anecdotally, a common fear for golfers is that conducting S&C training during competition weeks will result in muscle soreness, fatigue, and restriction in range of motion that would lead to an inability to execute the technical aspects of their golf swing and reduced overall performance. However, skilled S&C coaches can prescribe training in competi-tion weeks that reduces training volume load (the total amount of weight lifted across a session) and which also limits the amount of unfamiliar movements involving eccentric muscle actions, as these are contributors to muscle damage, soreness, and reduced muscle function (Hody et al., 2019), while still achieving

		Mon	Tue	Wed	Thu	Fri	Sat	Sun
Competition Week – Early Tee time	AM	Rest Day	Travel	Practice/Gym*	Competition	Practice	Competition/Gym*	Competition
	PM	Rest Day	Practice Round	Practice/Gym*	Gym	Competition	Competition/Gym*	Travel
Competition Week – Late Tee time	AM	Rest Day	Travel	Practice/Gym*	Practice	Practice/ Competition	Competition/Gym*	Competition
	PM	Rest Day	Practice Round	Practice/Gym*	Competition	Gym	Competition/Gym*	Travel
Competition Week – Missed Cut – Early Tee Time	AM	Rest Day	Travel	Practice/Gym*	Competition	Practice	Practice/Gym*	Rest
	PM	Rest Day	Practice Round	Practice/Gym*	Gym	Competition	Practice/Gym*	Travel
Competition Week – Missed Cut – Late Tee Time	AM	Rest Day	Travel	Practice/Gym*	Practice	Practice/ Competition	Practice/Gym*	Rest
	PM	Rest Day	Practice Round	Practice/Gym*	Competition	Gym	Practice/Gym*	Travel

Figure 8.2 Example week plan for an elite touring golfer
*Dependent on tee time for practice round.
Source: Taken from Bliss (2018).

a training stimulus that can maintain or even improve physical qualities. To ensure a well rationalised, appropriate programme is devised for the golfer in competition weeks, players are encouraged to seek S&C support from a qualified practitioner.

Case Study Examples of Support for Elite Golfers:

Case Study 1 – Elite Junior Female Amateur (Player A)s

Background

This case report details the physical development journey of a junior girl (Player A) progressing through the England Golf performance pathway. Support for the player began upon successful application to the England Golf regional performance programme in the autumn of 2017, at this point the player was 13 years of age with a handicap of 6.5 (stature: 167 cm, body mass 53 kg).

A Behavioural Approach to Athlete Development

The England Golf regional programme aims to "produce 12 players each year with the skills and capabilities to represent and win points for England at the European Team Championships". In order to pursue this ambitious goal, S&C coaches assume shared responsibilities with the golf coaches, and are then also assigned some further, discipline specific Key Performance Indicators (KPIs). These are outlined below:

Table 8.1 Regional coaching team responsibilities with S&C discipline specifics

Shared Responsibilities of Regional Coaching Team	S&C Discipline Specific Responsibilities
• H'cap improvements; • Participation in national tournaments; • # players transitioning to national squad over 3-year period; • Evidence of strong relationships fostered with players.	• Demonstrable progression of "Train Well" behaviours: warm up, gym, structure; • Demonstrable progression of "Eat Well" behaviours: nutritional prep; • Demonstrable progression of "Rest Well" behaviours: sleep, self-management, recovery strategies. • Development of clubhead speed.

Given these responsibilities largely centre around behaviour change, it made sense to use behavioural milestones to evaluate the progress of Player A. Consequently, development was driven through habit formation and

Table 8.2 Behavioural Milestones used to drive and evaluate progress (target to reach milestone 5 before exit)

Milestone	Mindset	In Session	Out of Session
1	Doesn't appreciate value of S&C. Receives a programme rather than participates	Arrives on time and follows instruction	Only performs S&C when timetabled for squad sessions. No engagement with coaching platform
2	Recognises value of S&C, but understanding is limited. Training misdirected through negative influences	Familiar with some exercises and basic programming variables like sets, reps, rest etc.	Independently does a warm up at least twice per week
3	Positively influenced and shows some appropriate S&C training behaviours	Can follow programme independently. Some compound exercise with ~50% body mass	Performs home DIY S&C sessions twice per week. Engages with coaching platform sporadically
4	Engaged, asks questions about exercises and goal setting and how this connects to golf	Some explosive strength development exercise (jumps, throws) and some compound movements with ~100% body mass	Can work safely with free weights or home set up. Effectively applying progressive overload. Regular contact on coaching platform
5	Makes requests around exercise and programming. Informs, active participant in training. Stable S&C habits	Can perform loaded movement, compound and explosive (Oly lift and derivative etc.). Compounds ~150% body mass	Has a variety of sessions available to them and knowledge of how to adapt them to tournament/ travel requirements. Regularly engaged with coaching platform

process goals as opposed to outcome goals (see Table 8.2), although these goals were intertwined with tangible physical development markers – namely the "Earn the Right to Rotate" criteria.

Years 1–2 – Build a robust chassis / Earn the Right to Rotate (13–15years)

The "Earn the Right to Rotate" concept was implemented to help reduce the risk of injury. With the increasing emphasis on young players to develop CHS, and the prevalence of spondylolysis in adolescents participating in high-velocity extension-rotation based sports (Brearley et al., 2021), S&C coaches have a responsibility to safeguard young players through such processes which harness swing speed development in a safe manner. Furthermore, any time loss from practice at such a critical stage in their technical development has the potential to significantly stall progress and prevent them from reaching their potential in the sport at senior level.

Therefore, the first two years of support with this player was focused on meeting the "Earn the Right to Rotate" criteria before moving onto dedicated speed training. The criteria is evolving with the evidence base but at the time it was as follows:

- Side plank capacity = >2mins
- Isometric anti-rotation trunk strength = >13kg
- Minimum of three months of gym-based loading (competent across gym-based fundamental movement skills and performing compound lifts with at least 50% bodyweight)

On reference to Table 8.2 you will see this to correspond to the tangible physical development markers embedded within milestone 3. The overarching rationale for tailoring training to these progress measures was to establish braking capabilities and a robust chassis, with a particular emphasis on the musculature of the hips and trunk. The side plank and isometric trunk test served to track progress in the local metabolic capacity and strength/static RFD of these muscle groups respectively. Additionally, given the evidence supporting the efficacy of general strength training to protect against overuse injury, it was decided the player should complete roughly three months of basic gym-based loading to allow time for the protein and collagen synthesis adaptations likely responsible for this apparent increased tissue resilience. Table 8.3 shows two typical gym-based sessions used to deliver these tangible objectives.

Years 3–4 – Build a bigger engine (16–17 Years)

Having established the requisite foundations to make every effort to safeguard the player against injury, the next step was to develop structure and neuromuscular capacities that would raise the potential for greater CHS longitudinally. This involved a major introduction of properly loaded, traditional barbell exercises or variants. On observation of the player executing heavy pulls from the floor (i.e. deadlift patterns) it was evident performance was limited by thoracic extensor strength and range as opposed to leg strength. Given the importance of thoracic spine function in the golf swing this therefore became a major focus of the programme and an inclined leg press was used concomitantly to avoid delay in lower limb muscle mass and extensor force development. For the upper body, chin up and bench press were primary tools used to drive muscle mass and

Table 8.3 Example programmes from years 1–2

Years 1–2 Establishing a Robust Chassis:
Typical gym session from winter training block

Session A

Strength Foundations & MSK Conditioning	Set	Rep	Rest	RPE	Wt	Notes
1 KB RDL	3	8–15	1.5	7		RDL = Romanian deadlift (loaded hinge)
2 Loaded Carry	3	20 m	1.5	8		Bilateral carry variations
3a Band lateral walkout (overhead)	3|3	4	1	7		1 rep = 1 lateral step
3b ECC Suspended row (2up/1down)	3|3	6–8	1	7		SLOW during lowering (~3–4 s)
3c Side Plank	3|3	TF	1	N/A		TF = To failure
3d Leg Plate Russian Twist	3|3	6–8	1	7		
4 wrist/neck loading						

Session B

Strength Foundations & MSK Conditioning	Set	Rep	Rest	RPE	Wt	Notes
1 KB Goblet Pause Squat	3	8–15	1.5	7		2 s pause at bottom
2 KB Split Squat	3|3	6–8	1.5	7		
3a Kneeling shoulder raise (asymmetric)	3|3	6–8	1	7		
3b Plank row / Crawling plank	3	10 m	1	7		Increase distance weekly
3c Side Plank	3|3	TF	1	N/A		TF = To failure
3d Band pullover ISO/ Eccentric Push Up	3	5–15	1	7		
4 wrist/neck loading						

strength development, while the programme had a supplementary focus on isolated development of the scapula musculature and posterior cuff due to compensatory movement patterns around the scapula exhibited during gym-based fundamental movement patterns (i.e. push up). Table 8.4 shows typical gym-based sessions from both the autumn–winter and spring–summer periods, with a shift in emphasis towards explosive strength development in the latter.

Year 5 – Application (17 years–present)

Although a proportion of the training year continued to be devoted to development of structure and neuromuscular capacities, this year now placed greater emphasis on developing the players ability to express their current (neuromuscular) potential, within the specific conditions of the golf swing task. Staying with the motor sport analogy, this could be considered refinement of driver skill, and/or likened to "polish and porting" the cylinder head, a process undertaken to facilitate a smoother delivery of fuel to the engine to reap further gains in performance. Regarding human performance, these would relate to training oriented towards the development of intra and inter-muscular coordination. Such training comprised a greater proportion of the allotted time across this year with a view to maximising opportunities for skill development. Explicitly, it was intended these learning opportunities would help the player realise and utilise her newfound physical qualities to encourage movement strategies to refine and evolve (towards a faster, more efficient swing). This block therefore included a higher proportion of both semi-specific exercises in the gym, as well as coordinative overload and speed-based drills on the range (see Table 8.5). Naturally, these drills were designed in close collaboration with the golf coach, and the key measure to evaluate progress was CHS itself, along with motion capture via high speed video (although not 3D, so limitations to interpretations of the latter).

In May 2019, Player A was selected for the England Girls under-18 squad and shortly after achieved international honours. Therefore, in this instance the support team was able to execute a development programme which delivered the scope of objectives set by the NGB, details of which are outlined/evidenced below.

High-Performance Behaviours

Table 8.6 shows a timeline of Player A moving through the behavioural milestones, supported by comments from the National u18 Girls coach below…

"Player A is a prime example of a player who reaped the benefits of S&C input in the regional programme; transitioning to the national

Table 8.4 Gym-based sessions from the autumn–winter training block in years 3–4 for Player A

Years 3–4 Upgrading the Engine:
Typical gym session from autumn–winter training block

Session A

Strength		Set	Rep	Rest	RPE	Wt	Notes
1a	Deadlift	4–6	3–5	1.5	7		Use variations to challenge thoracic extensor strength
1b	Cable woodchop	3|3	5–6	2.5	8		
2a	BB Bench Press	4–6	3–5	1.5	7		
2b	Suitcase Carry	3|3	20 m	2.5	8		
3a	FOW Lateral swing	3|3	6–10	1	N/A		FOW = foot on wall
3b	DB Prone T's	3|3	8–20	1	N/A		
3c	Plate overhead raise	3	8–20	1	N/A		

Session B

Strength		Set	Rep	Rest	RPE	Wt	Notes
1a	Leg Press	4–6	3–5	1.5	7		In with bent arms, out
1b	ECC Torso rotations	3|3	5–6	2.5	8		SLOW with straight arms
2a	Chins	4–6	3–5	1.5	7		
2b	Weighted side plank – 5 s hold	3|3	5	2.5	8		
3a	Band Step Up	3|3	5–8	1	7		
3b	Suspended Rear Fly complex	3	8–20	1	N/A		
3c	Neck / wrist loading						

Session C

Strength	Set	Rep	Rest	RPE	Wt	Notes
1a RDL	4–6	3–5	1.5	7		
1b Kneeling BB Russian Twist	3|3	5–6	2.5	8		
2a BB Z Press	4–6	3–5	1.5	7		
2b GHR Supine Trunk Rotations	3|3	6	2.5	8		
3a FOW Flywheel Lateral swing	3|3	6–10	1	N/A		FOW = foot on wall
3b Prone DB WTY's	3|3	8–20	1	N/A		
3c Swiss ball wall shrug	3	8–20	1	N/A		

Years 3–4 Upgrading the Engine:
Typical gym session from spring–summer training block

Session A

Explosive Strength	Set	Rep	Rest	RPE	Wt	Notes
1 MB OH Toss	4–5	3–5	3			
2 MB Punch Throw	4–6	3–5	3			2–3 reps per side
3 Trap Bar Jumps	3–6	2–3	3–5			
4 Bench Throws	3–6	2–3	3–5			use velocity targets

MSK Conditioning

	Set	Rep	Rest	RPE	Wt	Notes
5 TB/MB Circuit (braking emphasis)						TB = tornado ball
						MB = medicine ball
6 Isometric trunk circuit						
7 Neck/wrist loading						

(continued)

Table 8.4 Cont.

Session B

Explosive Strength	Set	Rep	Rest	RPE	Wt	Notes
1 BW CMJ	4–5	3–5	3			
2 MB Discus throw	4–6	3–5	3			2–3 reps per side
3 Trap Bar Deadlift	3–6	2–3	3–5	8		
4 DB 1-arm Push Press	4–6	2–3	3–5	8		2–3 reps per side

MSK Conditioning	Set	Rep	Rest	RPE	Wt	Notes
5 TB/MB Circuit (braking emphasis)						TB = tornado ball MB = medicine ball
6 Isometric trunk circuit						
7 Neck/wrist loading						

Table 8.5 Example Year 5 training plan for Athlete A

Year 5 – Application:
Typical gym session from autumn–winter training block

Session A

Speed / Coordination	Set	Rep	Rest	RPE	Wt	Notes
1 Speed Swing Aid						prescription guided via launch monitor – velocity threshold
2 Confirmation swings (driver)	3	3	FULL			

Speed / Explosive Strength	Set	Rep	Rest	RPE	Wt	Notes
1 MB OH Toss	4–5	3–5	3			2–3 reps per side
2 MB Punch Throw	4–6	3–5	3			CMJ = countermovement jump
3 180 CMJ	3–5	5	3			use velocity targets
4 Bench Throws	3–6	2–3	3–5			

MSK Conditioning	Set	Rep	Rest	RPE	Wt	Notes
5 TB/MB Circuit (braking emphasis)						TB = tornado ball MB = medicine ball
6 Isometric trunk circuit						
7 Neck & wrist loading						

Session B

Speed / Coordination	Set	Rep	Rest	RPE	Wt	Notes
1 Coordinative Overload Drill						coach-led
2 Confirmation swings (driver)	3	3	FULL			

(continued)

Table 8.5 Cont.

Explosive Strength	*Set*	*Rep*	*Rest*	*RPE*	*Wt*	*Notes*
1 DB Squat Jump	4–5	3–5	3			
2 MB Discus throw	4–6	3–5	3			2–3 reps per side
3 Trap Bar Deadlift	3–6	2–3	3–5	8		
4 DB 1-arm Push Press	4–6	2–3	3–5	8		
MSK Conditioning	*Set*	*Rep*	*Rest*	*RPE*	*Wt*	*Notes*
5 TB/MB Circuit (braking emphasis)						TB = tornado ball MB = medicine ball
6 Isometric trunk circuit						
7 Neck & wrist loading						

Year 5 - Application:
Typical gym session from spring-summer training block

Session A

Speed / Explosive Strength	*Set*	*Rep*	*Rest*	*RPE*	*Wt*	*Notes*
1 Heavy KB Swing	4–5	3–5	3			
2 MB Discus throw	4–6	3–5	3			
3 Speed Swing Aid						prescription guided via launch monitor – velocity threshold
4 Confirmation swings (driver)						coach-led
MSK Conditioning	*Set*	*Rep*	*Rest*	*RPE*	*Wt*	*Notes*
5 TB/MB Circuit (braking emphasis)						TB = tornado ball MB = medicine ball
6 Isometric trunk circuit						
7 Neck & wrist loading						

Session B

Speed / Explosive Strength	Set	Rep	Rest	RPE	Wt	Notes
1 Bench Throw	3–6	2–3	3–5			use velocity targets
2 MB Punch throw	4–6	3–5	3			2–3 reps per side
3 Speed Swing Aid						prescription guided via launch monitor - velocity threshold
4 Confirmation swings (driver)						coach-led

MSK Conditioning	Set	Rep	Rest	RPE	Wt	Notes
5 TB/MB Circuit (braking emphasis)						TB = tornado ball MB = medicine ball
6 Isometric trunk circuit						
7 Neck & wrist loading						

Table 8.6 Player A progress throughout regional performance system

Milestone	Mindset	In Session	Out of Session
1	Doesn't appreciate value of S&C. Receives a programme rather than participates **(Achieved Sep 2017)**	Arrives on time and follows instruction **(Achieved Sep 2017)**	Only performs S&C when timetabled for squad sessions. No engagement with coaching platform **(Achieved Oct 2017)**
2	Recognises value of S&C, but understanding is limited. Training misdirected through negative influences **(Achieved Oct 2017)**	Familiar with some exercises and basic programming variables like sets, reps, rest etc. **(Achieved Dec 2017)**	Independently does a warm up at least twice per week **(Achieved Oct 2017)**
2	Positively influenced and shows some appropriate S&C training behaviours **(Achieved Dec 2017)**	Can follow programme independently. Some compound exercise with ~50% body mass **(Achieved Mar 2018)**	Performs home DIY S&C sessions twice per week. Engages with coaching platform sporadically **(Achieved Dec 2017)**
4	Engaged, asks questions about exercises and goal setting and how this connects to golf **(Achieved Feb 2019)**	Some explosive strength development exercise (jumps, throws) and some compound movements with ~100% body mass **(Achieved Jan 2019)**	Can work safely with free weights or home set up. Effectively applying progressive overload. Regular contact on coaching platform **(Achieved Nov 2018)**
5	Makes requests around exercise and programming. Informes, active participant in training. Stable S&C habits **(Achieved May 2019)**	Can perform loaded movement, compound and explosive (Oly lift and derivative etc.). Compounds ~150% body mass **(Achieved Dec 2019)**	Has a variety of sessions available to them and knowledge of how to adapt them to tournament/ travel requirements. Regularly engaged with coaching platform **(Achieved Apr 2020)**

girls squad with improved perceptions and intentions/habits around "EatWell" and "TrainWell" components. I've noticed she is autonomous in her warm up and thoughtful with her on-course nutrition, as well as being evidently confident and competent to enter a gym and execute a purposeful programme. Even better she is able to adapt her training if equipment isn't available. When players enter with these behaviours it allows the national training to be an enrichment programme rather than the introductory experience it was 5 years ago."

Outcomes

Engine Size and Performance:

Figure 8.3 depicts the change in force characteristics and the subsequent development of clubhead speed during this period of performance support.

Summary / Conclusion

This case report supports a behavioural approach to physical development, which produced high levels of autonomy and effective progression through tangible physical criteria. Adopting a long-term strategy facilitated the development of elite levels of CHS (currently the highest out of both the u18 and women's national squad) while evading the overuse injuries highly prevalent in players during this crucial period of maturation and development. Time invested in education and developing

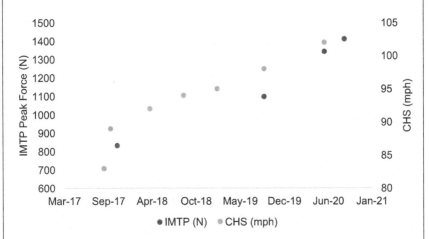

Figure 8.3 Force characteristics and CHS data for Player A over time.
Note: Handicaps were as follows: Sept 2017 = 6.5; April 2018 = 5.3; Sept 2018 = 3.0; Feb 2019 = 2.3; Sept 2019 = +0.4; January 2020 = +1.1

relevant self-management skills was likely key in facilitating the players transition to National team, and in the ongoing management of the psycho-social stress and pressures associated with golf at this level.

Case Study 2 – European Tour Winning Golfer (Player B)

Background

Golf affords its performers longer careers competing at the top level than most sports, meaning longevity is increasingly at the forefront of players' minds, particularly when it comes to their physical preparation. Although the opportunity is certainly there to continue as a tour professional well into the 5th and 6th decades of life, the golf swing action can be attritional and unfortunately injury does commonly disrupt and even prematurely end players' careers. This case report highlights how S&C can promote sustained readiness to perform by aiding in the management of two common musculoskeletal conditions seen in practice on the European Tour Physio unit, hip and lower back pain. The case in point, a 36 year-old European Tour player and previous winner who consulted the ETPI team for guidance on achieving his overriding goal to be fitter and more resilient than ever before by the time he reached 40 years of age. We detail a part of this "journey" from initial consultation through a subsequent review which saw a change in the focus of the S&C programme, while continuing to align to the players overarching goal of maintaining performance into his 40's.

Intervention

Initial Consultation & Intervention

The greatest threat to the player's week-to-week readiness was lower back pain and stiffness. This was secondary to a known pre-existing inflammatory condition. The player expressed how he'd previously found exercise effective for the management back pain and stiffness, and alleviating other associated symptoms, including fatigue and low mood. Discussions revealed that activities which significantly raised heart rate and involved a large excursion at all joints was found to be particularly helpful. Unsurprisingly, given the inflammatory nature of the player's condition, there was a particular affinity for performing this type of exercise on waking to alleviate prolonged morning stiffness and promote a sense of wellness. Therefore, the earliest component of his physical preparation programme to be established was the introduction of a morning "floor flow". This incorporated yoga but emphasised dynamic movement (this was important to the player) followed by a circuit (or a short interval running session) with a bias towards neuromuscular priming and work capacity. Example sessions are detailed below in Figures 8.4

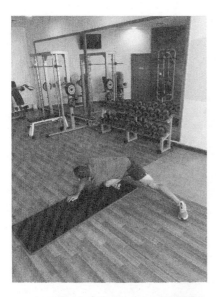

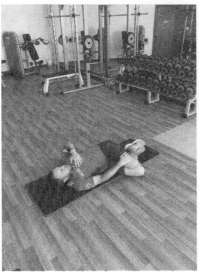

Figure 8.4 Example AM Floor Flow Routines

Outcomes and Ongoing Challenges

Given this intervention was led primarily through the player's previous insight, the benefits on general wellbeing and reduction of specific lower back symptoms in this individual were known. Reporting specific outcomes is therefore less applicable. However, the key challenge here was

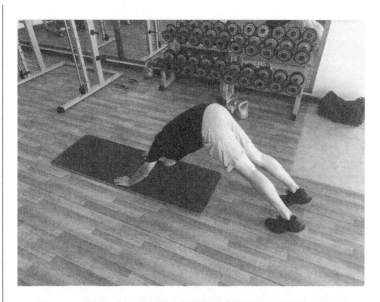

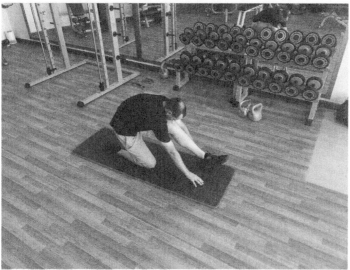

Figure 8.4 (Continued)

managing the consistency/variability balance. In order to be effective this routine needed to be daily and therefore avoiding tedium (See Chapter 3) was a challenge. A key strategy was to develop a bank of flow floors and circuits which although provided variability through content, consistently applied a target stimulus to achieve the responses and adaptations listed in Table 8.7

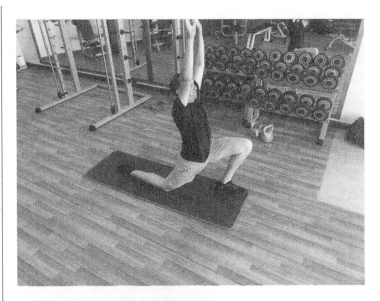

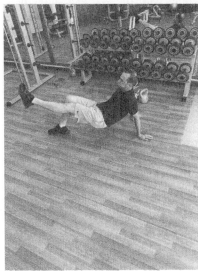

Figure 8.4 (Continued)

Review & Intervention 2

Within a later review it came to light that after years of mild discomfort, trail hip pain had now become the biggest threat to the player's readiness to perform on a weekly basis. Although this had not led to any missed tournaments, his golf swing action and general movement had become

Table 8.7 Intervention target responses and adaptations

Target Responses	Target Adaptations
• Increased synovial fluid production & restoration of "normal" joint ROM; • Increased body temperature / heart rate / blood flow; • Maximal neural drive and motor unit recruitment; • Boost mood and minimise fatigue.	• Maintenance of joint ROM (particularly lumbo-sacral, hip and thoracic spine) • Improve cardio-respiratory fitness and promote favourable changes in body composition; • Enhance RFD and rapid force expression; • Maintain sense of wellbeing.

affected and the player was seeking regular treatment post-round in an attempt to manage his symptoms. Imaging revealed CAM lesion of the right femoral head-neck junction and evidence of a labral tear which together with clinical assessment led to the diagnosis of femeroacetabular impingement (FAI) syndrome in keeping with the Warwick agreement (Griffin et al., 2016). With no clinical trials demonstrating the efficacy of certain interventions for this condition, the general guidance is to identify and target individual impairments that present.

S&C assessment utilised a hip force profile (see Table 8.8) which revealed marginally reduced active range of motion of the right hip, along with weakness and poor tissue capacity/muscular endurance (particularly inner range hip flexion, adduction, and abduction). Although hip flexion deficits were likely attributable to pain inhibition, the contralateral hip was also weaker than available norms (unpublished from the ETPI) for elite male golfers so an inter-disciplinary sports medicine decision was made to pursue these deficits over a relatively short period of time to assess what change could be made and whether that associated with a reduction in symptoms.

Regardless of short-term symptomatic relief, it was felt S&C input could also help offload the hip through longer term changes in neighbouring tissue properties and architecture since this would influence movement strategies (Newell, 1986) and associated costs (Prilutsky, 2002; Bertram, 2001). In particular, given that the trunk controls the pelvis, it was a priority to address the muscles and tissues of this region. Theoretically efficient muscle synergy will balance tension and distribute stressors to all interconnected tissues, while inefficiency will concentrate stress on certain tissues which may lead to overload and damage accumulation. With obvious anatomical connections between the muscles of the hip and trunk, and known important inter-muscular coordination strategies between the lateral hip and lateral trunk quadrant, any sub-optimal muscle

Table 8.8 Hip force profile using hand held dynamometry (ActivForce 2) for Player B. AROM= Active Range of Motion Asym= Asymmetry between left and right side

Hip Profile	Left	Right	% Asym
Flexion AROM (deg)	115	108	6.3
Inner Flexion (Mean kg)	12.1	8.6	33.8
Inner Flexion (Peak kg)	15.5	11.2	31.81
Outer Flexion (Mean kg)	28.2	25.6	9.66
Outer Flexion (Peak kg)	30.5	27.4	10.7
Adduction (Mean kg)	12.7	9.3	30.9
Adduction (Peak kg)	14.8	13	13
Abduction (Mean kg)	14.3	11.1	25.1
Abduction (Peak kg)	17.04	15.06	12.28
Extension (Mean kg)	29.1	26.7	8.6
Extension (Peak kg)	33	30	9.5
Add:Abd Mean Force (Ratio)	0.89	0.84	N/A

strength, coordination or tissue integrity may lead to inefficient strategies of dissipating force in the golf swing. Conversely, an increase in the active stiffness of the trunk muscles (particularly obliques and lateral quadrant) could reduce costs for given outputs due to more effective inter-muscular and inter-segmental force transmission. Therefore, the player's existing programme was reviewed with the addition of both stability challenges and high-tension strength exercises for the antero-lateral trunk quadrant. Additionally, the intervention was designed to develop work capacity, with a view to enabling the hip and trunk muscles to make repeated sub-maximal contractions without fatiguing, thus raising the tolerance threshold so that greater volumes of on course actions could be tolerated without a build-up of symptoms.

This hip and trunk directed intervention was embedded into the player's current existing strength and conditioning programme (Table 8.9) which included both "heavy" (trap bar deadlift) and "loaded explosive" jumps (BB squat jumps), medicine ball throws, and the floor flows and circuits previously discussed. Little modification was needed to this core strength/power programme as required ranges of hip flexion/internal rotation were already minimised and well tolerated.

Outcomes

Repeat hip profiling 4 weeks into the intervention demonstrated both mean and peak force improvements in the trail hip across all targeted movements: inner range hip flexion (+2.6 kg / 3.6 kg), hip adduction (+4.6 kg / 1.8 kg), and hip abduction (5 kg / 4 kg) (see Table 8.10).

Table 8.9 Example S&C content. Programme with hip and trunk conditioning bias

Series	Exercise	Prescription
AM Floor Flow / Primer circuit	see figures 1–3	
Hip Activation Menu	Thigh to wall lateral swing High Box Step ups Pulley / band standing deadbug Band 4-Point Deep Rotators	2–3 sets of 5–8 reps
Typical Strength / Power content	Barbell Jump squat Trap Bar Deadlift ISO (5 s) or ECC Trunk Rotation (varied degree's of rotation)	3–4 sets of 3–5 reps
Tissue capacity 1	Supported squat with hip turnout Lunge Hip Flexor ISO Swiss ball knee tucks Short lever adductor bridge	Time under tension 20–60 s × 3 rounds
Tissue capacity 2	Plank with hip abductions Band Psoas march Suitcase carry Tall kneeling pallof	Time under tension 20–60 s × 3 rounds
Tissue capacity 3	1-Leg Hip Thrusts Hanging knee raise Asymmetrical Trap bar hold Golfer pallof press	Time under tension 20–60 s × 3 rounds

Table 8.10 Post-intervention hip profile for Player B

Hip Profile	Left	Right	% Asym
Flexion AROM (deg)	115	112	2.64
Inner Flexion (Mean kg)	15.2	11.2	30.3
Inner Flexion (Peak kg)	17.9	14.8	18.9
Adduction (Mean kg)	14.2	13.9	2.13
Adduction (Peak kg)	15.4	14.8	3.97
Abduction (Mean kg)	17.5	16.1	8.3
Abduction (Peak kg)	22.2	19.1	15
Add:Abd Mean Force (Ratio)	0.81	0.86	N/A

AROM, Active Range of Motion; Asym, Asymmetry between left and right side

Additionally, hip flexion active range of motion increased by 5 degrees, a measure often used clinically to gauge improvement in FAI syndrome patients. Symptomatically the player reported little change, although this could have been attributed to the fact during this four-week period they had played back to back tournaments and subjected the hip to a high volumes of golf so arguably symptom stabilisation could be interpreted as a sign of increased load tolerance and overall improvement of the condition. Contralateral hip strength also improved but overall to a lesser extent (inner range hip flexion 13.1/2.4kg; hip adduction +1.5kg/0.6kg; hip abduction 3.2kg/5.16kg) meaning on the whole inter-limb asymmetries were reduced.

Given the high joint torques generated by the hip abductors in the golf swing (Chaudari et al., 2007, Callaway et al., 2012) a fatigue index protocol was used to assess changes in work capacity and muscular endurance of the hip abductors (see Figure 8.5). This consisted of 6x maximal 5 second isometric efforts with 10 seconds rest in between efforts. Interestingly, a greater decline in force was observed post intervention which may have been down to greater pre-intervention pain inhibition preventing the generation of sufficiently high forces to lead to fatigue on repeated efforts. This is supported by the fact that while a greater drop off in force was observed in repeat efforts post intervention, mean forces on single efforts did increase between pre and post.

The trunk training led to increased peak force on an isometric trunk rotation exercise used throughout (+3 kg / 3.5kg), along with observationally better control of rotary spinal torques, and increased work capacity in the antero-lateral quadrant as demonstrated by an ability to tolerate greater times under tension on training exercises such as side plank, suitcase carries and anti-rotational holds.

Summary / Conclusion

This case report highlights the diversity of physical preparation scope in golf at elite level, summarising two interventions directed towards optimising durability/readiness and availability. The benefits of exercise in both instances were probably largely general, particularly in the management of low back pain and stiffness. The encouraging early signs in the management of FAI syndrome adds to the evidence this condition can be managed conservatively with careful control of golf volume and S&C of individual deficits around the hip and trunk. However, ultimately longitudinal monitoring of the player is needed to determine whether improvements in hip function continued to correlate with a positive trend in symptoms in this individual case. As golf is a sport which can

Table 8.11 In–Tournament training example for Player C

Session A

Strength		Set	Rep	Rest	RPE	Wt	Notes
1a	Back squat	5	3		8		Smooth but heavy (don't grind)
1b	CMJ	5	3	3			As high as you can!
2a	Bench press	4	3		8		Smooth but heavy (don't grind)
2b	Explosive incline push up	4	4	3			As high as you can!
3	Romanian deadlift	3	6	3	8		
4	BB Russian twist	3	8–10	2	8–9		
5a	Banded neck iso anti–side flexion	3	30 s | 30 s		7–8		Keep arms straight
5b	Barbell wrist roller	3	4 up and downs	1	7–8		

Session B

Strength		Set	Rep	Rest	RPE	Wt	Notes
1a	Jump squat	4	3				Velocity target ~1 m/s
1b	MB punch throw	4	3|3	2.5		4 kg	As fast and hard as you can!
2	Trap bar DL (cluster 2:2)	4	4	3	8		Smooth but heavy (don't grind). ~20 s rest between doubles
3	Single arm DB push press	3	5	2.5	7		Heavy bust FAST
4	Single arm loaded carries	3	20 m	2	8		
5a	Banded neck iso anti–side flexion	3	30 s | 30 s		7–8		
5b	Barbell wrist roller	3	4 up and downs	1	7–8		

Session C

Strength	Set	Rep	Rest	RPE	Wt	Notes
1a 1/2 squat from pins	3-4	3	3	7		
1b 180 CMJ	3-4	3|3				As high as you can!
2a Explosive incline push up	3	4				As high as you can!
2b Rotational MB slam into floor	3	6	2		4 kg	As fast and hard as you can!
3 Pallof press (infront and overhead)	3	10|10	1	7		

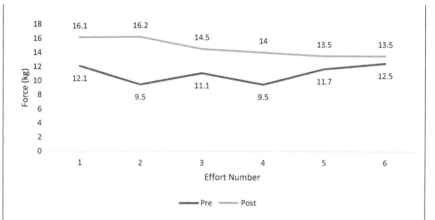

Figure 8.5 Pre-post hip abductor intervention fatigue index
Note: Higher force values for each effort post-test. Pre-intervention= 3% increase over time (peak= 12.1 kg. min= 12.5 kg). Post intervention= 16% decrease over time (peak 16.2 kg. min= 13.5 kg).

offer very long careers S&C has a lot to offer in the realms of both redu-cing the incidence of, and managing injury and illness which may be detrimental to their durability and subsequent readiness.

Case Study 3 – European Tour Golfer: S&C during tournaments

Background

One of the biggest S&C challenges facing the touring professional golfer is that of in tournament training. As with many sports, growing commer-cialisation and globalisation have resulted in long seasons where athletes chase the sun and compete all year round. All tours have full competition schedules throughout every month of the year. "In-season" breaks are also less common, and often short lived. There may be one or two mid-season breaks for two to three weeks, and if a player is fortunate, they may achieve early season success which allows them to take some additional one- or two-week breaks through the year. However, this only applies to the minority, and is often for the purpose of rest from a relentless string of events. Therefore, in all but the minority of cases, almost every tour-nament matters equally. Further to this, each tournament week is long. The player will often travel Monday or Tuesday morning, practice all day Tuesday, practice and compete in the "pro-am" Wednesday, and then compete for five hours per day for the next four (Thursday–Sunday) with practice interspersed between the competitive rounds. Spare time for S&C is lacking, and pressure on a player's time is significant. On Sunday, players will board a plane and fly home for one day or go straight onto the next event.

Despite these constraints, S&C practitioners need to support players to become bigger, stronger and faster while competing week to week. This case study follows a European Tour player (Player C), through the months of June–October (some of the busiest on the calendar). Player C is inside the top 100 in the World Rankings at the time of writing, has a good training history (although has had some recent inconsistency) and is in their 30s. They enjoy training, are competent in the gym and are experienced at training during events. They have no current injury history but have had minor wrist and neck issues in the past, all of which resolved over relatively short timespans. The player's primary objective was to remain healthy and reduce injury risk, with the aim of having a long and successful career. A secondary objective was to improve CHS by a meaningful amount (>3 mph).

Interventions

Approach to the Problem

When designing the interventions for this player, several key considerations were made. To achieve the goal of readiness, availability through injury and illness risk reduction and longevity in the game, a high degree of training consistency would be required. One of the key methods for achieving this was to make it an explicit and known goal, with a target of 70% compliance and above. This target was agreed by the player and coach prior to commencing the new season. Holding the team to account on this was an equally important aspect of success. During a busy tournament period, there are a lot of distractions for players and support staff, with regularly shifting targets, goals, and schedules. Therefore, the S&C coach had to take responsibility for maintaining regular contact with the player, appraising their consistency against the known target over the year and holding the team to account on the agreed target. Further to this, high-quality programming, player buy-in, building a training structure which lent into some of the players exercise preferences and upskilling the player to be able to adapt their programme to different training environments (e.g. a hotel gym with restricted equipment) would support success to maximise training consistency

The weekly tournament cycle had direct implications towards the programming approach. The cycle impacted aspects such as timing, volume and intensity of training through different days of the week, as well as other delayed onset muscle soreness (DOMS) and fatigue mitigation strategies as the player moved into the competitive days.

More intensive or higher volume training (session A) would take place on a Monday at home (or at the event when travelling straight over). On Wednesday, session B had a mild drop in volume and slight shift in exercise selection in line with points listed in the sections below. Session B was often completed in the morning, depending on pro-am commitments. Session C was the lowest volume session and took place on Friday or Saturday. Session B and C would finish at least two hours before a round, where this was not possible the session would be completed after the round.

Volume

Higher volumes of training were included in the start of the week, when the player had more available time and a lower requirement for "readiness to perform" (i.e. could take on more fatigue). Volume would be primarily controlled through number of exercises within the programme, repetitions, sets, time under tension (TUT) and range of movement (ROM) required for the exercise.

Intensity

Overall intensity remained high through the week, with fatigue primarily mitigated through control of volume. However, there was a shift towards more explosive exercises as the week progressed, equal intensity (e.g. weight on the bar/initial bar velocity) at lower reps led to lower overall rating of perceived exertion (RPE) scores, which were combined with the use of velocity drop-off to prevent excessive accumulation of fatigue within session.

DOMS Mitigation Strategies

Largely the above methods were used to control for both fatigue in events (while maintaining training intensity and progress) as well as mitigating risk of DOMS. High levels of training consistency through events (so less unaccustomed exercise), reductions in volume throughout the week – including reduction of variables such as TUT and ROM (e.g. avoiding eccentric dominant exercise such as Romanian Deadlifts (RDLs), using half squats etc.), and controlling intensity all helped to mitigate the risk of DOMS impacting play.

Outcomes

Consistency Through a Busy Period

Achieving a high level of training consistency through a dense competitive schedule was essential to achieve the player's primary and secondary objectives. Over the period of June–October the player completed 75% of the programmed three sessions per week.

Subjective Player Feedback

The player reported feeling healthy and injury free throughout the period of training. They suffered no known negative consequences as a result of the in-season training programme and often found training before play beneficial, stating it was a good distraction, made them feel more alert and improved the "feel" of their swing. The player was happy that he managed to achieve such a high level of consistency over this period.

Summary

This case has highlighted that professional tour players cannot rely on "off-season" training time to make progress in their physical preparation for performance, due to the long and dense tournament schedules and continual pressure to perform. Despite this, we have shown progress is still possible, even within the busiest periods of the year provided appropriate solutions are found. We proposed key areas for consideration, with suggested solutions (including consistency, weekly schedule, timing, volume, intensity and DOMS mitigation strategies). We have also given an example programme during this period to demonstrate these principles in action (Table 8.11).

Case Study 4 – Challenge Tour Golfer: S&C with a Hypertrophy Focus

Background

Unlike the European and PGA Tours, the Challenge Tour provides a reasonable off-season for its players, allowing time for them to focus on their winter training with minimal disruption. Every player coming through Challenge Tour is hoping to gain full status on the European Tour, through a top-20 finish in the overall standings. However, a European Tour card creates a long and relentless season with diminished opportunity for substantial off-season training. As a result, Challenge Tour players aim to take

Table 8.12 Key physical performance measures for the period of June–October

	June	October
Countermovement jump impulse (N.s)	352	378
IMTP peak force (N)	2252	2850
Isometric trunk strength (N)	L: 126	L: 137
	R: 128	R: 135
Isometric neck strength (N)	L: 432	L: 441
	R: 389	R: 428
CHS (mph)	116	120
Body mass (kg)	83	85

full advantage of any off-season afforded to them, knowing if things go well in the following year, it may be their last opportunity to do so.

This case follows a Challenge Tour player through the months of November – March. The player is in their mid-20s, has a good background in strength and conditioning and has maintained a high level of consistency throughout the season. Their overall goals are to ensure longevity throughout their career, as well as increase clubhead speed by a meaningful amount (>3 mph). They understand the benefits of a longer off-season and want to use it to increase mass as a primary goal, believing it will help in achieving both of their goals. The player and their coach are working on some swing changes over winter, which include minimising lateral movement of the pelvis during the downswing. While they believe this is mainly a technical issue, they've asked for some consideration in the programme.

Interventions

Approach to the Problem

When designing the interventions for this player, several key consider-ations were made (outlined below). As well as completion of the training plan, optimising nutrition was essential to player success. Therefore, the golfer worked with the ETPI nutrition team to ensure they maximised the off-season opportunity to add mass.

When designing a plan for the eight-week off-season, two key blocks were identified. Block 1 (November–January) and Block 2 (January–March). During Block 1, the player had more time to focus on resistance training, with relatively less focus on golf. However, moving into Block 2, golf practice volumes would increase and occasional events would be taking place leading into March where the Challenge Tour season started properly. As a result, Block 1 used an upper/lower split with four training sessions per week, whereas Block 2 was a three day per week full body

Table 8.13 Programme example for Case Study 4

November – January (Hypertrophy early off-season)

Session A (Monday & Thursday)

Strength		Set	Rep	Rest	RPE	Wt	Note
1	Front squat	6	4	3+	8 to 9		
2	Romanian deadlift	5	5	3+	8 to 9		
3	Supine trunk rotations	4	5 each side	2	8 to 9		
4a	Split squat	4	6 to 8 each side		8 to 9		
4b	Half kneeling overhead pallof	3	5 each side	90s	8 to 9		

Session B (Tuesday & Friday)

Strength		Set	Rep	Rest	RPE	Wt	Note
1a	BB overhead press	5	4		8 to 9		
1b	Weighted chin-ups	5	6 to 8	3+	8 to 9		
2a	Incline DB bench	4	6		8 to 9		
2b	Seated 1-arm cable pulldown	4	6 to 8 each side	3+	8 to 9		
3	Suitase carry	3	30 yards each side	2	8 to 9		
4	Seated hip abductor	4	8 to 10	2	8 to 9		

(continued)

Table 8.13 Cont.

January – March (Hypertrophy late off-season/pre-season)

Session A (Monday)

Strength		Set	Rep	Rest	RPE	Wt	Note
1a	Front squat	6	3		8 to 9		
1b	Countermovement jump	6	3	3+			Jump as high as you can!
2	Push press	5	4	3+	7	–	Heavy but FAST
3	Box step up	3	6 each side	2	8		
4a	Single arm bent over row	3	6 each side		8 to 9		Maintain trunk, hip and knee control
4b	Half kneeling overhead pallof	3	5 each side	2	8 to 9		

Session B (Wednesday)

Strength		Set	Rep	Rest	RPE	Wt	Note
1a	Romanian deadlift	5	4		8 to 9		
1b	Broad jump	5	3	3+			Jump as far as you can!
2a	Bench press	4	6		8 to 9		
2b	Medicine ball punch throw	4	5 each side	3+			Throw as fast & hard as you can!
3a	Split squat	3	6 each side	2	8 to 9		
3b	Weighted chin-ups	3	6 to 8		8 to 9		
4	Suitcase carries	3	30 yards each side	2	8 to 9		

Session C (Friday)

Strength		Set	Rep	Rest	RPE	Wt	Note
1a	Back squat	5	5		8 to 9		Cluster 2,2,1 with 20 seconds recovery {don't grind)
1b	Countermovement jump	5	3	3+			Jump as high as you can!
2	Half kneeling single arm overhead press	4	6 each side	2	8 to 9		
3	Box step up	3	6 each side	2	7		
4a	Pendlay row	3	5		7		Maintain trunk, hip and knee control
4b	Half kneeling overhead pallof	3	5 each side	2	8 to 9		Heavy but FAST

approach to balance the time commitments of the player over the two periods of time. Also, moving into Block 2, a higher focus was given to explosive strength training, so that the player could maximise transfer of their gym work to CHS transitioning into March (Table 8.13).

Despite common beliefs that to maximise hypertrophy, a programme should consist of lower load, higher repetition training (e.g. 4x8-12), more consideration should be given, based on an individual's training need (Schoenfeld et al., 2017). Challenge Tour golfers benefit from high levels of maximal strength (Wells et al., 2019), so the use of higher load and lower repetition training was utilised throughout both training blocks to support both hypertrophy and maximal strength gains. Although some lower load, higher repetition exercises were also used in the programme. Given training was conducted at relatively high loads, training to muscle failure was not encouraged, because it was unlikely to contribute any additional benefits (Lasevicius et al., 2022).

To support the player in their goals of minimising lateral pelvis movement in the downswing, a range of hip and trunk control exercises were included in the plan. The hip abductor machine was used in block 1 to drive structural change, in block 2 this transitioned to box step ups to develop strength and control of the hip through anti-adduction. Throughout both blocks, a range of anti-side flexion exercises (e.g. suitcase carries, half kneeling overhead Pallof, half kneeling single arm overhead press) were used to support trunk control throughout the swing.

Lastly, while not in the programme, the player was given some optionality at the end of the session. They were permitted to add isolated "bodybuilding" style exercises for enjoyment. Guidelines were to pick two different exercises of their choice (e.g. biceps curls and rope triceps extensions or lateral raises and dumbbell pullover) and complete a superset of three to four sets x 10-20 repetitions).

Outcomes

Table 8.14 Key physical performance measures during the off-season

	November	*March*
Countermovement jump impulse (N.s)	290	319
Isometric mid-thigh pull peak force (N)	2458	2862
Isometric trunk strength (N)	L: 134	L: 142
	R: 129	R: 138
Isometric hip abduction strength (N)	L: 232	L: 277
	R: 228	R: 276
CHS (mph)	112	117
Body mass (kg)	78	88

Summary

This case demonstrates how a longer off-season could be used for hypertrophy while continuing to develop swing-specific physical qualities, strength, and explosive strength.

References

Bertram, J., & Young-Hui, C. (2001). Mechanical energy oscillations of two brachiation gaits: Measurement and simulation. *American Journal Of Physical Anthropology*. 115: 319–326. 10.1002/ajpa.1088.

Bliss, A (2018). Hitting it far and going under par: The role of S&C. Dec, *PGA Professional*.

Brearley, S., Coughlan, D., & Wells, J.E.T. (2019). Strength and conditioning in golf: probability of performance impact. *Sportsperfsci.com*. 61–1.

Brearley, S, L., Buckley, O., Gillham, P., Clements, B., & Coughlan, D. (2021) Interdisciplinary conservative management of bilateral non-united lumbar pars defects in a junior elite golfer. *International Journal of Sports Physical Therapy*. 16(1): 236–247.

Callaway, S., Glaws, K., Mitchell, M., Scerbo, H., Voight, M., & Sells, P. (2012). An analysis of peak pelvis rotation speed, gluteus maximus and medius strength in high versus low handicap golfers during the golf swing. *International Journal of Sports Physical Therapy*. 7(3): 288–295.

Chaudhari, A. M., Lindenfeld, T. N., Andriacchi, T. P., Hewett, T. E., Riccobene, J., Myer, G. D., & Noyes, F. R. (2007). Knee and hip loading patterns at different phases in the menstrual cycle: implications for the gender difference in anterior cruciate ligament injury rates. *The American Journal Of Sports Medicine*. 35(5): 793–800. https://doi.org/10.1177/0363546506297537

Fowler, P, M., Knez, W., Crowcroft, S., Mendham, A, E., Miller, J., Sargent, C., Halson, S., & Duffield, R. (2017). Greater effect of east vesus west travel on jet lag, seep, and team sport performance. *Medicine and Science in Sports and Exercise*. 49(12): 2548–2561.

Griffin et al (2016) The Warwick Agreement on femoroacetabular impingement syndrome (FAI syndrome): an international consensus statement.

Hody, S., Croisier, J,L., Bury, T., Rogister, B., & LePrince, P. (2019). Eccentric Muscle Contractions: Risks and Benefits. *Frontiers in Physiology*. doi: 10.3389/fphys.2019.00536

Lasevicius, T., Schoenfeld, B. J., Silva-Batista, C., Barros, T. D. S., Aihara, A. Y., Brendon, H., ... & Teixeira, E. L. (2022). Muscle Failure Promotes Greater Muscle Hypertrophy in Low-Load but Not in High-Load Resistance Training. *Journal of Strength And Conditioning Research*, 36(2): 346–351. https://doi.org/10.1519/JSC.0000000000003454

Lauersen, J,B., Bertelsen, D,M., & Andersen, L,B. (2014). The effectiveness of exercise interventions to prevent sports injuries: a systematic review and meta-analysis of randomised controlled trials. *British Journal of Sports Medicine*. 48(11): 871–877.

Leatherwood, W.E., & Dragoo, J.L. (2013). Effect of airline travel on performance: a review of the literature. *British Journal of Sports Medicine*. 47(9): 561–567.

Newell, K. M. (1986). Constraints on the development of coordination'. In: M.G. Wade and H.T.A. Whiting (eds.), Motor Development in Children: Aspects of Coordination and Control, Boston: Martinus Nijhoff. pp. 341–360.

Pipe, A, L. (2011). International travel and the elite athlete. *Clinical Journal of Sports Medicine*. 21(1): 62–66.

Prilutsky, B. & Zatsiorsky, V. (2002). Optimization-Based Models of Muscle Coordination. *Exercise and sport sciences reviews*. 30(1): 32–38. 10.1097/00003677-200201000-00007

Schoenfeld, B. J., Grgic, J., Ogborn, D., & Krieger, J. W. (2017). Strength and hypertrophy adaptations between low-vs. high-load resistance training: a systematic review and meta-analysis. *The Journal of Strength & Conditioning Research*. 31(12): 3508–3523.

van Rensburg, D, J., van Rensburg, A,., Fowler, P., Fullagar, H., Stevens, D., Halson, S., Bender, A., Vincent, G., Claassen-Smithers, A., Dunican, I., Roach, G. D., Sargent, C., Lastella, M., & Cronje, T. (2020). How to manage travel fatigue and jet lag in athletes? A systematic review of interventions. *British Journal Of Sports Medicine*. 54(16): 960–968. https://doi.org/10.1136/bjsports-2019-101635

van Rensburg, D, C, J., van Rensburg, A, J., Fowler, P. M., Bender, A. M., Stevens, D., Sullivan, K. O., Fullagar, H., Alonso, J. M., Biggins, M., Claassen-Smithers, A., Collins, R., Dohi, M., Driller, M. W., Dunican, I. C., Gupta, L., Halson, S. L., Lastella, M., Miles, K. H., Nedelec, M., Page, T., Botha, T. (2021). Managing Travel Fatigue and Jet Lag in Athletes: A Review and Consensus Statement. *Sports Medicine*. 51(10): 2029–2050. https://doi.org/10.1007/s40279-021-01502-0

Vitale, K, C., Owens, R, O., Hopkins, S, R., & Malhotra, A. (2019). Sleep hygiene for optimizing recovery in athletes: review and recommendations. *International Journal of Sports Medicine*. 40(8): 535–543.

Wells, J. E., Charalambous, L. H., Mitchell, A. C., Coughlan, D., Brearley, S. L., Hawkes, R. A., ... & Fletcher, I. M. (2019). Relationships between Challenge Tour golfers' clubhead velocity and force producing capabilities during a countermovement jump and isometric mid-thigh pull. *Journal Of Sports Sciences*. 37(12): 1381–1386.

9 A Perspective on Injuries in Golf

Poora Singh and Alex Bliss

Introduction

Golf is, by comparison to other sports, a relatively moderate-risk activity (Cabri et al., 2009). There are a range of purported health and wellbeing benefits associated with regular participation in golf. A recent review of golf and health literature summarised that golfers will walk approximately four to eight miles when playing 18 holes, with a subsequent, approximate energy expenditure of 3–8 kcal / min or 531–2,467 kcal per round (Murray et al., 2017). In addition to the various physical benefits of playing golf, it has also been reported that golfers demonstrate greater feelings of personal and psychological well-being than non-golfers (Sorbie et al., 2021). However, like any physical activity, there are associated risks, although the low-moderate nature of this risk is likely outweighed by the benefits of being physically active when playing golf compared to being inactive. Notwithstanding, systematic reviews have highlighted that the main causes of injury in golfers are the high volume of repetitive practice and suboptimal swing mechanics (Murray et al., 2017). In both amateurs and professionals, the spine, and particularly the lumbar spine is the most frequently injured area of the body (Robinson et al., 2019 Edwards et al., 2020), followed by wrist and shoulder (McHardy et al., 2006). However, while there are more data available on injury epidemiology in the amateur game, high quality evidence from professional golf is lacking, with a recent systematic review of musculoskeletal injuries in professional golf concluding that there is a paucity of high-quality literature available (Robinson et al., 2019).

In a departure from the format of other chapters in this book, to gain insight and an applied viewpoint of injuries in golf, this section focuses on the perspectives and experiences of a member of the medical staff on the European and Challenge Tours. Poora Singh is the Lead Therapist for the PGA European Challenge Tour and provides support for the European Tour Performance Institute. He is also a senior osteopath for British Athletics. The chapter is a transcription of a semi-structured interview carried out between the two

DOI: 10.4324/9781003099321-9

chapter authors and focuses on a range of themes aligned to injuries in golf. It provides an experiential, first-hand account of being a professional therapist in golf, provides advice on how to minimise common injury risk factors for golfers and what to do should injury occur.

Interview:

ALEX BLISS (AB): **Please could you provide an overview of your current role and experience of supporting golfers?**

POORA SINGH (PS): I've been involved with the European Tour since 2008, having started originally on the Challenge Tour with the ETPI [European Tour Performance Institute] in 2008. It started off as just a therapy service and what we were doing was just dealing with players on a therapy level. After that, we've developed over the years into a full welfare and performance model. We've got osteopaths, physiotherapists, S&C, nutrition psychology, medicine, and we've got orthopaedic specialists on there. I've been involved with that ever since the beginning from 2008 Challenge Tour. Outside of that, I've got a background in all sorts of sports. I do a lot with football and also work in athletics.

AB: **Talk me through some of the common injuries that you see in golfers and in your professional practice. This will probably be a long list!**

PS: An important point to make [at this stage] is that we can separate injuries that are based upon three things:

- Anatomy and the way that you're made physically.
- Injuries based around players trying to swing at high speeds or issues with trying to get to a physical performance they're not actually physically prepared for.
- And then the last one, which are overuse injuries.

I think that if we if we actually break it down, most of the injuries or issues that we see are overuse, with overuse being "you're not conditioned for the amount of load that you want to put through the body over time". That's why we really push for players to get on a thorough, really robust, strong athletic programme because it allows for a much bigger volume of play [and practice].

What we tend to see, the classic one, if we start off with lower back, I think that's the one that we see most commonly amongst players. It usually comes on with players feeling they've got an ache or soreness. It's rare that it is acute [happens immediately] and we rarely see the guys come in bent over double in really, really acute pain. Players that are unable to move. That's very, very rare because before that point that would have easily been to see one of us [ETPI medical staff] before that with all the pre-issue pain that they get.

It's [players] usually reporting something like:

> I've played five events back-to-back. Today I was on the range and I just got up to my drive, first driver hit and my back just kind of felt like it went and I've felt really, really sore since then. I can't really rotate on it. Bending forward hurts and I feel like I need to rest it.

We will see a lot of that and so we have been using manual therapy, use the stuff that manages the pain and pain receptors, so we deal with their pain. We deal with that issue, then fight to get them moving better. But then we also have to educate them on why it happened. I'm a massive believer, and this is part of the stuff that we backed at my clinic is finding the "why?" It's not so much about "oh, this is the tissue that failed. Let's just strengthen that tissue or find the part of your anatomy that had a problem and let's deal with that." It's more about:

- "Why did your lower back go?"
- "What is it that you're doing or in your swing? Is it a coaching cue that we need or is it because you've got a deficit elsewhere?"
- "Is it something that you're not getting from your hip, which is why you're overloading your back?"
- "Or is it simply that you did too much of it and you bloody hurt it!"

We're always looking at "why?". What's the "why" behind your injury? I'm of a massive, massive proponent of that. I love to educate our players on anatomy. I love to educate them on how the kinematics of body movement work. I might say to them:

- "Why would your back go if your hip wasn't working?"
- "Why does your lumbar spine get affected by your thoracic spine?"
- "Why does hip flexor strength really support your back?"

All of these [questions] are really informing the player. We see a lot of lower back stuff. But lower back issues, for me, the muscles around the lower spine are transference tissues. You produce a lower limb force, you're passing it through your lumbar spine up, [into the rest of the] spine, your shoulders, through the arms to the clubface and the ball. If your lower back is having an issue and your anatomy has failed (e.g. let's just say that you've damaged the disc and for now you've got a loss of integrity of tissue), and you can't actually play or you can't actually swing because of it, then we have to allow the tissue to heal. We have to get you to move and then reload you get the tissue strong again, and then get you playing again.

If we don't have an anatomical issue, if we've got a biomechanical issue, so, for example, if you've got something going on in your hip that's not allowing you to turn into your hip, and for that reason you're then asking your lumbar spine to do a lot of that rotation, you're basically asking it to do something it's not anatomically made for and you're going to get an issue there.

Then tertiary to that, let's say you're trying to get an extra bit of distance on your shots, you're putting a lot more force through your lumbar spine, but your thoracic spine is stiff as ****, we're going to get a problem in the lumbar spine.

Always look for the "why". Let's have a look at your anatomy, then let's have a look at your physical capacity. I might ask [a golfer] could you move your spine through flexion/extension, side bend, and rotation and are there gains to be made by making you do some general stretching and mobility? If that's the case and the answer is yes, brilliant. Then the third question is, can we get you stronger? Are there gains to be made by making you stronger? If we can then basically we've covered all bases and you've got decent anatomy, with decent mobility, with some really good strength. Then you've also got decent coaching, which is giving you better technique.

I would summarise as we try to put you into a position where the chance of you getting injured is as minimal as we possibly get. All then we've got to teach you is really good habits. I think lumbar spine injuries or lumbar spine problems are classic for players, but for me, they're always secondary to something else going on.

AB: **There's one thing you mentioned that I thought was interesting to note, most of what you see is overuse in nature. Do you think players understand what that means and also understand what some of the potential triggers for overuse are? I think we talked previously about players using things like practice punishment. They have a bad round, then all of a sudden, they'll go and hit another 2–300 balls to try to work it out that they wouldn't have done otherwise. Do you think players understand the overuse side of things?**

PS: Well, I think the older ones do, yes. But the younger ones that are desperate to get on the [European/Challenge] Tour, and the younger ones who are desperate to make a difference, don't. They really do not understand the concept of playing on tour. It's four rounds! it's four rounds plus a practice round, plus the pro-am, plus practice. If you imagine that, how much does a normal amateur do compared to that? Also, that's one week on tour! If you don't hone your practice and your practice circuits to a point where you're hitting the minimal amount of balls to get the greatest amount of change, then basically all you're doing is you're adding to the [physical] load.

To add to that, if you're really poor with your pre and post recovery stuff, then we're just waiting for you to break. It's not *if*, it's *when*. We really tried to push the players to understand that playing for an amateur day-to-day compared to professional golf are completely different things.

AB: **And understanding that transition and how to go from successful amateur to successful professional. That transitional step is now, whether the EuroPro Tour and the Challenge Tour, or the other tours before European Tour or, before being on the PGA Tour in America, trying to understand that transition. Education that sometimes just doing more and more and more isn't always better.**

PS: Yeah, exactly. Then getting them to understand that their anatomy dictates it. I like to transfer that to an anatomical model as well. There are so many different anatomical systems. You get guys that have really, really strong bones, really thick joint capsules, but not much flexibility. Typically, they're fairly robust, but haven't got much range and can be quite strong. However, if they're going to get injured, they're going to *really* hurt something! Then you get other guys that are very, very elastic. They've got really loose joints, really loose skin, really loose muscle, but they're actually quite powerful. If you give them a power movement to do they're very powerful, but then you ask them to do 100 movements then they fatigue really quickly. They just haven't got the stiffness, the capacity to allow the joint to do that movement without getting tired, you know. You've got to really understand all of that in terms of how you train them and, that to me would also give me a profile of what sort of injuries that they would have.

For example, when it comes to those guys, if we move away from the lumbar spine down to the hip, which is for me the most important joint in golf, because all the movements are based around that rotation. That rotation is going to come from the ability for you to rotate through your femoral head. If you've got anatomically, let's just say you've been born with a little bit of dysplasia in the hips, where the acetabulum is a bit smaller and the joint doesn't fit that well. You haven't got great movement through the hip but you're asking your body to go for a movement which is asking for massive amounts of rotation through those hips. As you go into your backswing, you're really sitting internally into that hip. Then as you're driving through, you're asking that same hip to open up into a massive external rotation. Then you're driving forward into the anterior hip and asking that to control a massive internal rotation.

There's so much rotation happening through those hips, right? If you haven't anatomically got great hips, then how are you going to be able to play on the Tour consistently year-on-year without having any injuries? The only way for you to do that is to ensure that you understand what your anatomy is and understand that a certain type of training for you specifically is what you're going to have to do to keep yourself strong. Not that it [S&C] will stop you ever getting hurt. We can't ever say that. Will it reduce the likelihood of you getting injured? Yes, we can say that because there is evidence to support it.

AB: **A conversation I've been having with a coach that I work with who wants one of his players [that they have worked with for multiple years] to turn more into his into his right hip on the backswing.**

The coach is saying "he's not sitting deep enough into that hip and we need to get him turning further". I'm thinking. "Well, OK, I can look and see if there's any kind of muscular restriction or anything there, but it might just be that that's just anatomically how it is and there might not be any more movement in the hips so we might have to find a swing solution that doesn't involve that kind of huge rotation around the trail hip joint."

PS: Let's say that 80% of them will have that standard hip. However, if 20 percent that don't have it naturally, that we're going to have a problem with. I think that they'd like to have that sort of idea in your head that when you see them. Let's take it structure to function. That's a very that's a very osteopathic term, but structure governs function. Let's have a look at the structure first and see what function you want from it. Have a look at the capacity of the person to achieve that function and see where we can make improvement. If they've got really good hips, let's just say they've got great hips with really great movement, but they're still getting a back problem the first thing I would look at is the strength of the hip.

AB: **How strong that is and how mobile or stable that joint is as well is going to be crucial for diagnosing what some of the issues are going to be. Just moving back to S&C, how do you try and utilise S&C support to rehab your injured players?**

PS: What we had to do first was debunk some myths. There was this massive cultural thought process within the golf world that S&C makes you bulky, it makes you slow, it's going to change your golf swing. Originally, when we first started that's what was in everybody's head and we had to debunk that. The best way to debunk it was through having really good role models. Luckily for us, we had players like Tiger [Woods], we had players like Rory [McIlory], we had these guys at that same time who were able to do all their S&C and people are saying. "OK, they're doing it and still playing world class golf, then maybe it's not as bad as what people say."

The second thing we needed to do was implement some sort of research where we could actually own and justify the processes that we are putting in place. Show that you actually can get better. We started researching on the Challenge Tour and just tried to answer some very basic questions. I think you might have seen the study that Dan [Coughlan] did with us there [Wells et al., [2019]. Dr Dan Coughlan was a co-author on the study]. Using an isometric mid-thigh pull, countermovement jump, and clubhead speed, and then the distance the ball went. The question we simply answered was. "Who hits the ball further and who has the fastest clubhead speed?" Lo and behold, it was the guys that had the strongest mid-thigh pull. It's very simple. It was a small cohort. I think it was about 30 players, but it gave us a starter block. It told us that if you can produce high forces, guess what, you can swing it faster and you will hit it further. We tried to make it simple for golfers by taking away all the science talk and just say, in a nutshell, that's what happens.

As soon as we did that, it was like "bam!" The players were interested and they bought in. Then all we did was just got involved with two or three players and again, lo and behold, those players start to play really well and started to hit it a bit further. They also start to feel confident and actually look better in clothes as well, which is a really big seller [for S&C programmes]. We feel for their responses as well, and if me telling the player that they're going to look great in a T-shirt is one of the things that I have to tell them to get them to buy into the S&C, but I know in the back of my mind that what I'm actually doing is making sure you don't blow a spinal disc playing golf, I'm going to tell them they look right in the T-shirt!

AB: **Whenever I'm working with young athletes, that's a big selling point for S&C. Yes, I don't want them training in a way that's not going to be particularly conducive to good golf. But at the same time, I think if they stick to a good S&C programme their physical makeup will change and they will look more athletic. Again, it's not a main focus as such, but it is a big selling point.**

The other thing you mentioned, which I think is interesting is that one of the barriers we have from a research perspective in golf is often that we [the scientific community] will conduct research in population groups where we have greater access. Maybe with club level players or your lower level professionals as examples. However, one of the barriers to adopting or translating that research at a high level is. "Oh, well, you know, they're different to us, they're not elite players." That you guys [ETPI] are conducting research with high performance athletes, elite players, means that barrier is removed. It then leads to the perception that. "If it's being shown in your high-level Challenge Tour guys then it's probably a fairer reflection of elite golf."

PS: Yeah, absolutely. I think that that's a really key point that we actually. When Dan [Coughlan] got involved with us, that was one of the main things that we wanted to get across. We needed to have some really good, robust data where we can say. "guys, look!".

We know that it's not always going to be exercise-based. This is a high skill sport and there are going to be guys that come on Tour that say, "I'm not going to lift a single weight. I'm happy playing how I'm playing and I'm going to win championships." We still have players like that. Absolutely. Some players that do absolutely nothing [from a S&C perspective] for 15 years and don't have a single injury. They are your outliers, your n= 1. Really, they're the lucky b*****ds!

However, we want to offer some understanding and some backup to the fact that when you actually hit the Tour now, you've got to hit it 300 yards. The guys that hit it 300 plus tend to be the ones that are in the top 20. That's just the stats and what's been demonstrated in the research literature. The top 10 players in the world and how far are they are hitting it. So, maybe the golf that they want to play is one thing, but the golf that is being played at the "Premier League", at the top end of the sport is slightly different. We encourage them that you need to actually incorporate that [distance, and S&C training to support that] if you want to be in the top, top elite.

AB: **For golfers that are injured, do you have any suggestions to try and encourage a successful recovery? Are there things that you see players do that maybe get in the way of successful rehab?**

PS: Yeah, ignoring the injury. Number one. "I'm not injured." "This will go away." "I'm fine." If you get hurt, the very simple rule I give my players is this: if something bothers you for more than two or three days, ask. There's no harm in having a good person to go and ask, have a good therapist. I don't care what they're called, they could be called an osteopath, a physiotherapist, a sports therapist. Have someone that has some knowledge that you can go and ask and say "I've got this pain". Get it diagnosed for one.

Once it's diagnosed, always understand about injury, recovery and what you can do for it. The standard kind of [advice, such as] ice, good nutrition, and understand that rest is a really good repair tool. Once you've done that, also know that as you as you recover, you need to also start loading [through physical training] correctly as well. You need to be able to use your body and use it for the things that you want to do with it as well.

You need to be able to have someone that can guide you through that whole process if you manage an injury at the beginning for tissue modelling. Let's say you've damaged tissue. If you've got a really robust programme that allows you to remodel that tissue in a really good way, timely fashion, and then you've got someone that can give you advice on how to load it correctly, you'll be back playing way faster than someone that does and be in a better position than the one that doesn't.

Just have a good therapist or a good medical person that you rely on. Don't be afraid to ask, right? Just because it's golf doesn't mean that it doesn't have risks for playing. People think that it's OK when you play football if you get injured to go and get someone [a medical professional]. "I've got injured playing football, I've got to go and ask someone for help." But if somebody gets injured playing golf, it's as if like there's an embarrassment to it, like they don't want to say anything at all. "Look, he got injured playing golf the wuss!". No! It doesn't work like that. It's a high speed, high power sport, it has inherent risk. So, to summarise, [if you're injured] don't be afraid, just ask.

AB: **That's excellent advice. You touched upon this a little bit, actually, and this is going slightly left-field, but you talked about this at the England Golf Coaches Conference [in 2021] and I thought it was really fascinating. Are there any issues that you experience with golfers that are maybe not particularly well reported? A lot of what you have said so far corresponded nicely with findings from the scientific literature. We know that lower back injuries are very prominent for example. But at the conference you touched upon**

some of the more behavioural aspects of competing on the on the elite tours and some of the issues you face supporting golfers on those tours.

PS: Just to just go back a little bit, one injury people don't realise that golfers can get are neck injuries. Neck injuries, are massive. That's from travel, hotel pillows, etc. but also, it's the fact that you're swinging your shoulders left to right [for a right-handed golfer]. You're basically asking the cervical spine to go right to left as fast as possible. Players forget that your upper cervical and neck are really important areas to train. I love setting overhead presses. I love setting neck mobility exercise and all of that kind of stuff.

But now the outlying stuff. Obviously, there's mental health issues that we talked about [at the conference]. I think mental health with golf is massive because it's one of the only sports where if you make a mistake, you've got four hours to think about it. Your mental capacity throughout your game needs to be really, really, strong. As much as golf is fantastic for relieving stress and to help people to de-stress, it can also be a great cause of stress in golfers. Unless you've got really good mental strategies to get over that, it could be a problem.

Then there's the other part. You have golfers that when they're away, they try to look at areas to de-stress away from the game and we try to push that. Aspects such as "use the facilities where you are". By that we mean that if you're in a hotel and they've got a pool and they've got a gym and they've got, a cinema or whatever, use all of that.

Then you still get the others that just love a drink and they use alcohol to kind of de-stress. This is massive compared to other sports that I've been involved with, such as athletics. It's pretty much unheard of for an athlete having alcohol during season. When they're off season, loads! But in season, they will never touch it because they know it has such a detrimental effect on their performance.

I think one part of that isn't talked about is in golf is the players are inevitably going to events that are sponsored by high-profile sponsors. They've got sponsor's evenings, and pro-am dinners etc. where there's free flowing alcohol, and a lot of it. Yes, I'd say a lot of them do use alcohol as the de-stress tool. They might say. "I've had such a bad round. I need some beers tonight." How many times have I heard that, Alex? I've heard it more times than I've had hot dinners!

AB: **It's one of the idiosyncrasies of the sport. Historically, particularly at recreational level, they've always kind of gone hand-in-hand.**

PS: It's an accepted part of it. It's the 19th hole! Again, this is where we have to separate amateur golf from professional golf. Professional golf, if you want to play for the future then you need to understand you need to be like an athlete. To be like an athlete you need to live like an athlete. Recover and prepare well, you need to play well. You need to recover well. Alcohol interferes with recovery. Unless you're having half a pint, right, you know, you're going to interrupt your recovery from whatever training you did. All of these aspects of taking on board what elite athletes do and learning from other sports and other athletes, all of this stuff needs to be done.

AB: **As you said, if there are facilities at the hotel or facilities in the town that they're playing or the city they're playing to go and unwind that doesn't cause too much travel stress then maybe they could do that as an option?**

PS: It's about building good habits, isn't it? In football, they have on average, what, 15 years [for their careers at elite level], 20 to 35 years of age? You have a short window in which you can earn all your money and you can become successful and build a brand. Golf ain't like that! You can play until you're 50 and then guess what, from 50 to 75, you can play on the seniors. But also, you could be a 65-year-old and still play on the main tour! There's no age stop, there's nothing that can stop you. The only thing that will stop you is your own mentality, isn't it? If you have five years' bad play and the players says. "I'm done with this now, I'm going to start a hotel", or something like that and go do something else, you can do it. Golf is this beautiful game in which you have just years and years of the ability to play at the top level. If you've got bad habits of drinking and smoking and you don't really give a ****, then, you know, as long as you're making the money, then who cares?

I think that's one part of golf that, you know, quietly I respect. These guys who just enjoy life. Go there [on Tour], live fast, die young. But, professionally, if we're talking about creating an environment for an elite level of sport and moving golf to the next chapter, then we've got to talk about being athletic and we've got to talk about being fit and strong.

AB: **You've touched upon neck, lower back, and hip. Any other areas of the body you see frequently injured?**

PS: We see a lot of shoulder and wrist. Lower limb, we see very few ankle injuries. The ankle injuries that we see are more to do with people tripping over, falling over, sliding down a bank, sliding in the sand and similar. They're not necessarily to do with the actual act of the golf swing. However, if they do injure an ankle and the ankle then becomes a bit lax, it does affect the game. If it's the left ankle, let's just say you're right handed golfer, the actual brace that you had from the ankle to allow for that force transfer, you won't have that. They need a really robust, a good, strong programme when they're when they're injured to recover.

Knees, again, a classic injury area. That's again a force transference tissue. However, we don't see a lot knee issues. Hips, lots of injuries. Lower back, lots of injuries. Upper back and neck, lots of injuries from travelling. Then finally, shoulder and wrist. It's very weird that we don't see a lot of elbow injuries in golf. Professional golf that is, but in amateur golf, we see quite a bit, yeah, and I think that has to do with confidence in your swing.

AB: **Would you like to expand on that?**

PS: Yeah, so I think that the guys that injure their wrists and elbows are adjusting the clubhead from the point of coming down on their swing. They're making micro adjustments. For me, a micro adjustment that they're making is that they're set up and where they started from, they weren't happy with. You could see those guys that are happy with their coach and are happy with their swing because the swing is just fluid. There's no adjustment to it. They know where the starting point is and where they're going to be hitting the ball. And they're confident with their body, they're confident with their movement, they're able to do it.

The guys that aren't and are making adjustments with their wrists and with their shoulders have usually got something wrong elsewhere and they're trying to make compensation for poor control or anatomy.

AB: **And unfortunately, wrists are a really difficult area to treat as well.**

PS: That is the one injury, and I said this in my talk when I did the England Golf Conference, I really don't want to see on a player when they walk in to clinic because unfortunately it's the one that we have to allow Mother Nature to do what it's got to do. We cannot force it, there's no manipulation, there's no soft tissue, there's nothing manually you can do as an osteopath. Also, S&C-wise everything is about gripping. Everything's about holding a bar, or a medicine ball, or a kettlebell and therefore it restricts your training from that perspective. Also, the tissue and the bones are so delicate and so compacted that the tiniest amount of inflammation can cause a lot of pain. As they are quite small the chance of fracture is really high and a fractured wrist takes time to recover.

It's one of those areas we really don't like to see. However, if someone came in with wrist pain or wrist discomfort, it's the one that you would want them immediately to go see a specialist for. We would look for very good x-rays, and MRI scans, MRI scans to make sure that everything else in there is looking good.

AB: **Do you have any concluding remarks or any other top tips or anything for the readers?**

PS: Top tips are the same ones that you give someone who was going to come into the gym. Have a really good pre warm-up routine. Stretch and mobilisations and some activation stuff. I like people skipping. I like my players to bring a skipping rope and just skip a little bit. Five, six minutes of it. Great activation for your glutes, activation from your calves gets you a little bit warm. It's a really easily achievable thing. Chuck it in the golf bag. Have a really nice warm up, have a really nice mobility drill and then make sure you hydrate. Also, make sure you've got some food to eat on the round because a lot of people forget that. Four and a half, five hours, you're expending lots of calories. You want to take some protein too.

Then following that, when you recover, recover well. A good meal, do some stretching, go and use whatever gym facilities you've got and then train well. Just train for your game. That is a really good one to finish on. Train for your game.

References

Cabri, J., Sousa, J, P., Kots, M., & Barreiros, J. (2009). Golf-related injuries: a systematic review. *European Journal of Sports Sciences.* 9(6):353–366. https://doi.org/10.1080/17461390903009141.

Edwards, N., Dickin, C., & Wang, H. (2020). Low back pain and golf: a review of biomechanical risk factors. *Sports Medicine and Health Science.* 2(1): 10–18 https://doi.org/10.1016/j.smhs.2020.03.002

McHardy, A., Pollard, H., & Luo, K. (2006). Golf injuries: a review of the literature. *Sports Medicine.* 36(2): 171–187. https://doi.org/10.2165/00007256-200636020-00006

Murray, A, D., Daines, L., Archibald, D., Hawkes, R, A., Schiphorst, C., Kelly, P., Grant, L., & Mutrie, N. (2017). The relationships between golf and health: a scoping review. *British Journal of Sports Medicine.* 51: 12–19. doi:10.1136/bjsports-2016-09662

Robinson, P, G., Murray, I, R., Duckworth, A, D., Hawkes, R., Glover, D., Tilley, N, R., Hillman, R., Oliver, C, W., & Murray, A, D. (2019). Systematic review of musculoskeletal injuries in professional golfers. *British Journal of Sports Medicine.* 53:13–18. doi:10.1136/bjsports-2018-099572

Sorbie, G., Richardson, A. K., Glen, J., Hardie, S., Taliep, S., Wade, M., Broughton, L., Mann, S., Steele, J., & Lavallee, D. (2021). The association of golf participation with health and wellbeing: A comparative study. *International Journal of Golf Science.* 9(1).

Wells, J., Charalambous, L. H., Mitchell, A., Coughlan, D., Brearley, S. L., Hawkes, R. A., Murray, A. D., Hillman, R. G., & Fletcher, I. M. (2019). Relationships between Challenge Tour golfers' clubhead velocity and force producing capabilities during a countermovement jump and isometric mid-thigh pull. *Journal of Sports Sciences.* 37(12), 1381–1386. https://doi.org/10.1080/02640414.2018.1559972

10 Transfer of Training

Gym to Swing

Simon Brearley and Jamie North

Introduction

Transfer of training refers to the degree of crossover from a training exercise to a target task. Although a point of contention across many sports, it is particularly debated in golf where the benefits of strength and conditioning are less intuitive than in sports that have such an obvious physiological underpinning such as rowing or cycling. Such debates typically revolve around the principles of specificity and overload within exercise selection. The specificity principle in particular, is often misunderstood, with many assuming it can be assessed through intuition alone. This process typically consists of a brief visual comparison of the similarity between an exercise and the target task, yet in reality assessing specificity and forecasting transfer is far more complex.

Assessing specificity and transfer

Driving distance is one of the most important factors linked to success within golf (Broadie, 2014), and so increasing it is a common objective of coaching interventions. To control the variables associated with driving distance (centredness of strike, environmental conditions, friction of the landing area), we can use clubhead speed as an outcome variable as it is inextricably linked (Hume, Keogh & Read, 2005). This therefore becomes a measure of interest for the strength and conditioning coach, often tracked to determine the success of training interventions.

Various approaches and methods have been used to assess the potential for an exercise and its associated benefits to transfer positively to driving distance. Researchers have previously used cross-sectional (e.g., how does squat performance relate to clubhead speed?) (Parchman & McBride, 2011) and interventional (e.g. how does squatting for six weeks effect clubhead speed?) (Coughlan et al., 2019) study designs. Another approach is to examine the biomechanical profile of the exercise and compare it to the golf swing. Due to logistical barriers of experimental study design, this may be the most useful approach, since it can be inferred (based on the principles and theories proposed herein) that certain exercises possess higher fidelity. That is, they are more likely to facilitate transfer

DOI: 10.4324/9781003099321-10

since they represent either the golf swing action more closely, or develop the requisite physical qualities underpinning that action. This approach is employed infrequently, probably because collecting and examining biomechanical data is not an easy task, and there is a reliance on high-quality existing research. If this research is lacking, the practitioner may have to use research conducted in similar sports, or perhaps dissimilar participant groups (i.e. university students rather than elite golfers), thus diminishing how confidently the conclusion and recommendations can be applied to elite golfers. There are many biomechanical measures that one could collect, but most commonly researchers have examined ground reaction force characteristics, joint torque magnitudes, rate and timing of muscle activity (via surface electromyography), how joints and/ or segments are moving in relation to one another (3D motion capture) or a combination of kinetics (ground reaction forces) and kinematics (3D motion capture) via inverse dynamics analyses.

Training principle interplay: specificity, overload and individuality

Broadly, the overload principle states that training must exceed a performer's habituated level of stress to evoke an adaptive response. Within strength training, this is most commonly achieved through the addition of more external load. Ironically, specificity and overload are somewhat conflicting training principles in that you must often sacrifice some specificity to get some overload in return. For example, Olympic weightlifting (snatch/clean and jerk) will elicit a higher hip extensor moment than the golf swing, thus achieving overload, yet the movements have little similarity to the golf swing. In contrast, a weighted club swing has more similarity to the golf swing, but it achieves less overload in Newtonian terms, and the heavier you make the club, the less specific the exercise becomes. Given that we cannot apply mechanical overload to the global movement (without reducing specificity), this leaves us with four options to navigate the specificity-overload conflict (Figure 10.1):

i) remove mechanical overload altogether, and only use highly specific exercises. In other words, focus on skill learning;
ii) accept part-specificity, applying mechanical overload to one or two elements of the golf swing;
iii) disregard movement specificity and target structural adaptations (e.g., muscle mass and architecture) and general neuromuscular capacities (e.g., neural drive); and
iv) adopt a mixed methods approach navigating a balance between skill and neuro-musculoskeletal development, seeking to understand the interrelationships between the two.

Exercises with greater movement specificity, unsurprisingly, are often better received by players and coaches in comparison to those which bear less resemblance to actions performed on the course. However, a desired change to the

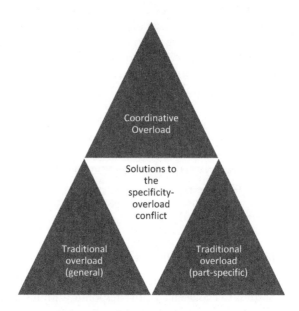

Figure 10.1 Solutions to the specificity–overload conflict. Adapted from Brearley & Bishop (2019). **Coordinative overload** = promote a change in movement strategy (coordination) believed to be favourable to the target task; **Traditional overload (part-specific)** = promote a change in local coordination (about a given joint) specific with the target task or develop neuromuscular capacities under locally/internally specific conditions; **Traditional overload (general)** = change structural qualities underpinning the target task

performance of one of these actions may be reliant on a change to an underpinning physical quality (Newell, 1986). Therefore, the best exercise to deliver this change may in fact not be the one which bears most resemblance, but rather the one which provides overload to produce the adaptations specific with the underpinning physical quality. The constraints on action framework (Newell, 1986) provides a theoretical basis for how altered organismic constraints (e.g. a change to underpinning physical qualities) can shape emergent behaviour (actions performed on the course). This ecological dynamics-based theory will be referenced throughout alongside best available evidence to guide how strength and conditioning should be delivered to golfers to maximise transfer of training benefits from the gym to the swing on the course.

Finally, it is important to appreciate any transfer of training benefits will be a product of an interaction between specificity–overload characteristics and individual factors, since responses to a given training stimulus are not homogenous. Such factors may include biological age (Radnor, Lloyd & Oliver, 2017), genetics (Jones et al., 2016), and training history (Suchomel et al., 2018) The latter is particularly significant as individuals who have accrued substantial structured strength and conditioning training may have fewer or less significant musculo-skeletal limitations constraining their actions on course and therefore reap more benefit from continued skill refinement rather than less-specific gym-based training. This highlights the importance of context when navigating specificity and overload in training design and exercise selection. Indeed, understanding the inter-relationships between a player's physical capacities and their swing tendencies will help optimise the impact of strength & conditioning. This means not viewing physical and technical development as separate entities, but as integrated and complementary processes.

Coordinative overload approach (overload via variation)

The ability to produce stable performance outcomes despite significant movement variability is a common feature of elite performers across all sports and is referred to as 'functional variability' (Robins et al., 2006; Koenig et al., 1994, Carson, Collins & Richards, 2014). Functional variability represents movement degeneracy which is required to deliver consistent performance outcomes despite ever changing context and conditions e.g. changes in wea-ther (environmental constraints) or individual fatigue (organismic constraints) (Newell, 1986, Scholz & Schoner, 1999). To illustrate, the top 50 golfers in the world would exhibit a degree of swing-to-swing (within trial) variability, even when playing the same shot, requiring the same ball flight outcome.

Exposure to variability is thought to be effective for learning skills as the performer learns to adapt to the variable constraints in which they may be required to perform the skill and find effective movement solutions (Kelso, 1995; Pekny, Izawa & Shedmehr, 2015; Ranganathan & Newell, 2013). The *uncontrolled manifold hypothesis* (Scholz & Schroner, 1999) would describe this as constraining the 'performance variables' (technical features of a movement that matter) while releasing the 'elementary variables' (those that do not). While mechanical overload (adding significant resistance to the golf swing) would stifle learning, applying overload through subtle variation can challenge the performer to diversify their movement solutions (Knight, 2004). This variation may be imposed through manipulation of the environment or the task itself to encourage the emergence of different/new motor behaviours. An example of task manipulation would be the swing plane gate drill where alignment sticks are placed in the ground, typically at ~45 degrees, to constrain the individual's swing plane. Likewise, high-pressure skills challenges would be a common way to manipulate the environment. Indeed, there are many (almost infinite) ways a golf coach can adopt a constraints-based approach for the purpose of skill learning or refinement. However, given the primary aim of this chapter is to provide a theoretical foundation for how strength and conditioning can influence an individual's golf swing action, from here on, the focus will remain largely on the manipulation of organismic constraints to remove neuromuscular-skeletal limitations on performance, and thus open up new action possibilities.

Individuals with different organismic constraints have different opportunities for action (defined as affordances) (Fajen, Riley & Turvey, 2008). As mentioned, there are many ways to swing a golf club, but some of those options are taken away in the absence of physical capacities (action-scaled affordances) or as a result of body dimensions and proportions (body-scaled affordances). While some of these organismic constraints are non-modifiable (i.e., arm span, stature), both physical capacities (mobility/strength) and other body-scaled affordances (i.e., body mass, segment mass) can be changed over time and that is how it is possible to support transfer from 'gym to swing' through strength and conditioning interventions which change physical capabilities, and thus alter the affordances available to the golfer (see Figure 10.2).

To summarise using the case of the resisted golf swing example, although some research supports the use of small deviations in the weight of striking implements to support learning (De Renne, 1995), attempts to overload the musculoskeletal determinants of performance without sacrificing movement specificity will likely lead to sub-optimal outcomes for two distinct reasons:

1) The emergent behaviours will differ too greatly to that of the unloaded golf swing and will not promote effective learning.
2) The overload stimuli will likely be inadequate to produce any significant change in organismic constraints/change to the biomechanical determinants of performance e.g. change the torque generating capacity at the hip joint.

Hopefully this makes it apparent why simply adding resistance to the golf swing is not effective strength and conditioning practice, nor is it a good 'coordinative overload' task to promote effective learning (at least beyond minor deviations in regular shaft/clubhead weight). The following section will focus on better 'mechanical overload' alternatives to modify relevant physical capacities.

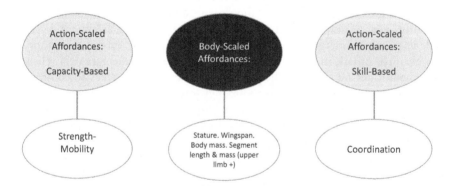

Figure 10.2 Barriers to affordances (action possibilities)
Source: adopted from Fajen, Riley & Turvey (2008).

Traditional overload approach: specificity and overload characteristics

An understanding of the neuromechanical determinants of performance in the golf swing is a crucial first step in the interrogation of the principles of overload and specificity within exercise selection for golfers. Only with a foundation of evidence can we make strength and conditioning recommendations which we are confident are more likely to enhance the likelihood of transfer.

As discussed, relying on crude visual comparison (of training task to golf swing action) to assess specificity is inadequate, and has in fact been shown to be unreliable. For example, Brazil et al. (2020) examined the intra-joint coordination patterns of commonly deemed specific and non-specific exercises in relation to a sprint start and found that the non-specific exercises had greater coordination similarity. An example of a visually (golf-) specific exercise is a downswing 'woodchop' performed on a cable machine. Such exercises are commonly rationalised as being 'functional', yet as we intend to convey here, function is a product of the adaptation elicited, not visual similarity.

Not only is visual comparison unreliable, but using the movement pattern as a sole criterion for specificity is also an oversight. This not only devalues the principle of overload, but also overlooks other factors which are potentially more important. In reality, exercises with little resemblance to the movement pattern may have similar neuromuscular activation or musculotendinous-unit (MTU) behaviour about a given joint, meaning they can offer overload while maintaining a degree of internal or 'local' specificity. To produce similar neuromuscular activation and MTU behaviour, a training task will need to demand a similar type, timing, rate and magnitude of muscle activity as the target task (Siff & Verkhoshansky, 1998).

Figure 10.3 illustrates how a degree of local specificity is possible without movement specificity, while highlighting how some of these factors are inextricably linked due to the mechanics of human muscle function. For example, joint angle and excursion will impact on magnitude of force production due to length-tension relationships, and both external load and movement velocity (linked due to the load-velocity relationship) will impact on contraction speed due to the force-velocity relationship. Using this model as a framework, the remainder of this section will consolidate the existing biomechanical research to evaluate the specificity and overload characteristics of a selection of exercises in relation to the different phases of the golf swing, shown in Figure 10.4. Note that in the interests of simplicity this section will refer to the respective phases using the same definitions and titles used by McCardy & Pollard's (2005) original electromyographic research, despite the movement phases commonly being further sub-divided in the more recent literature (Han et al., 2019). For clarity, Table 10.1 below defines these phases.

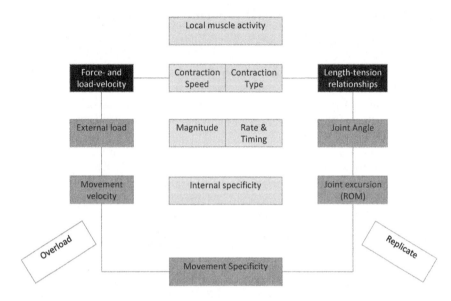

Figure 10.3 **Determinants of exercise specificity.** The model shows determinants of local coordination centrally (local specificity) and global coordination peripherally (movement specificity). In theory, specificity is maximised with similarity of both central and peripheral factors, but this is not possible when accommodating mechanical overload. Part-specific training tasks can overload the left-central and left-peripheral factors while maximising similarity of right-central and right-peripheral factors. This increases the possibility of evoking structural (contractile) and neural adaptations desirable to the target task

Table 10.1 Golf swing phases defined

Phase	Description
Back swing	Address to top of back swing
Forward swing	Top of back swing to club horizontal (early downswing)
Acceleration	Club horizontal to impact (late downswing)
Early follow through	Impact to club horizontal
Late follow through	Club horizontal to completion of swing

Barbell compound lifts

Researchers have provided evidence that low-handicap golfers regulate ground reaction force (to control shot distance) and that ground reaction force magnitude is a key determinant of high clubhead speed. This includes cross-sectional correlational (Read et al., 2013, Myers et al., 2008, Wells et al., 2018; 2019), interventional (Oranchuk et al., 2020, Doan et al., 2006, Gatt et al., 1998;1999) and cross-sectional biomechanical analysis study designs (Berrentine et al., 1994, Hume, 2005, McNitt-Gray et al., 2013, Myers et al., 2008, Keogh et al., 2009).

Traditional barbell compound lifts such as squats and deadlifts develop force generation capacity in the leg extensors which are highly active during the forward (early downswing) and acceleration (late downswing) phases of the golf swing (McNitt-Gray et al., 2013, Bechler et al., 1995, McCardy & Pollard, 2005) (see Figure 10.4). There is some contention surrounding the force-time integral in the golf swing, with researchers previously focusing on the duration of the downswing (time elapsed from top of backswing to impact) (~284ms) as an indicator of the available time for force production (Cochran & Stobbs, 1999; Tinmark et al., 2010). However, considering the downswing is initiated from the ground up while the upper body is still rotating away from the target, more time is likely afforded (Wells, 2018). Since maximal force expression becomes a greater influence in explosive force production with longer force-time integrals (Tillin, Pain & Folland, 2018) (Figure 10.5), this suggests that leg extensor force capacity may be more important than previously thought. The strong positive correlations between lower body strength and clubhead speed in the literature support this (Ehlert, 2020). Notwithstanding, we can consider the following variations to move towards a greater degree of specificity in relation to certain phases of the swing.

Quasi-isometric variants to support transition

Semi-static or 'quasi-isometric' would be a fitting description for many lower body muscle actions in the golf swing, which involves minimal change in hip or knee joint angle for the majority of its duration prior to acceleration/impact, despite significant interaction with the ground to generate angular momentum (Hume et al., 2005., Lynn & Wu, 2017, McCardy & Pollard, 2005, McNally, 2014). For example, the lower body initiates the transition from backswing to downswing, creating pelvic rotation through a combination of posterior and anterior directed ground reaction forces (McNitt-Gray et al., 2013), before the knee is maintained in a flexed position while energy is transferred up the kinetic chain (Bechler et al., 1995, Nesbitt & Serrano, 2005). This is an important consideration in training programme design since strength gains are contraction mode specific (Vikne et al., 2006), meaning strengthening a muscle in an isometric manner transfers better to isometric muscle actions (Siddique et al., 2020, Vikne et al., 2006). Accordingly, an isometric mid-thigh pull (Figure 10.6a) could deliver adaptations specific to the muscle actions of the lower body bracketing the transition from backswing to forward swing (downswing).

RAPID ISOMETRIC-ECCENTRIC VARIANTS TO SUPPORT DOWNSWING

Although there are contrasting perspectives surrounding the 'weight-transfer' principle (Burden, Grimshaw & Wallace, 1998; Wallace, Grimshaw & Ashford,

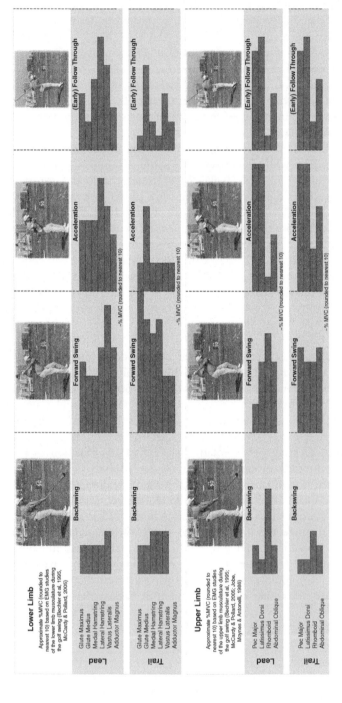

Figure 10.4 Muscle EMG during the phases of the golf swing. A limitation of EMG is while we know what muscles are active it doesn't provide information on how they are acting (i.e. muscle activity type). More research is needed to obtain this information through joint kinetics analysis

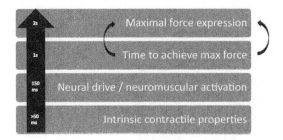

Figure 10.5 Determinants of explosive force production with increasing force-time integrals (Tillin, Pain & Folland, 2018). Note the increasing influence of maximal strength and how time to achieve max force (RFD) scales to maximal strength

1994), most of the evidence suggests greater transference of the centre of pressure towards the target is favourable for clubhead speed generation (Berrentine et al., 1994; Okuda, Gribble & Armstrong, 2010; Williams & Cavanagh, 1983; Wallace, Graham & Bleakley, 1990; Koenig, Tamres & Mann, 1994). Further, some research has identified a greater rate of change of centre of pressure from trail to lead leg during the downswing as a differentiator of high and low-handicap players (Wallace, Grimshaw & Ashford, 1994; Okudo, Armstrong & Tsunezumi, 2002; Wallace, Graham & Bleakley, 1990). While some players load the trail side more than others, it is generally accepted that low-handicap golfers produce considerable vertical ground reaction force (Hume et al., 2005) shifting their centre of pressure towards the lead leg in the downswing after significant unweighting in the backswing, to achieve greater frontal plane torque and therefore clubhead speed through impact (Burden, Grimshaw & Wallace, 1998). Accordingly, the high activity of the lead leg knee extensors during the downswing (see Figure 10.4) likely reflects the quadriceps serving a net force dissipation role as they accept force transfer from the trail leg and act as a fulcrum around which the pelvis rotates (Bechler et al., 1995). Given that the degree of unweighting and centre of pressure shift has been linked to greater clubhead speed at impact, it is recommended that players develop these isometric-eccentric qualities to support such techniques. Research has reported average vertical, antero-posterior and medio-lateral ground reaction forces during this phase to be in the region of 1.6–2, 0.4–0.6 and 0.2–3 x bodyweight respectively (Berrentine et al., 1994, Gatt et al., 1999, Koenig, 1994). It is therefore important that selected exercises exceed this habituated level of stress/strain.

There are many exercises which could overload the lead leg lower limb joints by mirroring the intention of preventing hip and knee flexion. Barbell variants could include trap bar jumps (Figure 10.6b) with minimal displacement on landing impact to overload the rate and magnitude of muscle activity in the sagittal plane. Band or flywheel resistance could also be added to further increase the rate demand on the downward phase.

(a)

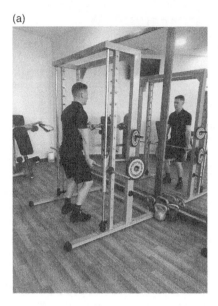

Figure 10.6a Isometric Pull

(b)

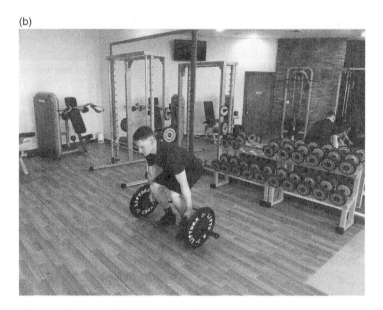

Figure 10.6b Set up for trap bar jump

Despite overcoming some of the limitations of conventional barbell lifts in relation to replicating the local coordinative state, many of the proposed solutions do not satisfy specificity in respect of force direction, intra-and inter-muscular coordination and contraction speed. Research has previously suggested both intention to exert force explosively (early phase neural drive) and actual movement velocity (inter-muscular coordination) contribute to strength velocity-specificity (Blazevich, 2012; Tillin, Pain & Folland, 2012, Brearley & Bishop, 2019). These specificity characteristics are best pursued via other exercises discussed below.

Jumps and throws

With similar force-time integrals to the golf swing (~1second), and minimal external resistance to overcome, bodyweight jumps and medicine ball throws (see Figure 10.7) have potential to support the acceleration phase of the golf swing. During this phase the glutes and hamstrings of the lead leg and the large muscles of the shoulder (pectorals and latissimus dorsi) exhibit short duration, explosive contractions (McCardy et al., 2005, Gorman, 2001, McNally, Yontz & Chaudhari, 2014). The pectorals work bilaterally during the downswing to maintain a triangle between the grip on the shaft and the sternum, creating a central rotational hub for 'one-piece acceleration' (Hume et al., 2005) before contributing to the summation of force pre-impact, likely similar to their role in rotational medicine ball throw variants. With this local specificity there is potential for transfer through adaptations such as increases in early phase neural drive (Balshaw et al., 2016, Tillin, Pain & Folland, 2012; Tillin & Folland, 2014). Moreover, performance in most of these variants requires effective proximal to distal force summation like the golf swing. Therefore, medicine ball throws may also exhibit part-movement specificity in regards to contraction speed, patterns of force production and force vector.

Efficient transfer and summation of force from the ground to the upper extremity (shoulder) and into the clubhead is achieved via a stiff/braced torso. Like the golf swing, many medicine ball throw variants demand trunk stiffness to transmit the force from lower to upper extremities and resist centrifugal force to maintain stability over their base of support. Indeed, swinging a standard-length driver at a clubhead speed of 112 mph produces a centrifugal force of almost 60 kg (Jones & Stevenson, 2015) so roped medicine ball exercises such as a hammer throw may offer benefit through enhancing rotational stability.

Beyond stabilisation, the trunk also contributes to the summation of forces through exploiting stretch shortening cycle mechanisms (Hume, Keogh & Reid, 2005) (where a pre-stretch augments the subsequent concentric contraction). Okuda et al. (2002) described how the eccentric action of the trunk muscles (abdominal obliques) initiates the downswing sequence while the arms continue to rotate away from the target to complete the backswing (Gatt et al., 1998; Bechler et al., 1995; Okuda et al., 2002), a concept often

(a)

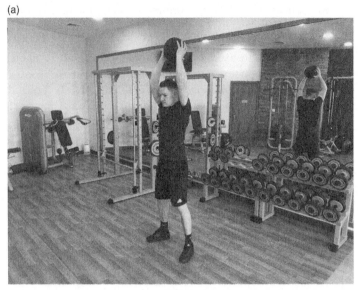

(b)

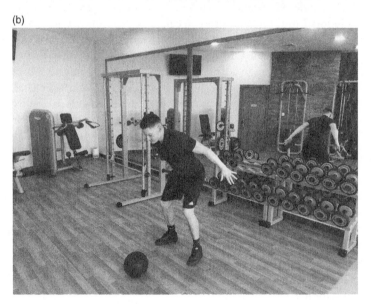

Figure 10.7a and b Medicine ball slam

referred to as the 'X-Factor stretch'. The lead shoulder muscles also experience stretch tension in the backswing and therefore also use passive force production via the series elastic component to contribute to force generation (Gorman, 2001, Pink, Jobe & Perry, 1990). Since stretch shortening cycle force augmentation increases with greater rates of stretch, players who utilise a long, fast backswing (and importantly a fast transition) in particular exploit this. Many rotational medicine ball throws involve a rapid separation of the shoulders from the pelvis which can develop these elastic qualities around the shoulder and trunk.

Supplementary exercises

During the downswing, the trail hip extensors (glute max, hamstrings) and abductors (glute med, deep rotators) work synergistically to rotate as well as extend the trail hip while the adductor magnus of the lead leg facilitates pelvis rotation (Bechler et al., 1995). One of the few studies examining individual joint kinetics in the golf swing was conducted by Foxworth et al. (2013) who found that the trail hip exhibited the greatest extensor moment and differentiated clubhead speed in young and senior healthy male amateurs. Additionally, Foxworth (2013) and Callaway et al. (2012) showed strong relationships between hip torques produced during the swing and clubhead speed, with the latter reporting glute medius and maximus strength to be correlated with lower handicap scores. Therefore, hip extensor strength is a probable musculoskeletal determinant of performance in golf and should be overloaded through an array of posterior chain exercises.

In addition to their apparent role in phases of power generation, the hamstrings are also thought to be important power dissipators, playing an important role in both pelvic and knee stability, which is crucial when exploiting a longer hand path to maximise clubhead speed (Maddalozzo, 1987). Given this important rotational and stabiliser role it is logical to supplement classic posterior chain exercises such as the barbell hip thrust and kettlebell swings (Figure 10.8 a–d) with variations outside the sagittal plane. This could be any exercise which requires the hamstring to rotate or stabilise the pelvis, thus offering a greater similarity of timing and neuromuscular activation. Furthermore, considering the hip abductors (together with the deep rotators) contribute 2.5 times the torque during a golf swing than in sagittal plane jumping (Chaudari et al., 2007), supplementary exercises for this muscle group may be warranted to ensure the player has the capabilities to maintain a stable base. Single leg vertical push exercises like step ups (Figure 10.8 e–f) are an excellent choice as it places the performers' CoM medial to their base of support thus creating a large hip abductor moment arm and therefore a very large increase in the activity of the hip abductors (Neumann, 2010). Many of the supplementary exercises discussed in this section also challenge rotary trunk stability, a welcomed secondary training effect. This section has offered a guideline for exercise selection when looking to apply overload to neuromuscular-skeletal determinants of performance, while retaining internal (local) and movement specificity where possible or appropriate. While it is theoretically possible to find exercises that offer both overload and part-specificity, exercises in this category should primarily be shortlisted based on their ability to produce the desired biological adaptation

(a)   (b)

(c)   (d)

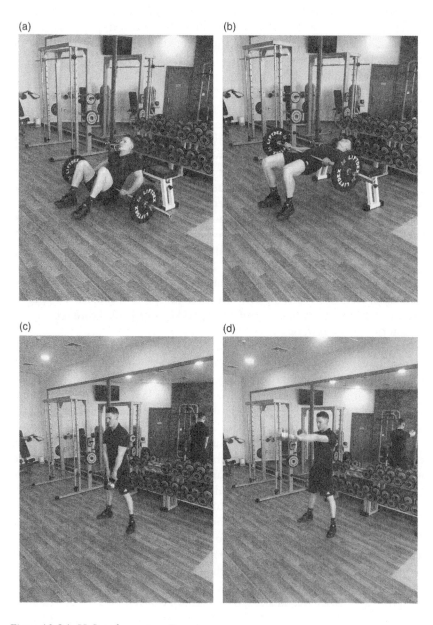

Figure 10.8A–H Supplementary Exercises

(e)

(f)

(g)

(h)

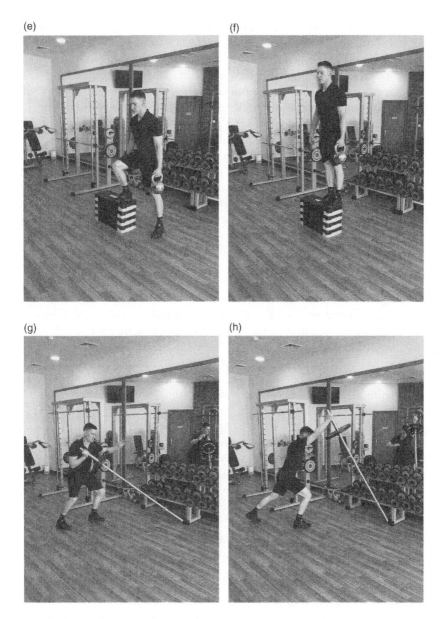

Figure 10.8A–H (Continued)

rather than improve coordination (Brazil, 2020). However, overloading a joint in a manner which produces similar activity of all the muscles crossing that joint (local coordination) will improve the likelihood of promoting adaptations which are favourable to the target task, so specificity remains a consideration.

More research is needed to advance our biomechanical understanding of the neuromuscular-skeletal determinants of performance in the golf swing (particularly single limb joint kinetics and kinematics). Notwithstanding, this section can help practitioners ensure their exercise selection is based on best available evidence, first principles and logical inference, rather than intuition. Similarly, it will also help coaches recognise the value in what may be perceived as non-specific gym-based exercises. Given the known complexity of force production during the swing, future research analysing the overload and specificity characteristics of the exercises discussed herein would be of great value to either challenge or corroborate existing evidence and make guidelines more robust.

Mixed methods approach

The previous section highlighted different ways in which exercises can be 'specific', so it is logical to consider the combined transfer potential of multiple exercises (i.e. the programme as a whole) to avoid targeting too much with a single exercise. In other words, transfer should be considered an interlinked process. This can include general exercises to develop relevant adaptations specific with the musculoskeletal determinants, and more specific exercises to develop coordination and an ability to apply force favourably (patterns of force production/force vector). By understanding the underpinning adaptations and mechanisms, training tasks can be loosely categorised in line with the model previously proposed by Brearley & Bishop (2019) (Figure 10.1). A host of factors then need to be considered when deciding on the proportion of the programme (across a training cycle) which should comprise exercises from each respective category. These will include (but are not limited to) the individual player's:

- existing technique/movement strategy;
- biological age;
- existing physical qualities;
- physical training history; and
- performance support team personnel/dynamics.

The 'training status' of an individual is a key factor. As discussed, little specificity is required to simply make a muscle bigger, change its architecture or develop general neuromuscular capacities. However, transfer of traditional strength training will reduce over time and an increased emphasis on part-specificity may be needed to maximise transfer from gym to swing. One need only look at the movement strategies of the longest hitters on tour or long-drive competitors to see how technique has evolved to deliver greater clubhead speed. While general overload in the gym may help develop the physical qualities underpinning such techniques, part-specific exercises and overload via variation may also promote coordinative structures associated with the golf swing action, helping the player utilise their newfound capacities through stimulating changes in intermuscular coordination as a result of their altered organismic constraints (Burnie et al., 2017). It is for this reason that a mixed-methods approach is always recommended. However, this should not be confused with selecting or designing training tasks which are thought to offer both specificity and overload, and thus blur the boundaries between the exercise classification in Figure 10.1. The reader can be assured by fundamental principles of strength and conditioning science and motor learning that the best exercise for producing local or global coordination is unlikely to be the best exercise for inducing biological adaptation.

Practical applications

The purpose of this section is to consolidate concepts discussed above through case study illustrations. Specifically, we demonstrate how inter-disciplinary interpretation (performance, medical, therapy, PGA professional) of both qualitative and quantitative analysis provides insight into strategies for individualisation. To aid understanding of the assessments referenced in the interpretations, the reader is advised to refer back to the 'Needs Analysis and Physical Profiling' section. Additionally, performance ratings on such assessments are informed by research (Wells et al., 2018, Wells et al., 2019) and unpublished standards obtained by the European Tour Performance Institute (ETPI).

Case comparison 1

Player A and B are both junior players struggling for distance off the tee (clubhead speed of 81 mph and 87 mph respectively). They have both previously consulted with a biomechanist. Player A is a 15-year-old female (179 cm, 63 kg) identified by the coach to exhibit a 'slide' characteristic in her golf swing (excessive lateral movement of the pelvis towards the target line in the downswing). This is supported by kinematic data. Player B is a 16-year-old male (172 cm, 80 kg) exhibiting an 'early extension' pattern (hips and spine extend too early in the downswing). 3D force plate analysis reveals low antero-posterior (heel-toe) force through the lead leg during the downswing, limiting the transverse plane torque.

PLAYER A INTERPRETATION

Physical profiling shows a lack of leg extensor force capacity (isometric mid-thigh pull – 1431 N) and anti-rotational trunk strength (combined isometric trunk rotation = 162 N). She also frequently displays hip hike/drop and knee valgus during single leg movements in the gym, indicative of poor lateral hip stability and inter-segmental control. Lateral hip stability (hip abductor and deep rotator strength) and trunk anti-rotation strength are both necessary qualities to allow a golfer to create a large distance between their centre of pressure and centre of mass during the backswing, generating a large moment arm in the frontal plane for torque production. The 'slide' movement decreases this moment arm, thereby reducing the demand on both the hip abductors, trunk musculature and other inter-segmental stabilisers. Intervention should therefore be directed towards removing the physical limitations currently constraining the player's technique/ movement strategy. It is important player expectations are managed by setting out a realistic timeline for a more favourable movement strategy to emerge.

INTERVENTION OBJECTIVES/EXAMPLE S&C CONTENT

- Develop trunk strength and progress to stiffness/static RFD drills – heavy anti-rotation bracing, loaded carries → roped medicine ball drills, Powerbag © figure of eight swings, and other trunk stability challenges;
- Develop hip stability and inter-segmental control – single leg work i.e. step ups → overhead single leg tasks, hamstring work in transverse plane;
- Establish a long-term strategy to develop the structural foundations upon which to build leg extensor force capacity.

PLAYER B INTERPRETATION

Physical profiling reveals a polarised profile to that of player A, with good leg extensor force capabilities (as indicated by a peak of 2650 N during an isometric mid-thigh pull). Further, a countermovement jump impulse of 360N.s suggests the vertical ground reaction force potential to generate higher swing speeds. Given that there are no major restrictions in joint range of motion (or limitations in further isolated assessments of strength) intervention should be directed towards patterns of force production (skill component). Effective manipulation of antero-posterior ground reaction forces is essential for torque generation in the transverse plane. In other words, to create rotation towards the target there must be a force couple where the lead foot must push backwards (reaction force pushes forwards) and the trail foot must push forwards (reaction force pushes backwards). Therefore, facilitating player B to push the lead foot backwards during the downswing should help 'clear the hips'; thereby omitting the early extension move and affording the opportunity to maximise lead leg propulsion during the acceleration phase. Given player B's shorter stature and lever system than player A, they will need to generate greater hip angular velocity to achieve the same angular momentum (since angular momentum = moment of inertia x angular velocity), thus further increasing their reliance on transverse plane torque. Although this intervention may be somewhat conceptual, the strength and conditioning coach may be able to offer valuable support through the development of explosive strength in the antero-posterior plane. Jumps and throws with a rotational component may help develop the skill of proximal to distal torque summation as well as RFD qualities. If successful, the player and coach could expect relatively fast improvements in clubhead speed, but if short-term improvements are not observed this should be recognised quickly so that other technical interventions can be trialled.

INTERVENTION OBJECTIVES/EXAMPLE S&C CONTENT

- Challenge RFD under conditions of similar local muscle activity and through part-specific pattern of force production – MB rotation throws, shot put style throws and landmine split jerk (Figure 10.8 g–h);
- Work with the technical coach to complement the above with coordinative overload/application drills and devoted range-based speed sessions to maximise opportunity for learning.
- Above drills form part of a wider coaching intervention to encourage greater horizontal torque production/omit early extension patterns.
- Ensure the above is integrated with low volume traditional strength work to maintain force generating capacities and tissue robustness.

Case comparison 2

Players C & D are both male early career professionals with similar maximal swing speeds (115 mph) playing on the European Challenge Tour. Player C is 20 years of age (183 cm, 75 kg), renowned for his high clubhead speed as a junior (which has decreased marginally since he was an u16 amateur). He has a notably long and fast hand path, and is described by his coach as 'wired' and 'elastic'. Prior to stopping all other sports aged 15 he also competed in athletics (multi-events). The player has been hampered by injury throughout his junior career (neck, shoulder and lumbar spine) which has deterred him from engaging in gym-based training in fear of aggravating these issues. Rather, his training history is akin to that of a 'chronic rehabber', hopping from therapist to therapist, exploring different treatment modalities. However, he has and continues to use speed sticks/swing aids extensively with a view to honing his inherent speed asset or 'super strength'. Player D (23 years of age, 177 cm, 88 kg) has a comparably short backswing, with his recent physical training history directed towards increasing his range of motion. This intervention made no change in ~6 weeks to either passive or active range of motion at the shoulder/thoracic spine or hip and he continued to have technical issues at impact when adopting a longer backswing arc. Over the last 2 years the player has worked with a personal trainer and made significant improvements in 'gym-strength', but with little carryover to clubhead speed.

PLAYER C INTERPRETATION

Physical profiling reflected the lack of structured strength training history. The player was in the 20th percentile for leg extensor force capabilities (isometric mid-thigh pull) according to ETPI standards (see Figure 10.9). Additionally, although the forces generated in the countermovement jump resulted in a respectable jump height, his impulse ranked only moderately (40th percentile), and by the same standards he exhibited similarly modest isometric trunk

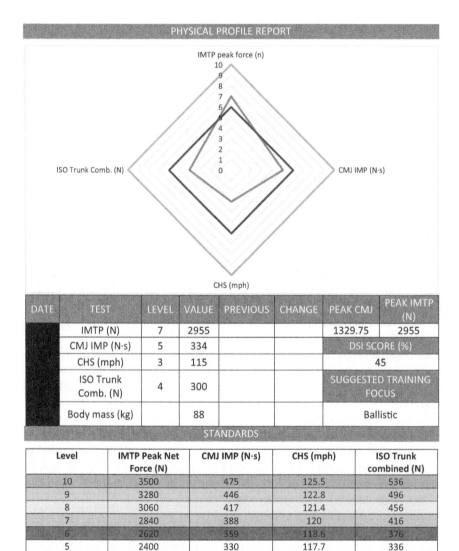

DATE	TEST	LEVEL	VALUE	PREVIOUS	CHANGE	PEAK CMJ	PEAK IMTP (N)
	IMTP (N)	7	2955			1329.75	2955
	CMJ IMP (N·s)	5	334			DSI SCORE (%)	
	CHS (mph)	3	115			45	
	ISO Trunk Comb. (N)	4	300			SUGGESTED TRAINING FOCUS	
	Body mass (kg)		88			Ballistic	

STANDARDS				
Level	IMTP Peak Net Force (N)	CMJ IMP (N·s)	CHS (mph)	ISO Trunk combined (N)
10	3500	475	125.5	536
9	3280	446	122.8	496
8	3060	417	121.4	456
7	2840	388	120	416
6	2620	359	118.6	376
5	2400	330	117.7	336
4	2180	301	116.4	296
3	1960	272	114.6	256
2	1740	243	113.2	216
1	1520	214	108	176

Figure 10.9 Physical Profiling Report – Player D

rotation strength. Medical investigations confirmed no serious pathology at the cervical or lumbar spine, and the only noteworthy finding from a physio-led musculoskeletal assessment was some anterior capsule laxity of the lead shoulder (greater than normal for a right-handed golfer).

This player evidently had the ability to create tremendous whip and 'hand speed' but is doing so over a somewhat unstable base. Accordingly, a structured strength training programme orientated towards muscle mass development in the lower body and hip/trunk was recommended. As well as raising the force generating capacity of the muscles, the additional body mass would also create a greater anchoring effect to enable him to exploit his inherent speed qualities/elastic capabilities. An array of dynamic trunk stability tasks would also be programmed to support this. Finally, it is possible the player may be 'holding back' due to fear avoidance created by his injury history. Therefore, isolated progressive loading for the posterior trunk/chain (lumbar spine), and an upper limb health programme (neck and shoulder) would also be recommended in an attempt to make these structures more robust, increase tissue tolerance while reducing nociceptive activity and sensitisation. Whether to target weaknesses or turn strengths into 'super-strengths' is a common philosophical dilemma when performance strategizing. The above approach does not intend to dampen this player's 'super-strength' but rather unlock co-existing musculoskeletal and psychological constraints so that it can be exploited further. For buy-in, it is essential this is explained to the player and packaged as a long-term strategy.

PROPOSED S&C INTERVENTION

- Develop structure to provide a stable base on which to rotate – explore trap bar deadlift, leg press, safety-bar squat, belt squats and loaded carries;
- Additional posterior trunk/chain loading – deadlifts, Romanian deadlifts, bent over rows, weighted back extensions to reduce fear avoidance (lumbar spine);
- Trunk stability challenges - roped medicine rotations, roped medicine ball hammer throw;
- Neck loading - Isometric →isotonic →static RFD;
- Holistic shoulder health programme; upward rotators, cuff loading, end-range eccentric strength (i.e., pullovers);
- Continue with, but reduce (volume and frequency), range-based speed development sessions.

PLAYER D INTERPRETATION

Receipt of player D's previous programmes quickly offered some explanation as to the disconnect between rising gym-based strength levels and clubhead speed progression. With over two years following what was essentially a body-building programme, this player had developed significant muscle mass which had increased his ability to express maximal leg extensor force, but as a side effect he had developed a significant explosive strength deficit identified via force diagnostics (see Figure 10.9) revealing:

- High but shallow isometric pull force-time trace (high peak force but low RFD);
- low-moderate countermovement jump impulse;
- Dynamic strength index of 0.45 (< 0.60 thought to indicate a dynamic strength deficit, Sheppard et al., 2011).

Dynamic strength index is a common means to objectify an athletes' ability to access their maximal force generation capacity in a ballistic (time-constrained) task. Player D's peak forces achieved in the countermovement jump was compared to that achieved in the isometric pull to obtain the dynamic strength index (Sheppard et al., 2011). Although similar diagnostics were not carried out on the upper limb, it was assumed a similar deficit would be present. Since the player and coach were not looking to further pursue a longer hand path, intervention is principally directed towards reducing the player's explosive strength deficit to enable greater impulse to be generated within the existing, limited force-time integral (afforded by their current backswing length).

PROPOSED S&C INTERVENTION

- Replace high volume bodybuilding routine with explosive strength development;
- Short duration, explosive muscle contractions – band assisted explosive push ups, medicine ball throws (slams, overhead toss, kneeling chest pass), bodyweight jumps;
- Loaded explosive lifts – trap bar jumps, push/split jerks, jump shrugs, bench throws and pulls;
- Isometric RFD challenges (intent to develop force as quickly as possible) – isometric pulls/squats, hip thrusts and Pallof pressing both in neutral and towards end-range torso rotation;
- Concomitant, dedicated range-based speed development sessions.

References

Balshaw, T. G., Massey, G. J., Maden-Wilkinson, T. M., Tillin, N. A., & Folland, J. P. (2016). Training-specific functional, neural, and hypertrophic adaptations to explosive- vs. sustained-contraction strength training. *Journal of Applied Physiology*, *120*(11): 1364–1373. https://doi.org/10.1152/japplphysiol.00091.2016

Barrentine, S. W., Fleisig, G. S., Johnson, H. and Woolley, T. W. (1994) Ground reaction forces and torques of professional and amateur golfers, In: A. Cochran & M. Farraly (Eds.), *Science and Golf II: Proceedings of the World Scientific Congress of Golf*, London: E & FN Spon: 33–39.

Bechler, J. R., Jobe, F. W., Pink, M., Perry, J., & Ruwe, P. A. (1995). Electromyographic analysis of the hip and knee during the golf swing. *Clinical Journal of Sport Medicine: Official Journal of the Canadian Academy of Sport Medicine*, *5*(3): 162–166.

Bosch, F. (2015) Strength training and coordination: an integrative approach, uitgevers. 2010publishers ISBN 978 94 90951 27 6

Blazevich, A. J., & Jenkins, D. G. (2002). Effect of the movement speed of resistance training exercises on sprint and strength performance in concurrently training elite junior sprinters. *Journal of Sports Sciences*, *20*(12): 981–990. https://doi.org/10.1080/026404102321011742

Blazevich, A. (2012). Are training velocity and movement pattern important determinants of muscular rate of force development enhancement? *Eur J Appl Physiol*, 112: 3689–3691. https://doi.org/10.1007/s00421-012-2352-66.

Bradshaw, E. J., Keogh, J. W., Hume, P. A., Maulder, P. S., Nortje, J., & Marnewick, M. (2009). The effect of biological movement variability on the performance of the golf swing in high- and low-handicapped players. *Research Quarterly for Exercise and Sport*, *80*(2): 185–196.

Brazil, A., Exell, T., Wilson, C., & Irwin, G. (2020). A biomechanical approach to evaluate overload and specificity characteristics within physical preparation exercises. *Journal of Sports Sciences*, *38*(10): 1140–1149.

Brearley, S. and Bishop, C. (2019) Transfer of training: How specific should we be?, *Strength and Conditioning Journal*, *41*(3): 97–109.

Broadie, M. (2014). *Every Shot Counts*. New York: Avery Publishing Group.

Burden, A.M., Grimshaw, P.N. and Wallace, E.S. (1998) Hip and shoulder rotations during the golf swing of sub-10 handicap players, *Journal of Sports Sciences*, *16*(2): 165–176.

Burnie, L, Barratt, P, Davids, K. Stone, J, Worsfold, P. and Wheat, J. (2017) Coaches' philosophies on the transfer of strength training to elite sports performance. *International Journal of Sports Science and Coaching*, *13*(5). https://doi.org/10.1177/1747954117747131

Callaway, S., Glaws, K., Mitchell, M., Scerbo, H., Voight, M., & Sells, P. (2012). An analysis of peak pelvis rotation speed, gluteus maximus and medius strength in high versus low handicap golfers during the golf swing. *International Journal of Sports Physical Therapy*, 7(3): 288–295.

Carson, H. J., Collins, D., & Richards, J. (2014). Intra-individual movement variability during skill transitions: a useful marker?. *European Journal of Sport Science*, *14*(4): 327–336. https://doi.org/10.1080/17461391.2013.814714

Chaudhari, A. M., Lindenfeld, T. N., Andriacchi, T. P., Hewett, T. E., Riccobene, J., Myer, G. D., & Noyes, F. R. (2007). Knee and hip loading patterns at different phases in the menstrual cycle: implications for the gender difference in anterior cruciate ligament injury rates. *The American Journal of Sports Medicine*, *35*(5): 793–800. https://doi.org/10.1177/0363546506297537

Cochran, A. and Stobbs, J. (1999) '*Search for the Perfect Swing*', 2nd ed., Chicago: Roundhouse Publishing Ltd.

DeRenne, C., Buxton, B.P., Hetzler, R, K., Ho, K, W. (1995). Effects of Weighted Bat Implement Training on Bat Swing Velocity, *Journal of Strength and Conditioning Research*, *9*(4): 247–250.

Doan, B.K., Newton, R.U., Kwon, Y. and Kraemer, W.J. (2006) Effects of physical conditioning on intercollegiate golfer performance, *Journal of Strength and Conditioning Research*, *20*(1): 62–72.

Ehlert, A. (2020). The correlations between physical attributes and golf clubhead speed: A systematic review with quantitative analyses. *European Journal of Sport Science*, 1–24. 10.1080/17461391.2020.1829081

Fajen, B. R., Riley, M. A., & Turvey, M. T. (2008). Information, affordances, and the control of action in sport. *International Journal of Sport Psychology*, *40*: 79–107.

Foxworth, J.L., Millar, A,L., Long, B, L., Way, M., Vellucci, M, W., Vogler, J, D. (2013). Hip joint torques during the golf swing of young and senior healthy males. *Journal of Orthopaedic & Sports Physical Therapy*, *43*(9): 660–665

Gatt CJ, Pavol MJ, Parker RD, et al. (1998) Three dimensional knee joint kinetics during a golf swing: influences of skill level and footwear. *American Journal Sports Medicine*, *26*(2): 285–294.

Gatt CJ, Pavol MJ, Parker RD, et al. A kinetic analysis of the knees during a golf swing (1999) In: Farrally MR, Cochran AJ, editors. Science and golf III. Proceedings of the 1998 World Scientific Congress of Golf. Champaign (IL): Human Kinetics, pp. 20–28.

Gorman J. (2001) In the swing: the shoulder's role in this complex golf stroke. *Sport Med Update*, *15*(3): 7–12.

Ki Hoon Han, Christopher Como, Jemin Kim, Cheng-Ju Hung, Mohammad Hasan & Young-Hoo Kwon (2019) Effects of pelvis-shoulders torsional separation style on kinematic sequence in golf driving. Sports Biomechanics, 18(6): 663-685, DOI: 10.1080/14763141.2019.1629617

Hume, P. A., Keogh, J., & Reid, D. (2005). The role of biomechanics in maximising distance and accuracy of golf shots. *Sports medicine (Auckland, NZ)* , *35*(5): 429–449. https://doi.org/10.2165/00007256-200535050-00005

Jones, B., & Stevenson, G. (2015). Strength and power training for golf players. *Professional Strength and Conditioning*, 38: 17–26.

Jones N, Kiely J, Suraci B, Collins DJ, de Lorenzo D, Pickering C, Grimaldi KA. . (2016 Jun). A genetic-based algorithm for personalized resistance training. *Biol Sport*, *33*(2):117–126. doi: 10.5604/20831862.1198210. Epub 2016 Apr 1. PMID: 27274104; PMCID: PMC4885623.

Kelso, J.A.S. (1995) Dynamic patterns: The self organisation of brain and behaviour. Cambridge, MA: MIT Press.

Keogh, J.W.L., MSarnewick, M.C., Maulder, P.S., Nortje, J.P., Hume, P.A. and Bradshaw, E.J. (2009). Are anthropometrics, flexibility, muscular strength, and endurance variables related to clubhead velocity in low- and high-handicap golfers?, *Journal of Strength and Conditioning Research*, *23*(6): 1841–1850.

Knight, C.A. (2004). Neuromotor issues in the learning and control of golf skill. *Research Quarterly for Exercise and Sport*, *75*: 9–15.

Koenig G, Tamres M, Mann RW. The biomechanics of the shoe-ground interaction in golf. In: Cochran AJ, Farrally MR. Science and golf II. Proceedings of the 1994 World Scientific Congress of Golf; 1994 Jul 4–8; St Andrews. London: E & FN Spon, 1994: 40–45.

Kok, A (2016). Het Hiërarchisch Brein. Inleiding tot de Cognitieve Neurowetenschap. Tweede herziene uitgave. Januari 2016. ISBN 978-94-92182-75-3.

Lynn, S.K. & Wu, W. (2017). The use of ground reaction forces and pressures in golf swing instruction, In Toms, M. (ed.), Routledge International Handbook of Golf Science, (1st 412 ed., pp. 413 15–25). Oxford: Routledge.

Maddalozzo, G.F. (1987). SPORTS PERFORMANCE SERIES: An anatomical and biomechanical analysis of the full golf swing. *National Strength & Conditioning Association Journal*, *9*(4): 6–9.

McHardy, A., & Pollard, H. (2005). Muscle activity during the golf swing. *British Journal of Sports Medicine*, *39*(11): 799–804.

McNally, M. P., Yontz, N., & Chaudhari, A. M. (2014). Lower extremity work is associated with club head velocity during the golf swing in experienced golfers. *International Journal of Sports Medicine*, *35*(9): 785–788. https://doi.org/10.1055/s-0034-1367010

McNitt-Gray, J.L., Munaretto, J., Zaferiou, A., Requejo, P.S. and Flashner, H. (2013) Regulation of reaction forces during the golf swing, *Sports Biomechanics*, *12*(2): 121–131.

Myers, J., Lephart, S., Tsai, Y.S., Sell, T., Smoliga, J. and Jolly, J. (2008) The role of upper torso and pelvis rotation in driving performance during the golf swing. *Journal of Sports Sciences*, *26*(2): 181–188.

Nesbit, S.M. and Serrano, M. (2005) Work and power analysis of the golf swing. *Journal of Sports Science and Medicine*, *4*(4): 520–533.

Newell K,M. Constraints on the development of coordination. (1986) In: Wade M, Whitling H, editors. Motor Development in Children: Aspects of Coordination and Control (pp. 341–360). Lancaster: Martinus Nijhoff.

Neumann D. A. (2010). Kinesiology of the hip: a focus on muscular actions. *The Journal of orthopaedic and sports physical therapy*, *40*(2): 82–94. https://doi.org/10.2519/jospt.2010.3025

Okuda, I., Gribble, P. and Armstrong, C. (2010) Trunk rotation and weight transfer patterns between skilled and low skilled golfers. *Journal of Sports Science and Medicine*, *9*(1): 127–133.

Okuda I., Armstrong C.W., Tsunezumi H., et al. (2002) Biomechanical analysis of professional golfer's swing: Hidemichi Tanaka. In: Thain E, editor. Science and golf VI. Proceedings of the 2002 World Scientific Congress of Golf; 2002 23-26 July, St Andrews. London: E & FN Spon: 19–27.

Oranchuk, DJ., Mannerberg, J., Robinson, T., Nelson, and Megan C. (2020) Eight Weeks of Strength and Power Training Improves Club Head Speed in Collegiate Golfers. *Journal of Strength and Conditioning Research*, *34*(8): 2205–2213.

Parchmann, C. J., & McBride, J. M. (2011). Relationship between functional movement screen and athletic performance. *Journal of strength and conditioning research*, *25*(12): 3378–3384. https://doi.org/10.1519/JSC.0b013e318238e916

Penner, A. R. (2003). The physics of golf. *Reports on Progress in Physics*, *66*, 131–171.

Pink, M., Jobe, F.W., & Perry, J. (1990). Electromyographic analysis of the shoulder during the golf swing. *The American Journal of Sports Medicine*, *18*(2): 137–140. https://doi.org/10.1177/036354659001800205

Pekny, S. E., Izawa, J., & Shadmehr, R. (2015). Reward-dependent modulation of movement variability. *Journal of Neuroscience*, *35*(9): 4015–4024. https://doi.org/10.1523/JNEUROSCI.3244-14.2015

Radnor, J. M., Lloyd, R. S., & Oliver, J. L. (2017). Individual Response to Different Forms of Resistance Training in School-Aged Boys. *Journal of strength and conditioning research*, *31*(3): 787–797. https://doi.org/10.1519/JSC.000000000000152740.

Ranganathan, R., & Newell, K. (2013). Changing Up the Routine: Intervention-Induced Variability in Motor Learning. *Exercise and Sport Sciences Reviews*, *41*, 64–70.

Read, P.J., Lloyd, R.S., De Ste Croix, M. and Oliver, J.L. (2013) Relationships between field-based measures of strength and power and golf club head speed. *Journal of Strength and Conditioning Research*, *27*(10): 2708–2713.

Robins, R. Wheat, J., Irwin, G. & Bartlett, R.M. (2006) The effect of shooting distance on movement variability in basketball. *Journal of Human Movement Studies*, 50(4) 217–38.

Scholz, J. P., & Schöner, G. (1999). The uncontrolled manifold concept: identifying control variables for a functional task. *Experimental brain research*, *126*(3): 289–306. https://doi.org/10.1007/s002210050738

Sheppard, J.M. and Chapman, D.W. (2011) An Evaluation of a Strength Qualities Assessment for the Lower Body. *Journal of Australian Strength and Conditioning, 19*: 14–20.

Siddique, U., Rahman, S., Frazer, A. K., Pearce, A. J., Howatson, G., & Kidgell, D. J. (2020). Determining the Sites of Neural Adaptations to Resistance Training: A Systematic Review and Meta-analysis. *Sports medicine (Auckland, N.Z.), 50*(6): 1107–1128. https://doi.org/10.1007/s40279-020-01258-z

Siff, M., & Verkhoshansky, Y. (1998). Supertraining 4th Edition. Denver, USA

Suchomel, T. J., Nimphius, S., Bellon, C. R., & Stone, M. H. (2018). The Importance of Muscular Strength: Training Considerations. *Sports medicine (Auckland, N.Z.), 48*(4): 765–785. https://doi.org/10.1007/s40279-018-0862-z

Tillin, N.A. and Folland, J.P. (2014) Maximal and explosive strength training elicit distinct neuromuscular adaptations, specific to the training stimulus. *European Journal of Applied Physiology, 114*(2): 365–374.

Tillin, N. A., Pain, M. T., & Folland, J. P. (2012). Short-term training for explosive strength causes neural and mechanical adaptations. *Experimental Physiology, 97*(5), 630–641. https://doi.org/10.1113/expphysiol.2011.063040

Tillin, N. A., Pain, M., & Folland, J. P. (2018). Contraction speed and type influences rapid utilisation of available muscle force: neural and contractile mechanisms. *The Journal of Experimental Biology, 221*(Pt 24), jeb193367. https://doi.org/10.1242/jeb.193367

Tinmark, F., Hellström, J., Halvorsen, K. and Thorstensson, A. (2010) Elite golfers' kinematic sequence in full-swing and partial-swing shots. *Sports Biomechanics, 9*(4): 236–244.

Vikne, H., Refsnes, P. E., Ekmark, M., Medbø, J. I., Gundersen, V., & Gundersen, K. (2006). Muscular performance after concentric and eccentric exercise in trained men. *Medicine and science in sports and exercise, 38*(10): 1770–1781. https://doi.org/10.1249/01.mss.0000229568.17284.ab

Wallace E.S., Graham, D., Bleakley, E.W. (1990) Foot-to-ground pressure patterns during the golf drive: a case study involving a low handicap player and a high handicap player. In: Cochran AJ, editor. Science and golf I. Proceedings of the First World Scientific Congress of Golf; 9–13 July, St Andrews. London: E & FN Spon: 25–29.

Wallace E.S., Grimshaw P.N., Ashford R.L. (1994) Discrete pressure profiles of the feet and weight transfer patterns during the golf swing. In: Cochran AJ, Farrally MR, editors. Science and golf II. Proceedings of the 1994 World Scientific Congress of Golf; 1994 4–8 July, St Andrews. London: E & FN Spon: 26–32.

Wells, J.E.T., Mitchell, A.C.S, Charalambous, L.H. and Fletcher, I.M. (2018) Relationships between highly skilled golfers' clubhead velocity and force producing capabilities during vertical jumps and an isometric mid-thigh pull. *Journal of Sports Sciences, 36*(16), 1847–1851.

Wells, J.E.T., Charalambous, L.H., Mitchell, A.C.S., Coughlan, D., Brearley, S.L., Hawkes, R.A., Murray, A.D., Hillman, R.G. and Fletcher, I.M. (2019) Relationships between Challenge Tour golfers' clubhead velocity and force producing capabilities during a countermovement jump and isometric mid-thigh pull. *Journal of Sports Sciences, 37*(12): 1381–1386.

Williams, K. R., & Cavanagh, P. R. (1983). The mechanics of foot action during the golf swing and implications for shoe design. *Medicine and Science in Sports and Exercise, 15*(3): 247–255.

11 Speed Training for Golf

Alex Ehlert and Alex Bliss

Introduction

Analyses of golf performance statistics are beginning to highlight the potential value of increased driving distance. For example, using the strokes gained approach, Broadie (2014) suggested a 20-yard distance increase gains a PGA Tour professional ~0.75 strokes per round, while a similar increase would gain even more for a recreational golfer. It is now common for golfers to seek increased driving distance. For example, Bryson Dechambeau recently made headlines by drastically increasing body mass, engaging in concerted speed training, and by changing his swing technique. The primary factor for increasing distance is clubhead speed (CHS) (Hume et al., 2005). If all else remains constant (strike quality, equipment, environmental conditions, etc.), a faster CHS at impact will result in greater post-impact ball speed (BS) and greater shot displacement (Hume et al., 2005). Numerous factors influence CHS, including the physical capacity of the golfer. As such, many golfers are employing S&C coaches as part of a team-based approach to maximise performance (Farrally et al., 2003; Smith, 2010).

This chapter will summarise the literature related to training with the goal of increased CHS or BS (which will be termed "speed training"). The first section will provide a background on the topic. This will cover themes such as the mechanics that underpin speed in the golf swing, the physical attributes associated with faster speed, and a review of training studies. The second section will focus on practical considerations for speed training, including how to structure training in a way that will maximise increases in CHS and BS. The chapter will culminate in recommendations for speed training and several examples of how this can be implemented into a golfer's preparation schedule.

The Mechanics Underpinning CHS

Mechanical determinants of performance during movements such as jumping, throwing, or striking are commonly explained from either an impulse-momentum or work-energy perspective (Turner et al., 2020; Winter & Fowler, 2009). According to Newton's Second Law of Motion, a body's change in

DOI: 10.4324/9781003099321-11

momentum is dependent on the direction and size of forces applied, and the duration over which that force is applied (Winter & Fowler, 2009). Specifically, there is a direct proportional relationship between impulse, quantified as force x time, and momentum, quantified as mass x velocity (Turner et al., 2020; Winter & Fowler, 2009). Given that there is no substantial change in the mass of an athlete or implement (i.e., the golf club) during a given movement, increases in impulse should result in proportional increases in velocity. Greater impulses can be generated by either producing more force during a specific time period, or by producing equivalent forces over longer periods of time (Turner et al., 2020). Similarly, there is a direct proportional relationship between work and energy. Changes in kinetic energy are a function of the work performed during the action, with work being the product of the force applied and the displacement through which the force is applied (Turner et al., 2020). This suggests that an athlete could enhance the transfer of kinetic energy by either increasing force application over a given displacement, or by applying force across a greater displacement.

Despite differences in how movement performance is defined, each of these theorems present similar implications in terms of the mechanical determinants of CHS. For example, considering the impulse-momentum relationship, a golfer could theoretically increase CHS by generating larger impulses during the golf swing. This could be accomplished by either increasing force production during the duration of the golf swing, increasing the duration of the golf swing to allow more time for force production, or some combination of each. Indeed, recent studies have found that positive impulse generated during countermovement jumps is a strong predictor of CHS in skilled amateur and professional golfers (Wells et al., 2018; Wells et al., 2019). Similarly, CHS can be maximised by enhancing transfer of kinetic energy through the body and into the club (Kenny et al., 2008; Nesbit & Serrano, 2005). Given the work-energy relationship, the golfer could enhance CHS by applying greater forces during the swing, increasing the displacement over which force is applied, or a combination of each. Evidence for this proposition was recently demonstrated in a sample of 76 amateur golfers (Mackenzie et al., 2020). The authors quantified total linear work during driver swings and found that it accounted for 90% of the variance in CHS. They also quantified the subcomponents of linear work, and reported that both the force applied along the hand path (the force component of work) and hand path length (the displacement component of work) were significant predictors of CHS. These results suggest that a golfer could potentially achieve a faster CHS by either applying more force in the hand path direction, or by extending the timeframe or displacement over which that force is applied.

Force production during the swing can be affected by several factors (i.e., swing coordination or technique, exertion levels, etc.), however most relevant to speed training is the force generating capabilities of the muscles that accelerate the clubhead (Mackenzie et al., 2020). Notably, work analyses of the golf swing have suggested that work performed by the lower extremity is a significant contributor to CHS (McNally et al., 2014), and that specific areas of the body such as the lumbar spine, right hip, and thoracic spine perform a substantial proportion of total work during the swing (Nesbit & Serrano, 2005). From the perspective of muscle activation (assessed via electromyography), the gluteus complex (maximus and medius), hamstrings, and lead side adductor magnus of the lower extremity, and the obliques, latissimus dorsi, and pectoralis major of the upper extremity, are all highly active during the downswing (Cole & Grimshaw, 2016; McHardy & Pollard, 2005). Taken together, the major muscle groups of the lower extremity, trunk, and upper extremity contribute to accelerating the clubhead, and improving the force potential from these muscles could increase CHS.

However, as noted by Goodwin and Cleather (2016), force production in the context of sport is a function of both 1) the force generating potential of the contributing muscles and connective tissues and 2) the skill of being able to use this force potential optimally within the specific movement context of the sport or action. As such, while enhancing the force generating capabilities of the muscles can increase a golfer's speed potential, the ability to utilise that force in the skill of the golf swing is an important consideration (see Transfer of Training chapter). Beyond force production, a longer backswing or hand path may be valuable as it could increase displacement and time over which to produce force, ultimately increasing linear work, impulse, and subsequently CHS (Turner et al., 2020).

Several specific aspects of swing kinetics and kinematics are associated with CHS and may also contribute to useful work performed or impulse generated during the golf swing. Notably, it is possible that some of these factors could be either directly or indirectly influenced by speed training (Ehlert, 2020). This includes changes in pressure patterns (Ball & Best, 2007), the magnitude and timing of ground reaction forces (McNitt-Gray et al., 2013; Pataky et al., 2015), sequencing muscle contributions in a proximal-to-distal pattern during the downswing (Mackenzie & Sprigings, 2009), and the relative difference between torso and pelvis rotation both at the top of the backswing ("X-Factor"; Myers et al., 2008) and during the early downswing as the pelvis begins to rotate ("X-Factor Stretch"; Cheetham et al., 2001; Joyce, 2017a). For example, rapid shifts in pressure patterns toward the target and greater magnitudes of ground reaction forces in the target direction are associated with faster CHS (Ball & Best, 2007; Pataky et al., 2015). Further, skilled golfers tend to generate larger magnitudes of vertical ground reaction force in the lead foot and have this force peak at an earlier time point than less-skilled golfers (Barrentine et al., 1994; Lynn et al., 2012). By rapidly shifting pressure and generating large magnitudes of ground reaction forces, golfers use the ground to generate impulse (and ultimately momentum) during the downswing. While a golfer's interaction with the ground is heavily influenced by their swing mechanics and technical prowess, golfers that can produce high forces with the lower body during the timeframe of the golf swing may be better equipped to generate large ground reaction forces in a shorter timeframe than a less powerful golfer.

It is common for the golf downswing to be initiated with the lower extremity and subsequent body segment contributions to be sequenced in a proximal-to-distal fashion (Nesbit & Serrano, 2005; Lamb & Glazier, 2017). This finding is not exclusive to golf swings, as similar proximal-to-distal sequences have been observed in actions such as tennis serving (Fleisig et al., 2003; Martin et al., 2013), javelin throwing (Antti et al., 1994), baseball pitching (Naito, 2021), and cricket fast bowling (Ferdinands et al., 2013). There is considerable inter-individual variation in the sequence patterns used, even at elite levels of golf, but evidence from modeling studies and the literature as a whole has suggested that proximal-to-distal sequencing is likely advantageous for CHS (Lamb & Glazier, 2017; Mackenzie & Sprigings, 2009; Neal et al., 2008). Increased force applied at each segment of the kinetic chain and enhanced transfer of energy throughout the entire chain would increase the amount of usable work performed during the downswing (Mackenzie et al., 2020; Nesbit & Serrano, 2005). By increasing the force generating capabilities of the muscles spanning the kinetic chain, speed training could theoretically increase CHS (Read et al., 2014), assuming that the golfer is able to effectively use that force potential within the context of the golf swing.

Finally, several studies have found that CHS is associated with greater X-Factor and X-Factor stretch (Cheetham et al., 2001; Myers et al., 2008; Joyce, 2017a). It has been suggested that the backswing provides a "pre-stretch" of the muscles, increasing force production during the downswing through a stretch-shortening cycle (SSC) mechanism (Hume et al., 2005). However, it is not clear whether SSC can explain the associations between CHS and X-Factor/X-Factor Stretch, given that assessments that are dependent on concentric components tend to correlate strongly with CHS (Read & Lloyd, 2014). An alternative explanation is that a larger X-Factor and X-Factor Stretch may be associated with a more proximal-to-distal sequence, which is considered advantageous for accelerating the clubhead (Lamb & Glazier, 2017; Mackenzie & Sprigings, 2009). Specifically, large X-factor stretch values are often achieved when the golfer initiates the downswing by rotating the hips towards the target. This not only creates a larger degree of separation between the pelvis and torso, but also promotes the use of a proximal-to-distal sequence of body segment contributions. Additionally, individuals with greater relative torso rotation (and as such greater X-Factor and X-Factor Stretch) could have longer backswings and hand paths (Mackenzie et al., 2020), the benefits of which are outlined above. Regardless, these findings suggest that the ability to rotate the torso efficiently is associated with faster CHS.

Summary of Mechanical Underpinnings of Speed

Figure 11.1 displays a theoretical framework through which speed training could enhance CHS through increases in force production during the swing and the displacement or time over which force production occurs. The key points from this section are summarised below:

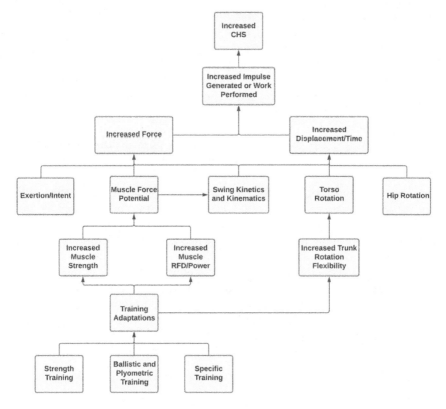

Figure 11.1 A simple theoretical framework of how speed training may increase CHS. *CHS = clubhead speed, RFD = rate of force development. Swing kinetics and kinematics include factors such as rapid shifts in center of pressure, rapid generation of ground reaction forces, proximal-to-distal sequencing during the downswing, and X-Factor/X-Factor Stretch. Additional factors are likely involved, and the precise associations and causal relationships between these factors require further clarification

- The mechanical underpinnings of CHS can be described from either an impulse-momentum or work-energy perspective.
- Impulse (force x time) is directly related to changes in momentum (mass x velocity). Given that mass remains relatively stable during the golf swing, generating larger impulses during the golf swing should result in increased velocity (and CHS). Similarly, changes in kinetic energy are directly related to the work performed (force x displacement). As such, golfers that perform more useful work during the golf swing should have enhanced transfer of kinetic energy, and ultimately faster CHS than those that perform less work (Kenny et al., 2008; Mackenzie et al., 2020).

- Taken together, golfers could theoretically increase CHS by 1) increasing force production during the golf swing, 2) increasing the distance or time over which force is produced, or 3) some combination of each.
- Force production during the swing is a function of both the force generating potential of the relevant musculature and connective tissue and the golfer's skill in using that force potential within the context of the golf swing. As such, both physical and technical factors will contribute to CHS.
- Speed training could enhance the force generating capabilities of the muscles by increasing muscle strength, power, and rate of force development (RFD). This could then result in faster CHS if that force can then be applied in the direction of the hand path during the timeframe of the golf swing.
- Speed training could also influence additional kinetic and kinematic variables that are associated with CHS, including the ability to rapidly shift centre of pressure patterns, generate large magnitudes of ground reaction forces earlier in the downswing, and increased force and torque application at each segment of the kinetic chain.
- An increase in hand path length can also enhance linear work and impulse by increasing the time and displacement through which force can be applied to the golf swing. This can be influenced by the ability to rotate the hips and torso. Addressing physical limitations that restrict the ability to rotate effectively (torso rotation flexibility, pelvis stability) could allow a golfer to lengthen their hand path, and potentially increase X-Factor and X-Factor Stretch.

The following section will discuss the available research on speed training for golf, and the potential role of muscle strength, power/RFD, and torso rotation flexibility. Additionally, body mass will be discussed given recent attention on the changes that Bryson Dechambeau has made to his body in the pursuit of speed (Pennington, 2020).

Muscle Power and RFD

Muscle power is defined as the work rate that can be performed (work x time), while RFD is change in force divided by change in time (Suchomel & Comfort, 2018). Given that most sporting actions must be performed in a limited amount of time, power and RFD are considered critical to athletic performance (Cormie et al., 2011). The short duration of the downswing (<0.30 seconds) has led several authors to suggest that improving power and RFD should be a priority for golfers (Smith, 2010; Sheehan et al., 2019b;). This is supported by a recent meta-analysis that found large correlations between CHS and measures such as estimated power during jumps ($r = 0.51$) and outcomes from seated ($r = 0.57$) and rotational ($r = 0.60$) medicine ball throws (Ehlert, 2020b). Further, Torres-Ronda et al. (2014) found that load that resulted in maximal power output for the bench press ($r = 0.68$) and back squat ($r = 0.70$)

had large correlations with BS in skilled amateur golfers. Taken together, golfers with higher levels of power and RFD tend to also have faster CHS. Developing greater muscle power and RFD in the downswing muscles could influence the linear work performed or impulse generated during the swing by enhancing the force generating capabilities of the muscles (Mackenzie et al., 2020).

Muscle Strength

Muscle strength is defined as the ability to exert force on an external resistance (Stone et al., 1993). There are several reasons that strength could either directly or indirectly influence CHS. First, while the downswing duration is <0.3 seconds (McTeigue et al., 1994), golfers begin pushing into the ground and generating ground reaction force during the backswing (McNitt-Gray et al., 2013; Tinmark et al., 2010). As such, the force generating timeframe may not be restricted to only the 0.30 second timeframe of the downswing. From a mechanical standpoint, a strong and stable lower body could provide a stable base for the trunk to rotate upon, while strength throughout the body could facilitate transfer of kinetic energy (Hume et al., 2005; Sheehan et al., 2019a). This would be expected to increase linear work and impulse by increasing hand path length (through increased torso rotation) and increasing average force in the hand path direction (Mackenzie et al., 2020; Turner et al., 2020). Muscle strength could also indirectly benefit CHS through its positive associations with power and RFD (Suchomel et al., 2016). Stronger athletes tend to be able to express more power and respond more readily to power or velocity-oriented training (Behm et al., 2017; Cormie et al., 2011; Suchomel et al., 2016). Indeed, strength has been described as a vehicle to drive gains in other attributes (DeWeese et al., 2015; Suchomel et al., 2018).

Torso Flexibility

The role of flexibility for achieving fast CHS likely depends on the area and type of movement. For example, two studies have found that internal hip rotation range of motion is lower in more skilled golfers (Keogh et al., 2009) and golfers with faster CHS (Sheehan et al., 2019a) than their less skilled and slower CHS counterparts. This is perhaps related to the fact that many modern golf swings rotate the torso upon a relatively stable pelvis (Cole & Grimshaw, 2016). As mentioned previously, torso rotation flexibility could allow a golfer to increase the length of their backswing and hand path (Hume et al., 2005; Mackenzie et al., 2020). Greater torso rotation upon a relatively stable pelvis would also result in higher levels of X-Factor and X-Factor stretch, which is positively associated with CHS (Cheetham et al., 2001 Hume et al., 2005). However, research findings so far have been mixed and inconclusive. One study found a significant correlation between seated trunk rotation and CHS (Brown et al., 2011), but three others did not (Gordon et al., 2009; Keogh et al., 2009; Sheehan et al., 2019a). However, it is worth noting that many of these studies had relatively small sample sizes (n $\leq$ 22), which may have impacted the ability to detect a statistically significant correlation. Several training studies have suggested that interventions such as yoga (Sorbie et al., 2019) and plyometric training (Bull & Bridge, 2012) can increase X-factor variables, however CHS was not assessed in either study. One potential explanation for the inconclusive results is that the assessments of seated trunk rotation do not reflect the dynamic demands of the golf swing. For example, the golf swing relies heavily on the interaction between the golfer and the ground (Lamb & Glazier, 2017). Indeed, skilled golfers often begin pushing into the ground and rotating their hips while the club is still moving away from the target in the backswing (McNitt-Gray et al., 2013; Tinmark et al., 2010). This early rotation of the hips creates additional separation between the torso and pelvis (i.e., greater X-factor Stretch) during the downswing, which is thought to "stretch" the muscles, and ultimately enhance CHS (Cheetham et al., 2001 Hume et al., 2005). This quality is unlikely to be reflected in seated assessments of trunk rotation flexibility, given that dynamic interaction with the ground is largely removed.

Alternatively, torso rotation flexibility could possibly be important on an individual basis, in that it may be a limiting factor for some golfers, but not others. For example, a golfer that has particularly poor torso rotation flexibility may not be able to rotate far enough to complete a full backswing, and thus are limited in terms of their ability to accelerate the clubhead during the downswing, though there is currently limited evidence to either support or refute this proposition. Another potential explanation is that possessing higher levels of trunk rotation flexibility may not necessarily mean that a golfer will utilise it in the golf swing, as a recent study found that axial rotation flexibility was not significantly associated with X-Factor variables (Joyce, 2017b). This could indicate that golfers with high levels of trunk rotation flexibility must learn to use it in the swing through coaching or practice.

Body Mass and Anthropometrics

The anthropometric characteristics of a golfer could theoretically influence their performance and ability to achieve fast CHS. A recent and notable example is Bryson Dechambeau, who substantially increased his body mass over the last year or two and appears to have increased CHS as a result (Pennington, 2020). Notably, when comparing the 2019 and 2020 seasons, his average strokes gained off the tee increased from 0.421 to 1.039 per round, while mean CHS increased from 118.2 mph to 125.0 mph (PGA Tour Stats, 2021). Ehlert (2021) pooled the correlation coefficients from 6 samples of golfers (n = 192 golfers) and found that body mass had a moderate correlation with CHS (r = 0.44). While body mass may not directly influence the golf swing *per se*, larger individuals tend to have more fat-free mass and increased force output (Lieber & Friden, 2000), which would be advantageous for CHS. This hypothesis is supported by Keogh et al. (2009), who found that CHS had stronger correlations with fat-free mass (r = 0.43) vs total body mass (r = 0.27). There is also less potential downside of increasing muscle mass in golf than other sports. For example, the golfer does not need to perform activities such as jumping and sprinting where body mass is a critical determinant of performance. Further, absolute strength appears to be more important than relative strength for golf CHS (Hellstrom, 2008). It appears that increasing muscle mass could be a viable strategy for enhancing speed. Notably, certain phases of training could aim to increase cross-sectional area to help contribute to increased strength, and in turn drive improvements in other attributes (Suchomel & Comfort, 2018).

Review of the Golf S&C Speed Research

Effects of S&C Interventions on Speed

The volume of published training studies focusing on S&C for golf is relatively low, particularly in comparison to other sports. Early S&C studies in golf had significant limitations such as small sample sizes, the lack of control groups, samples of untrained and recreational skill level golfers, and dated training methods that made it difficult to identify cause and effect relationships, and to generalise findings to other skill levels of golfers. However, there has been a recent surge in published studies on golf S&C across different golfer populations. For example, a recent systematic review found that S&C interventions have tended to increase CHS, and BS by a mean of 4.1 and 5.3% respectively across many golfer subgroups (Ehlert, 2020). In some cases, improvements have been quite large, even in skilled golfers. For example, the low handicap golfers recruited by Alvarez et al. (2012) experienced a 10.4% mean increase in BS after 18-weeks of a periodised strength and power programme. However, there has been inconsistency across studies in terms of the interventions used. Most studies have used multi-modal interventions consisting of various combinations of strength training, ballistic or plyometric exercises, and flexibility exercises. This is problematic as combining interventions does not allow for the attribution of any effects observed to a particular training modality. Further, there is limited information about the underlying mechanisms and training adaptations that produced the improvements, which has made identifying optimal training approaches a challenge. Finally, there is limited information available about the training status of golfers recruited for the studies. This is an important consideration as less-well trained or untrained golfers will likely experience an improvement in physicality from any training undertaken, as where highly-trained golfers will require a tailored, well-rationalised programme to improve physical performance.

Effects of S&C Interventions on Golf Swing Kinetics and Kinematics

Only a few studies have evaluated the effects of training on swing kinematics or kinetics. Bull and Bridge (2012) had golfers engage in an eight-week plyometric programme consisting of various lower body jumps and bounds, and rotational medicine ball exercises. They found that the plyometric programme increased maximal X-Factor during the downswing, X-Factor Stretch recoil, and increased speed of the hand and wrist. Choi et al. (2017) had a group of novice golfers perform a periodised medicine ball throwing programme prior to playing golf for eight-weeks. They reported large improvements in CHS (15.9%) and increases in the percentage of bodyweight shifted to the lead foot at impact (+34.3%). This suggests that medicine ball throws performed in a manner like the golf swing could positively influence centre of pressure patterns. However, it is unclear whether such an intervention would have similar effects in experienced golfers. Parker et al. (2017) found that the addition of isokinetic squats and standing rotation exercises to a strength training programme resulted in changes such as increased lead arm speed and acceleration, X-Factor stretch, and the rate at which the shoulder was stretched during the backswing. Finally, a pilot study by Sorbie et al. (2019) found that a six-week yoga programme that targeted inflexible areas of the shoulders, hips, and torso increased X-Factor compared to a control group. They also reported increased pelvic rotation at the top of the swing and when the club was parallel to the ground, and just before impact. In sum, the limited available research suggests that training programmes can impact golf kinematics though more data is needed to determine if these effects would generalise to a variety of golfer populations and whether these changes in kinematics result in increased CHS.

Comparison of Training Interventions

While most studies compared effects of interventions to a control group or used single group designs, a few studies compared different training interventions. Hegedus et al. (2016) compared the effects of a traditional resistance training programme versus golf-specific resistance exercises in recreational female golfers. The results suggested that benefits were similar between the groups. Parker et al. (2017) found that the addition of isokinetic standing rotations and squat exercises resulted in greater increases in BS compared to a standard isotonic training programme (3.5% vs 1.1%) in intercollegiate golfers. This may have been related to increases in X-factor stretch and lead arm speed in the isokinetic group. Finally, intercollegiate golfers assigned to a periodised strength and power programme had improvements in CHS (3.2%; $p < 0.05$), while those assigned to a low-load programme did not (Oranchuk et al., 2020).

Acute Changes in Speed

A recent systematic review found that warm-up interventions that include dynamic and/or resistance exercises can acutely increase golf performance measures (Ehlert & Wilson, 2019). Alternatively, warm-up programmes consisting of large quantities of static stretching can impair performance measures (Gergley, 2009). Two studies have found that post-activation potentiation in the form of countermovement jumps can acutely enhance speed (Bliss et al., 2021; Read et al., 2013). The recent study by Bliss et al. (2021) showed that acute increases in CHS can be obtained by maximally swinging a weighted implement prior to golf performance testing, though the benefits were similar to the jumps. Overall, dynamic exercise, resistance exercise, and post-activation potentiation in the form of jumping or swinging a weighted implement can acutely enhance speed prior to golf play.

Gaps and Limitations

The current research suggests that focusing on a combination of muscle strength, power/RFD, and flexibility can increase speed and impact certain swing kinematic variables (Ehlert, 2020). However, most studies have utilised multi-modal interventions, and have compared the results to golfers that are not engaged in training. This has made it difficult to ascertain the exact training modalities and adaptations that are most likely to enhance speed. The limited evidence available suggests that traditional resistance training yields similar results as golf-specific resistance training (Hegedus et al., 2016), that high load strength and power training is more effective than low load training programmes (Oranchuk et al., 2020), and that the addition of isokinetic squats and standing rotations to a S&C intervention can increase BS and X-Factor stretch (Parker et al., 2017).

Practical Applications

Structuring Speed Training

Both general and specific factors contribute to increased CHS. For example, while some exercises elicit "primary transfer" through high specificity, others can benefit an athlete through "secondary transfer," which occurs when training improves the physical attributes that underpin the sport movement (Goodwin & Cleather, 2016). Notably, the use of exercises that drive improvements through secondary transfer early in a training programme can facilitate greater improvements when focus is shifted towards more direct transfer. For example, strength training exercises may be expected to have less direct transfer to improved clubhead speed than those that have greater similarity to the swing (e.g. weighted implement training), but a stronger golfer will be in a better position to exploit the potential benefits from the more specific modalities in the future, resulting in greater long-term development (Deweese et al., 2015; Goodwin & Cleather, 2016). As such, not all training must be highly specific, skill-based exercises to effectively increase CHS. Instead, it is important to build up a foundation of general physicality before (or at least in addition to) maximising output during the skill itself.

Baker (1996) discussed methods of improving vertical jump performance by categorising resistance training exercises as 1) general, 2) special, or 3) specific. General exercises seek to increase the strength of relevant muscles. Special exercises aim to translate that increased strength into power and RFD. Finally, specific exercises are meant to apply a stimulus that is highly specific to the movement pattern. DeRenne et al. (2001) applied a similar categorisation system to baseball throwing velocity. The categorisation of training focuses into general and specific is a useful way of conceptualising speed training for golf as well, particularly given the similarities with baseball and throwing athletes. Within this broad framework, exercise selection and training can be progressed in a way that addresses limitations to speed and enhances transfer of training to performance over time.

General Preparation: Strength Training and Ballistic or Plyometric Training

General preparation training phases aim to develop the force generating capabilities of the muscles so that the golfer can increase CHS and be put in a position to benefit maximally from future specific training. The golf swing involves the activation and coordination of most major muscle groups to accelerate the clubhead during the downswing (McHardy & Pollard, 2005). This suggests that training should focus primarily on compound exercises that emphasise the transfer of energy through the kinetic chain.

Maximal strength development should be emphasised during general preparation periods. Raising a golfer's maximal strength provides a foundation upon which to build CHS and other attributes. Strength training exercises that have been used successfully with golfers include squat variations, deadlifts, lunges, shoulder and bench press, and rows (Alvarez et al., 2012; Fletcher & Hartwell, 2004; Oranchuk et al., 2020). Bodyweight exercises may be a suitable option for those with limited training experience or those returning from injury (Suchomel et al., 2018). However, they also have limitations in the degree to which they can be progressively overloaded. Strength training can also promote muscle hypertrophy (Schoenfeld et al., 2017) and body mass is positively associated with CHS (Ehlert, 2021). As strength training can increase muscle cross-sectional area, this will also influence body mass and the potential for force production (Suchomel & Comfort, 2018).

Strength training elicits significant benefits in power among relatively weak individuals (Cormie et al., 2010). However, once a strength foundation has been established, further gains in power and RFD are likely made by training exercises that emphasise rapid force expression, such as ballistic, plyometric, or explosive strength training exercises (Baker, 1996). Ballistic exercises involve accelerating throughout the entire concentric phase, and is characterised by exercises such as medicine ball throws, ballistic push-ups and weightlifting exercises and their derivatives (Newton et al., 1996; Lake et al., 2012). This training style has several distinct advantages, including lowering of the recruitment threshold for high-threshold motor units (van Cutsem et al., 1998). This efficient and preferential recruitment of high-threshold motor units is considered crucial for maximising power and RFD adaptations from training (Duchateau & Hainaut, 2003; Suchomel & Comfort, 2018). Ballistic training also enhances motor unit firing frequency, which is a major contributing factor to increased RFD and power during explosive activities (Leong et al., 1999; Saplinska et al., 1980; van Cutsem et al., 1998).

Weightlifting exercises and their derivatives may be particularly effective for enhancing power, as they involve using ballistic intent to move moderate-heavy loads (Suchomel et al., 2017). Additionally, the use of weightlifting derivatives (variations that exclude the catch phase) can be a useful method of improving power and RFD, while being less technically demanding (Suchomel et al., 2015). Similarly, plyometric exercises are explosive movements that involve a rapid pre-stretch of muscles before a ballistic-type contraction (Suchomel & Comfort, 2018). Both plyometric and ballistic exercises have been utilised successfully with golfers, either in isolation (Bliss et al., 2015; Choi et al., 2017), or in combination with strength training exercises (Alvarez et al., 2012; Fletcher & Hartwell, 2004; Oranchuk et al., 2020). In addition to ballistic and plyometric exercises, power and RFD could also be enhanced by manipulating load and velocity of traditional strength training exercises. By lowering the load, the athlete can focus on maximising the velocity of the movement, resulting in greater power output. Notably, the load that resulted in maximal power output for the back squat and bench press had very large correlations with BS in skilled golfers ($r = 0.68 - 0.70$; Torres-Ronda et al., 2014).

For well-trained golfers, greater transfer may result from advanced or tailored methodologies. For example, complex training involves performing a high-force or high-power exercise immediately before a ballistic exercise that is similar biomechanically (i.e. a squat followed by a squat jump; Robbins et al., 2005). The preceding exercise is thought to potentiate performance during the ballistic exercise and could create a superior stimulus by allowing the athlete to increase their output (Docherty & Hodgson, 2007). Though it is worth noting that the effects may depend on many factors and is likely more suitable for well-trained individuals (Suchomel et al., 2016b). Further, within general preparation phases, manipulating certain variables to achieve higher correspondence could facilitate transfer in advanced athletes. For example, strength exercises can be periodically performed at a partial range of motion that is more specific to the sport's joint angles (Suarez et al., 2019).

Specific Training

Many golfers use over and under-weighted speed sticks with the goal of increasing CHS. Other than a couple of studies on the acute effects of swinging speed sticks (Bliss et al., 2021; Hébert-Loisier & Wardell, 2021), there has been no published literature on the effects of these specific modalities in golf. However, there is research from throwing and striking sports that may be useful to golf speed training. Weighted implement training involves swinging or throwing a slightly modified version of the actual sport implement (DeRenne & Szymanski, 2009). Former Soviet coaches and researchers have been using this method with track and field throwers for decades (Jarver, 1973; Vasiliev, 1983). The use of underweight implements is thought to increase joint segment movement velocities, while overweight implements slow the movement pattern down and allow for greater impulses due to higher forces applied over longer durations. The Soviet coaches and researchers generally believed this method to be effective for increasing speed-strength and posited that the implement weights should be modified within 5–20% of the standard weight, and that the weighted implements (heavy and light) should be used in a ratio of 2:1 compared to the standard weight implement (Jarver, 1973; Konstantinov, 1979; Kuznetsov, 1975; Vasiliev, 1983; Verkhoshansky & Tatyan, 1973).

Drawing inference from baseball research, acute enhancement of swing velocity has been noted when swinging weighted implements that are within 12% of a standard bat weight during a warm-up (DeRenne & Branco, 1986; DeRenne et al., 1992; Montoya et al., 2009), while bats that are significantly heavier than a standard bat increase moment of inertia and decrease swing velocity (Southard & Groomer, 2003). From a chronic training perspective, both overweighted training (DeRenne & Okasaki, 1983; Sergo & Boatwright, 1993) and a combination of over and underweighted training (DeRenne et al., 1995; Sergo & Boatwright, 1993) can increase swing velocity. Interestingly, Sergo and Boatwright (1993) found that a group that simply swung a standard weight bat an additional 300 times per week (100 swings per day, 3 days per week) significantly increased swing velocity as well. Though DeRenne et al. (1995) did not find a similar finding with a group swinging a standard 30 oz bat.

Syzmanski and DeRenne (2009) reviewed the literature related to both general and specific training modalities for increasing bat velocity. They concluded that general resistance training can increase swing velocity, and benefits can be enhanced by including explosive medicine ball training and/or specific training with weighted implements. They suggested that swinging a standard bat with intent can increase velocity in relatively untrained individuals, while weighted implement training may benefit well-trained players. Notably, they cautioned that players should be benefit well-conditioned before using such intensive specific training. Therefore, golfers should develop a foundation of general physical capacity with traditional S&C approaches. This can then be progressed to incorporate exercises that are more specific to the movement patterns of the swing in those that possess a strong foundation of physical capacity. This could include exercises such as explosive medicine ball throws or weighted implement training. Lastly, given that overuse injuries are common in golf (Gosheger et al., 2003), it is important to strategically utilise specific modalities so that there is not an increased risk of overtraining and injury.

Recommendations for Golf Speed Training

Based on the evidence outlined in this chapter, the following recommendations are provided for golfers and coaches that wish to implement speed training.

- An effective speed training programme will 1) increase the force generating capabilities of the downswing muscles, 2) address physical limitations that may affect the ability to rotate effectively (i.e. torso rotation flexibility, pelvic stability), and 3) strategically manipulate training variables and the degree of specificity during training phases to facilitate transfer of training to CHS.

- Increasing the force generating capabilities of the muscles can be accomplished by enhancing muscle strength, power, and RFD through traditional S&C training approaches. Compound, dynamic strength training exercises (variations of squats, deadlifts, lunges, pressing, and pulling) can serve to increase a golfer's maximal strength, drive improvements in power and RFD, and promote hypertrophy if desired. Power and RFD can be further enhanced using ballistic, plyometric, and explosive strength training. Exercise selection and loading depends on the specific aspect of the force-velocity curve being targeted. For example, weightlifting derivatives can be a useful means of targeting greater strength-power, whereas an unloaded jump can target velocity characteristics.
- Specific modalities such as weighted implement training may be useful for increasing CHS. However, the lack of golf-specific research and the high rates of overuse injury in golf warrants a cautious approach. Golfers should develop underlying physical attributes before engaging in intensive specific training, with consideration given to avoid large spikes in training volume.
- A mixed methods approach is likely beneficial, through sequencing training phases so that attributes are emphasised in a logical fashion. For example, developing a foundation of hypertrophy and strength may increase CHS in a relatively weak individual while also potentiating gains during subsequent phases focused on explosive strength.
- A flexible approach to periodisation is needed in-season. The golfer may wish to avoid intensive training during competition, and they are likely to have equipment limitations when traveling. However, avoiding all intensive training may lead to detraining that will limit performance across the season. Training should be structured so that more intensive training can be scheduled at times that allow for adequate recovery (i.e. earlier in the week), and coaches should be prepared to design programmes that deliver an effective stimulus with limited equipment options.

Conclusions

This chapter has summarised the available literature related to speed training. The golf-specific research was supplemented by findings from similar throwing and striking sports such as baseball. Based on these findings, speed training should focus on 1) developing the force generating capabilities of the down-swing muscles, 2) address physical limitations that affect torso rotation, and 3) strategically use specificity to maximise training transfer by integrating the developed neuromuscular capacity with the skill of swinging fast. Young (2006) conceptualised many of these principles related to improving sprint performance by using the analogy of developing a racecar. In this analogy, general strength training (e.g., loaded squats) is used to develop engine capacity through training adaptations such as increased muscle cross-sectional area. Exercises that focus on rapid force production (ballistic or plyometric exercises) are used to develop "engine power output" through adaptations such as increased motor unit recruitment and firing frequency. Finally, specific training modalities are used to convert that engine capacity and power output to the road by targeting output during the task itself. A similar analogy could be used with golf CHS. For example, strength training could develop a golfer's "engine capacity" by promoting training adaptations that contribute to muscle strength and hypertrophy, while ballistic or plyometric training may increase "engine output" by RFD or power adaptations. More specific modalities such as weighted implement training or swinging a golf club with maximal intent could potentially be a useful means of targeting output from the muscles within the specific movement context of the golf swing.

References

Alvarez, M. A. R. Í. A., Sedano, S., Cuadrado, G., & Redondo, J. C. (2012). Effects of an 18-week strength training program on low-handicap golfers' performance. *The Journal of Strength and Conditioning Research, 26*(4), 1110–1121.

Antti, M., Komi, P. V., Korjus, T., Navarro, E., & Gregor, R. J. (1994). Body segment contributions to javelin throwing during final thrust phases. *Journal of Applied Biomechanics, 10*(2): 166–177.

Baker, D. (1996). Improving vertical jump performance through general, special, and specific strength training. *Journal of strength and Conditioning Research, 10*, 131–136.

Ball, K. A., & Best, R. J. (2007). Different centre of pressure patterns within the golf stroke II: Group-based analysis. *Journal of Sports Sciences, 25*(7): 771–779.

Barrentine, S. W., Fleisig, G. S., Johnson, H., & Woolley, T. W. (1994). Ground reaction forces and torques of professional and amateur golfers. In *Science and Golf II: proceedings of the World Scientific Congress of Golf* (pp. 33–39). London: E & FN Spon.

Behm, D. G., Young, J. D., Whitten, J. H., Reid, J. C., Quigley, P. J., Low, J., & Granacher, U. (2017). Effectiveness of traditional strength vs. power training on muscle strength, power and speed with youth: a systematic review and meta-analysis. *Frontiers in Physiology, 8*, 423.

Bliss, A.; Livingston, H., & Tallent, J. (2021). Field-based and overspeed potentiated warm-ups increase clubhead speed and drive carry distance in skilled collegiate golfers. *The Journal of Sport and Exercise Science. 5*(2): 107–113 https://doi.org/10.36905/jses.2021.02.03

Bliss, A., McCulloch, H., & Maxwell, N. (2015). The effects of an eight-week plyometric training program on golf swing performance characteristics in skilled adolescent golfers. *International Journal of Golf Sciences, 4*(2): 120–135.

Broadie, M. (2014). *Every Shot Counts*. New York: Avery Publishing Group.

Brown, S. J., Nevill, A. M., Monk, S. A., Otto, S. R., Selbie, W. S., & Wallace, E. S. (2011). Determination of the swing technique characteristics and performance outcome relationship in golf driving for low handicap female golfers. *Journal of Sports Sciences, 29*(14): 1483–1491.

Bull, M., & Bridge, M. W. (2012). The effect of an 8-week plyometric exercise program on golf swing kinematics. *International Journal of Golf Science, 1*(1): 42–53.

Cheetham, P. J., Martin, P. E., Mottram, R. E., & St Laurent, B. F. (2001). The importance of stretching the "X-Factor" in the downswing of golf: The "X-Factor Stretch". *Optimising Performance in Golf*, 192–199.

Choi, W. J., Kim, T. H., & Oh, D. S. (2017). Effect of Weight Ball Throw Training on Weight Shifting of Lower Body, Head Speed of Club, and Driving Distance of Amateur Golfers. *Korean Society of Physical Medicine*, *12*(3): 111–117.

Cole, M. H., & Grimshaw, P. N. (2016). The biomechanics of the modern golf swing: implications for lower back injuries. *Sports Medicine*, *46*(3): 339–351.

Cormie, P., McGuigan, M., & Newton, R. (2010). Influence of strength on magnitude and mechanisms of adaptation to power training. *Medicine & Science in Sports & Exercise*, *42*(8): 1566–1581.

Cormie, P., McGuigan, M. R., & Newton, R. U. (2011). Developing maximal neuromuscular power. *Sports medicine*, *41*(1): 17–38.

DeRenne, C., & Branco, D. (1986). Overload or underload in your on-deck preparation. *Schol Coach*, *32*: 69.

DeRenne, C., Buxton, B. P., Hetzler, R. K., & Ho, K. W. (1995). Effects of weighted bat implement training on bat swing velocity. *Journal of Strength and Conditioning Research*, *9*: 247–250.

DeRenne, C., Ho, K. W., Hetzler, R. K., & Chai, D. X. (1992). Effects of warm up with various weighted implements on baseball bat swing velocity. *The Journal of Strength and Conditioning Research*, *6*(4): 214–218.

DeRenne, C., Ho, K. W., & Murphy, J. C. (2001). Effects of general, special, and specific resistance training on throwing velocity in baseball: a brief review. *Journal of Strength and Conditioning Research*, *15*(1): 148–156.

DeRenne, C., & Okasaki, E. (1983). Increasing bat velocity (Part 2). *Athletic J*, *63*: 54–55.

DeRenne, C., & Szymanski, D. J. (2009). Effects of baseball weighted implement training: a brief review. *Strength & Conditioning Journal*, *31*(2): 30–37.

DeWeese, B. H., Hornsby, G., Stone, M., & Stone, M. H. (2015). The training process: Planning for strength–power training in track and field. Part 1: Theoretical aspects. *Journal of Sport and Health Science*, *4*(4): 308–317.

Docherty, D., & Hodgson, M. J. (2007). The application of postactivation potentiation to elite sport. *International Journal of Sports Physiology and Performance*, *2*(4): 439–444.

Duchateau, J., & Hainaut, K. (2003). Mechanisms of muscle and motor unit adaptation to explosive power training. *Strength and Power in Sport*, 315.

Ehlert, A., & Wilson, P. B. (2019). A Systematic Review of Golf Warm-ups: Behaviors, Injury, and Performance. *The Journal of Strength and Conditioning Research*, *33*(12): 3444–3462.

Ehlert, A. (2020). The effects of strength and conditioning interventions on golf performance: A systematic review. *Journal of Sports Sciences*, *38*(23): 2720–2731.

Ehlert, A. (2021). The correlations between physical attributes and golf clubhead speed: A systematic review with quantitative analyses. *European Journal of Sport Science*, *21*(10): 1351–1363. https://doi.org/10.1080/17461391.2020.1829081

Farrally, M. R., Cochran, A. J., Crews, D. J., Hurdzan, M. J., Price, R. J., Snow, J. T., & Thomas, P. R. (2003). Golf science research at the beginning of the twenty-first century. *Journal of Sports Sciences*, *21*(9): 753–765.

Ferdinands, R. E., Kersting, U. G., & Marshall, R. N. (2013). Kinematic and kinetic energy analysis of segmental sequencing in cricket fast bowling. *Sports Technology*, *6*(1): 10–21.

Fleisig, G., Nicholls, R., Elliott, B., & Escamilla, R. (2003). Tennis: Kinematics used by world class tennis players to produce high-velocity serves. *Sports Biomechanics*, *2*(1): 51–64.

Fletcher, I. M., & Hartwell, M. (2004). Effect of an 8-week combined weights and plyometrics training program on golf drive performance. *The Journal of Strength and Conditioning Research*, *18*(1): 59–62.

Gergley, J. C. (2009). Acute effects of passive static stretching during warm-up on driver clubhead speed, distance, accuracy, and consistent ball contact in young male competitive golfers. *The Journal of Strength and Conditioning Research*, *23*(3): 863–867.

Goodwin, J. E., & Cleather, D. J. (2016). *The Biomechanical Principles Underpinning Strength and Conditioning* (pp. 36–66). New York: Routledge.

Gosheger, G., Liem, D., Ludwig, K., Greshake, O., & Winkelmann, W. (2003). Injuries and overuse syndromes in golf. *The American Journal of Sports Medicine*, *31*(3): 438–443.

Gordon, B. S., Moir, G. L., Davis, S. E., Witmer, C. A., & Cummings, D. M. (2009). An investigation into the relationship of flexibility, power, and strength to club head speed in male golfers. *The Journal of Strength and Conditioning Research*, *23*(5): 1606–1610.

Hébert-Losier, K., & Wardell, G. L. (2021). Acute and persistence of the effects of the SuperSpeed Golf™ weighted-club warm-up on golf driving performance and kinematics. *Sports Biomechanics*: 1–19. DOI: 10.1080/14763141.2021.1887344

Hegedus, E. J., Hardesty, K. W., Sunderland, K. L., Hegedus, R. J., & Smoliga, J. M. (2016). A randomized trial of traditional and golf-specific resistance training in amateur female golfers: benefits beyond golf performance. *Physical Therapy in Sport*, *22*: 41–53.

Hellström, J. (2008). The relation between physical tests, measures, and clubhead speed in elite golfers. *International Journal of Sports Science & Coaching*, *3*(1_suppl): 85–92.

Hume, P. A., Keogh, J., & Reid, D. (2005). The role of biomechanics in maximising distance and accuracy of golf shots. *Sports Medicine*, *35*(5): 429–449.

Jarver, J. (1973). Varied resistance in power development. *Mod Athlete Coach*, *10*(6): 5–8.

Joyce, C. (2017a). The most important "factor" in producing clubhead speed in golf. *Human Movement Science*, *55*: 138–144.

Joyce, C. (2017b). An examination of the correlation amongst trunk flexibility, x-factor and clubhead speed in skilled golfers. *Journal of Sports Sciences*, *35*(20): 2035–2041.

Kenny, I. C., McCloy, A. J., Wallace, E. S., & Otto, S. R. (2008). Segmental sequencing of kinetic energy in a computer-simulated golf swing. *Sports Engineering*, *11*(1): 37–45.

Keogh, J. W., Marnewick, M. C., Maulder, P. S., Nortje, J. P., Hume, P. A., & Bradshaw, E. J. (2009). Are anthropometric, flexibility, muscular strength, and endurance variables related to clubhead velocity in low- and high-handicap golfers?. *The Journal of Strength and Conditioning Research*, *23*(6): 1841–1850.

Konstantinov, O. (1979). Training program for high level javelin throwers. *Sov Sports Rev*, *14*(3): 130–4.

Kuznetsov, V. (1975). Speed and strength. *Yessis Rev*, *10*(3): 78–83.

Lake, J., Lauder, M., Smith, N., & Shorter, K. (2012). A comparison of ballistic and nonballistic lower-body resistance exercise and the methods used to identify their positive lifting phases. *Journal of Applied Biomechanics*, *28*(4): 431–437.

Lamb, P. F., & Glazier, P. S. (2017). The sequence of body segment interactions in the golf swing. In *Routledge International Handbook of Golf Science* (pp. 26–34). Abingdon: Routledge.

Leong, B., Kamen, G., Patten, C., & Burke, J. R. (1999). Maximal motor unit discharge rates in the quadriceps muscles of older weight lifters. *Medicine and Science in Sports and Exercise*, *31*(11): 1638–1644.

Lieber, R. L., & Fridén, J. (2000). Functional and clinical significance of skeletal muscle architecture. *Muscle & Nerve: Official Journal of the American Association of Electrodiagnostic Medicine, 23*(11): 1647–1666.

Lynn, S. K., Noffal, G. J., FW Wu, W., & Vandervoort, A. A. (2012). Using principal components analysis to determine differences in 3D loading patterns between beginner and collegiate level golfers. *International Journal of Golf Science, 1*(1): 25–41.

MacKenzie, S., McCourt, M., & Champoux, L. (2020). How Amateur Golfers Deliver Energy to the Driver. *International Journal of Golf Science, 8*(1).

MacKenzie, S. J., & Sprigings, E. J. (2009). A three-dimensional forward dynamics model of the golf swing. *Sports Engineering, 11*(4): 165–175.

Martin, C., Kulpa, R., Delamarche, P., & Bideau, B. (2013). Professional tennis players' serve: correlation between segmental angular momentums and ball velocity. *Sports Biomechanics, 12*(1): 2–14.

McHardy, A., & Pollard, H. (2005). Muscle activity during the golf swing. *British Journal of Sports Medicine, 39*(11): 799–804.

McNally, M. P., Yontz, N., & Chaudhari, A. M. (2014). Lower extremity work is associated with club head velocity during the golf swing in experienced golfers. *International Journal of Sports Medicine, 35*(09): 785–788.

McNitt-Gray, J. L., Munaretto, J., Zaferiou, A., Requejo, P. S., & Flashner, H. (2013). Regulation of reaction forces during the golf swing. *Sports Biomechanics, 12*(2): 121–131.

McTeigue, M., Lamb, S. R., Mottram, R., & Pirozzolo, F. (1994, July). Spine and hip motion analysis during the golf swing. In *Science and Golf II: Proceedings of the World Scientific Congress of Golf* (pp. 50–58). E & FN Spon: London.

Montoya, B. S., Brown, L. E., Coburn, J. W., & Zinder, S. M. (2009). Effect of warm-up with different weighted bats on normal baseball bat velocity. *Journal of strength and conditioning research, 23*(5): 1566–1569.

Myers, J., Lephart, S., Tsai, Y. S., Sell, T., Smoliga, J., & Jolly, J. (2008). The role of upper torso and pelvis rotation in driving performance during the golf swing. *Journal of Sports Sciences, 26*(2): 181–188.

Naito, K. (2021). Time-varying motor control strategy for proximal-to-distal sequential energy distribution: Insights from baseball pitching. *Journal of Experimental Biology. 224*(20): jeb227207. https://doi.org/10.1242/jeb.227207

Neal, R. J., Lumsden, R. G., Holland, M., Mason, B., Crews, D., & Lutz, R. (2008). Segment Interactions: Sequencing and timing in the downswing. In *Science and Golf V: Proceedings of the World Scientific Congress of Golf* (pp. 21–29).

Nesbit, S. M., & Serrano, M. (2005). Work and power analysis of the golf swing. *Journal of Sports Science & Medicine, 4*(4): 520.

Newton, R. U., Kraemer, W. J., Häkkinen, K., Humphries, B. J., & Murphy, A. J. (1996). Kinematics, kinetics, and muscle activation during explosive upper body movements. *Journal of Applied Biomechanics, 12*(1): 31–43.

Oranchuk, D. J., Mannerberg, J. M., Robinson, T. L., & Nelson, M. C. (2020). Eight weeks of strength and power training improves club head speed in collegiate golfers. *The Journal of Strength and Conditioning Research, 34*(8): 2205–2213.

Parker, J., Lagerhem, C., Hellström, J., & Olsson, M. C. (2017). Effects of nine weeks isokinetic training on power, golf kinematics, and driver performance in pre-elite golfers. *BMC Sports Science, Medicine and Rehabilitation, 9*(1): 21.

Pataky, T. C. (2015). Correlation between maximum in-shoe plantar pressures and clubhead speed in amateur golfers. *Journal of Sports Sciences, 33*(2): 192–197.

Pennington, B. (2020, June 24). Bryson DeChambeau's Latest Physics Experiment? Himself. Retrieved July 02, 2020, from www.nytimes.com/2020/06/24/sports/golf/bryson-dechambeau-weight.html

PGA Tour Stats (2021, Jan 17). *Bryson DeChambeau PGA Tour Profile* PGATour. (n.d.). Retrieved January 17, 2021 from www.pgatour.com/players/player.47959.bryson-dechambeau.html.

Read, P. J., Miller, S, C., & Turner, A, N. (2013). The effects of postactivation potentiation on golf club head speed. *Journal of Strength and Conditioning Research*, 27(6): 1579–1582.

Read, P. J., & Lloyd, R. S. (2014). Strength and conditioning considerations for golf. *Strength & Conditioning Journal*, 36(5): 24–33.

Robbins, D. W. (2005). Postactivation potentiation and its practical applicability: A brief review. *Journal of Strength and Conditioning Research*, 19(2): 453.

Saplinskas, J. S., Chobotas, M. A., & Yashchaninas, I. I. (1980). The time of completed motor acts and impulse activity of single motor units according to the training level and sport specialization of tested persons. *Electromyography and clinical neurophysiology*, 20(6): 529–539.

Schoenfeld, B. J., Grgic, J., Ogborn, D., & Krieger, J. W. (2017). Strength and hypertrophy adaptations between low-vs. high-load resistance training: a systematic review and meta-analysis. *The Journal of Strength and Conditioning Research*, 31(12): 3508–3523.

Sergo, C., & Boatwright, D. (1993). Training methods using various weighted bats and the effects on bat velocity. *The Journal of Strength and Conditioning Research*, 7(2): 115–117.

Sheehan, W. B., Bower, R. G., & Watsford, M. L. (2019a). Physical Determinants of Golf Swing Performance: A Review. *Journal of Strength and Conditioning Research*. Epub ahead of print.

Sheehan, W. B., Watsford, M. L., & Pickering Rodriguez, E. C. (2019b). Examination of the neuromechanical factors contributing to golf swing performance. *Journal of Sports Sciences*, 37(4): 458–466.

Smith, M. F. (2010). The role of physiology in the development of golf performance. *Sports Medicine*, 40(8): 635–655.

Sorbie, G. G., Low, C., & Richardson, A. K. (2019). Effect of a 6-week yoga intervention on swing mechanics during the golf swing: a feasibility study. *International Journal of Performance Analysis in Sport*, 19(1): 90–101.

Southard, D., & Groomer, L. (2003). Warm-up with baseball bats of varying moments of inertia: Effect on bat velocity and swing pattern. *Research quarterly for exercise and sport*, 74(3): 270–276.

Stone, M. H., Stone, M., & Lamont, H. (1993). Explosive exercise. *National Strength and Conditioning Association Journal*, 15(4): 7–15.

Suarez, D, G., Wagle, J, P., Cunanan, A, J., Sausaman, R, W., Stone, M, H. (2019). Dynamic Correspondence of Resistance Training to Sport: A Brief Review, Strength and Conditioning Journal: 41(4) 80–88. DOI: 10.1519/SSC.0000000000000458

Suchomel, T. J., & Comfort, P. (2018). Developing muscular strength and power. In Turner, A., & Comfort, P (Eds.) *Advanced Strength and Conditioning-An Evidence-based Approach* (pp. 13–38). Oxon: Routledge.

Suchomel, T. J., Comfort, P., & Stone, M. H. (2015). Weightlifting pulling derivatives: Rationale for implementation and application. *Sports Medicine*, 45(6): 823–839.

Suchomel, T. J., Nimphius, S., & Stone, M. H. (2016). The importance of muscular strength in athletic performance. *Sports medicine*, 46(10): 1419–1449.

Suchomel, T. J., Nimphius, S., Bellon, C. R., & Stone, M. H. (2018). The importance of muscular strength: training considerations. *Sports medicine*, 48(4): 765–785.

Suchomel, T. J., Sato, K., DeWeese, B. H., Ebben, W. P., & Stone, M. H. (2016b). Potentiation following ballistic and nonballistic complexes: The effect of strength level. *Journal of Strength and Conditioning Research*, 30(7): 1825–1833.

Szymanski, D. J., DeRenne, C., & Spaniol, F. J. (2009). Contributing factors for increased bat swing velocity. *The Journal of Strength and Conditioning Research*, 23(4): 1338–1352.

Tinmark, F., Hellström, J., Halvorsen, K., & Thorstensson, A. (2010). Elite golfers' kinematic sequence in full-swing and partial-swing shots. *Sports Biomechanics*, 9(4): 236–244.

Torres-Ronda, L., Delextrat, A., & Gonzalez-Badillo, J. J. (2015). The relationship between golf performance, anthropometrics, muscular strength and power characteristics in young elite players. *International SportMed Journal*, 15(2): 156–164.

Turner, A. N., Comfort, P., McMahon, J., Bishop, C., Chavda, S., Read, P., ... & Lake, J. (2020). Developing powerful athletes, part 1: Mechanical underpinnings. *Strength & Conditioning Journal*, 42(3): 30–39.

Van Cutsem, M., Duchateau, J., & Hainaut, K. (1998). Changes in single motor unit behaviour contribute to the increase in contraction speed after dynamic training in humans. *The Journal of physiology*, 513(1): 295–305.

Vasiliev, L. A. (1983). Use of different weight to develop specialized speed-strength. *Sov Sports Rev*, 18(1): 49–52.

Verkhoshansky Y, Siff MC. (2009) Supertraining. Verkhoshansky SSTM: Rome, Italy, 241–248.

Verkhoshansky, Y., & Tatyan, V. (1973). Speed-strength preparation of future champions. *Legkaya Atleika*, 2, 12–13.

Wells, J. E., Charalambous, L. H., Mitchell, A. C., Coughlan, D., Brearley, S. L., Hawkes, R. A., ... & Fletcher, I. M. (2019). Relationships between Challenge Tour golfers' clubhead velocity and force producing capabilities during a countermovement jump and isometric mid-thigh pull. *Journal of Sports Sciences*, 37(12): 1381–1386.

Wells, J. E., Mitchell, A. C., Charalambous, L. H., & Fletcher, I. M. (2018). Relationships between highly skilled golfers' clubhead velocity and force producing capabilities during vertical jumps and an isometric mid-thigh pull. *Journal of Sports Sciences*, 36(16): 1847–1851.

Westcott, W. L., Dolan, F., & Cavicchi, T. (1996). Golf and strength training are compatible activities. *Strength & Conditioning Journal*, 18(4): 54–56.

Winter, E. M., & Fowler, N. (2009). Exercise defined and quantified according to the Systeme International d'Unites. *Journal of Sports Sciences*, 27(5): 447–460.

Young, W. B. (2006). Transfer of strength and power training to sports performance. *International Journal of Sports Physiology and Performance*, 1(2): 74–83.

Zatsiorsky VM. (1995) Science and practice of strength training. Champaign: Human Kinetics.

Index

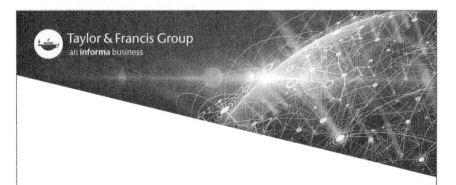